D1565018

Therapeutic Hypnosis with Children and Adolescents

Edited by

William C. Wester, II, EdD, ABPP, ABPH
&
Laurence I. Sugarman, MD, FAAP, ABMH

Crown House Publishing Limited
www.crownhouse.co.uk
www.chpus.com

First published by

Crown House Publishing Ltd
Crown Buildings, Bancyfelin, Carmarthen, Wales, SA33 5ND, UK
www.crownhouse.co.uk

and

Crown House Publishing Company LLC
6 Trowbridge Drive, Suite 5, Bethel, CT 06801-2858, USA
www.CHPUS.com

British Library Cataloguing-in-Publication Data
A catalogue entry for this book is available
from the British Library.

10-digit ISBN 1845900375
13-digit ISBN 978-1845900373

LCCN 2006939033

Printed and bound in the USA by
Versa Press

Dedication

This book is dedicated to my wife, Sally, whose love, encouragement, advice, and support have given me the inner strength necessary to complete this book. I wish that my children, William, Lori, and Scott, and Sally's children, Brian and Chris, always be blessed with self-understanding and compassion for others. I know that our grandchildren will continue to use their imagination and creative minds to guide them throughout their lives.

William C. Wester, II, EdD, ABPP, ABPH

Our accomplishments start with the faith of friends. For her faith, loving criticism, and selfless encouragement, I dedicate this text to my best friend, Laurie Hunt. I am grateful to my almost-grown-up children Emily and Nathan, who have given their time, listening ears, and honesty. The most valued contributors to this book are all those young people who validate this work by using it every day.

Laurence I. Sugarman, MD, FAAP, ABMH

Contents

Contributors

Ran D. Anbar, MD, FAPP
Professor of Pediatrics and Medicine
Director, Pediatric Pulmonary and Cystic Fibrosis Center
SUNY Upstate Medical University
Syracuse, NY

Rosalind E. H. Catchpole, MA
Doctoral Candidate, Simon Fraser University
Psychology Intern, British Columbia Children's Hospital
Doctoral Scholar, Social Sciences and Humanities Research Council
Senior Graduate Trainee, Michael Smith Foundation for Health
    Research
Vancouver, Canada

Gary Elkins, PhD, ABPP, ABPH
Professor
Director, Mind-Body Research Program
Department of Psychology and Neuroscience
Baylor University
Waco, TX

Charles G. Guyer, II, EdD, ABPP
Diplomate in Counseling and Family Psychology
Fellow, American Psychological Association
Past President, American Board of Family Psychology
Private Practice
Jacksonville, NC

Daniel P. Kohen, MD, ABMH
Director, Developmental-Behavioral Pediatrics Program
Clinical Director, KDWB University Pediatrics Family Center
Division of General Pediatrics & Adolescent Health
Professor, Departments of Pediatrics and Family Medicine and
    Family Health
University of Minnesota
Minneapolis, MN

Leora Kuttner, PhD (RegPsyc)
Clinical Professor of Pediatrics
University of British Columbia and BC Children's Hospital
Vancouver, Canada

Julie H. Linden, PhD
Clinical Psychologist
President, American Society of Clinical Hypnosis (2006–2007)
Private Practice
Philadelphia, PA

Thom E. Lobe, MD, NMD, ABMH
Pediatric Surgeon
Blank Children's Hospital
Des Moines, IA

Michelle M. Perfect, PhD
Assistant Professor
Department of Special Education, Rehabilitation, and School
    Psychology
University of Arizona
Tucson, AZ

Andrew E. Roffman, LCSW
Assistant Director – Family Studies Program
New York University Child Study Center
Clinical Instructor in the Department Of Psychiatry
New York University School of Medicine
Member, Center for Psychotherapy Cybernetics
Private Practice
New York, NY

Laurence I. Sugarman, MD, FAAP, ABMH
Clinical Associate Professor in Pediatrics
University of Rochester School of Medicine and Dentistry
General and Behavioral Pediatrics
Lifetime Health Medical Group
Rochester, NY

John A. Teleska, MEd
Member, Center for Psychotherapy Cybernetics
The Springs, Integrated Health Department,
Clifton Springs Hospital & Clinic, Clifton Springs, NY
Private Practice
Rochester, NY

Linda Thomson, PhD, MSN, CPNP
Adjunct Assistant Professor, University of Vermont
Nurse Practitioner and Approved Consultant in Clinical
    Hypnosis
Pioneer Valley Pediatrics
Enfield, CT and Longmeadow, MA
Greater Falls Family Medicine
Bellows Falls, VT

Thomas W. Wall, PhD, ABPP, ABPH
Clinical Psychologist
Clinical Associate Professor, University of Washington
Department of Psychiatry and Behavioral Sciences/
    Department of Clinical Psychology
Adjunct – Seattle Pacific University
Department of Graduate Psychology
Private Practice
Seattle, WA

William C. Wester, II, EdD, ABPP, ABPH
Clinical Psychologist
Clinical Professor, Wright State University
School of Professional Psychology
Recent – Adjunct Professor of Psychology, The Athenaeum of
    Ohio
Past President, American Society of Clinical Hypnosis
Forensic Hypnosis Consultant to ATF and FBI
Cincinnati, OH

Foreword

Separation of disciplines is an epidemic problem of our times. This has been especially true between the fields of physical and mental illnesses. For too long, clinicians have practiced in separate silos and did not talk the talk with each other. In the past few decades, several pioneers have made progress in bringing the fields together. Dr. George Engel of Rochester, New York coined the term "biopsychosocial" to emphasize that all health disorders have elements of each of the three factors inherent in them. Several research workers have demonstrated that psychological stress can lead to several different traditional medical illnesses, and many traditional psychological illnesses have been shown to have, in part, a physical basis. Psychological factors can alter immunological, endocrine, and other physiological processes. While this recognition of the interrelation of biopsychosocial factors in health and illness has been recognized, what has been lacking is a therapeutic skill to deal effectively with the interrelation of biopsychosocial factors. While hypnosis has been used for over a century to ameliorate physical symptoms, its use in children has become evident only in the past three decades. The authors of this collection of chapters have brought together leading practitioners and researchers who work with children to assemble a state of the art book on the uses of hypnosis in children.

As the authors point out, helping children deal with their emotional and physical symptoms by the use of hypnosis, cannot be learned from books alone. It requires training and practice. But readers of this fine book will come to understand that this therapeutic technique should be one of the skills of clinicians who care for children. The book goes far to break down the walls that have, for too long, separated clinicians who come from different disciplines to come together to better help children.

This text includes a review on the ethics of hypnosis with children and adolescents by Dr. Thomas W. Wall, a psychologist who is also past President of the American Society of Clinical Hypnosis (ASCH) and a chapter on how understanding child development impacts on teaching hypnosis to adults by Dr. Julie H. Linden, the current president of the ASCH. The first pediatric surgeon to integrate hypnosis into his daily practice, Dr. Thom E. Lobe, has written a chapter on pre-operative hypnosis. These authors represent the breadth and depth of the many who have contributed chapters and who represent just how far the application of hypnosis in child health has come. During the past five years there have been numerous functional MRI studies in adults which demonstrate actual brain changes during hypnosis. While this type of data impresses those who have been skeptical about hypnosis, the clinicians represented in this book have now offered much practical guidance to former skeptics which, we trust, will benefit thousands of children in the future.

Karen N. Olness, MD
Kenyon, MN
Robert J. Haggerty, MD
Canandaigua, NY

I think he does better at this because he doesn't know that he can't.
Father of an 8-year-old boy
who uses hypnosis for procedures

You can't give me my needle stick until I numb my arm with my magic quarter.
Tommy, age 8

I used my "control meter" and turned down the anxiety.
Anthony, age 12

Hypnosis teaches you things other people don't know. I like it a lot.
Abby, age 9

That was really cool. I went home on my magic carpet, got my glove, and now I am back at the family picnic.
Roger, age 9

Mom, I taught the doctors how I can turn off switches and the stitches didn't even hurt.
Emma, age 10

Learning to breathe away my headaches and worries has been very important to me. Now I want to get through every day without wasting one breath.
Brianna, age 17

I know how to turn off the headaches before I have them.
Allison, age 12

It's a powerful feeling.
Matthew, age 16

Preface

Our deepest fear is not that we are inadequate. Our deepest fear is that we are powerful beyond measure.[1]

Children are developmentally in motion both physiologically and psychologically. They live in a land of discovery where ideas realize themselves and imagination prevails. Children are always in a creative and imaginative trance-like state. They epitomize the truism that all hypnosis is self-hypnosis. We see this in their on-going play and as mommy or daddy kiss the "boo-boo" to make it better. In our therapeutic encounters with them, our goal is to interact with this on-going process, go with the flow and the child, and begin a journey of allowing children to do whatever is necessary to heal themselves. Those of us in this specialized field of human interaction have been strongly influenced by Milton Erickson whose utilization of naturally occurring psychophysiological responses makes it clear that our role as therapist and healer is to use whatever the child brings to the therapeutic encounter as we semantically work with the child to accomplish his goal.

We have brought together a cadre of distinguished authorities in the field of hypnosis with children and adolescents. These experts examine ways in which a variety of medical and psychological problems can be treated with this wonderful therapeutic interpersonal process. The reader will clearly begin to understand the significant differences between treating adults and children and will be exposed to marvelous varieties of approaches by these leaders in the field. Individual styles may vary, but the underlying premise of a creative patient-centered approach will be obvious. It's not a matter of using a direct or indirect approach. It's not a matter of developing highly creative metaphors since children will bring

---

[1] M. Williamson, *A Return to Love: Reflections on the Principles of a Course in Miracles.* New York: Harper Collins, 1992, p. 190.

their own. It's not a matter of asking children to remove symptoms. It's a matter of joining therapeutically with a children who are already well on their way to using their own creative imaginative processes to help themselves. We offer them guidance and confidence while having fun, being playful, and watching them develop their capacities for resilience.

Each chapter includes clinical vignettes, definitions of terms, working diagnoses, a review of relevant literature, a description of clinical strategies, and important caveats. We intend this book to be both well-grounded and clinically practical. The clinical examples are designed to illustrate the principles derived from literature and the authors' experiences. These vignettes are more than illustrations. We hope they enthuse the reader to interact creatively with the young people in therapy.

Of course, one cannot learn to implement clinical skills from a textbook. This volume is designed to stimulate or augment professional clinical training in hypnosis. The reader is also referred to the excellent texts cited in the list of references, many of which provide basic information on the fundamentals of hypnosis. Before clinicians can introduce hypnosis into their practices, they are advised to participate in professional courses, workshops, and supervision. In addition to university sponsored curricula and courses, The Society for Clinical and Experimental Hypnosis and The American Society of Clinical Hypnosis (with its component sections) provide superb training for licensed professionals in the US. Around the world, professional training is sponsored by national hypnosis societies, which are brought together by their affiliation with the International Society of Hypnosis. These organizations regularly include advanced workshops with a special focus on hypnosis with children and adolescents as part of their annual and regional meetings. Since 1987, the Society for Developmental and Behavioral Pediatrics has offered workshops in hypnosis with children at basic, intermediate, and advanced levels as part of its annual meeting. We encourage readers who have not availed themselves of such training opportunities to do so not only to develop the necessary clinical skills but also to enjoy the camaraderie and encouragement of like-minded professionals.

This collection of clinical exploration and discussion comes at a time when psychobiology is blossoming. In the nearly 250 years since Franz Anton Mesmer began using what he termed "Magnetisme Animal,"[2] the conjoined fields of psychophysiology and hypnosis have been evolving with accelerated speed. Over the past fifty years, increasing evidence of brain-body interactions with the peripheral immune, endocrine, and other somatic systems have begun to provide the intercellular evidence for what we have always known: the brain and body are powerfully connected. Even more, we are beginning to understand the neuroscience of consciousness and the psychobiology of gene expression explicated by Rossi's "psychosocial genomics."[3] This new information about how our experiences and memories structure our brains and psychophysiological reflexes supports novel therapies that promote brain plasticity and growth. Clinical hypnosis is proving to be such a therapeutic probe. This new science holds its greatest promise for its preventive potential with young people. It will inform our clinical work in helping children and adolescents develop resiliency and physiological self-regulation. In a sense, we are in the process of learning a better way to help children "mind."

A note about Clinician-Therapists: Many clinicians (physicians, surgeons, nurse practitioners, physician assistants) are not regarded as therapists. Similarly, mental health therapists (psychologists, social workers, marriage and family therapists) do not work in clinical settings as such and are not characterized as clinicians. Hypnotherapy, however, is a skill set and strategy that bridges both physiological and psychological in both intent and outcome. Therefore, to be inclusive, we will use the terms *clinician* and *therapist* interchangeably throughout this text.

We liken this text to a well-documented cookbook with no recipes, only enticing combinations of ingredients and descriptions of

[2] M. Mesmer, "Memoir sur la Decouverte du Magnetisme Animal," [Notes on the Discovery of Animal Magnetism] (1779). In *Foundations of Hypnosis from Mesmer to Freud*, M. M. Tinterow (Ed.). Springfield, IL: Charles C. Thomas, 1970, p. 32.
[3] E. L. Rossi, *The Psychobiology of Gene Expression: Neuroscience and Neurogenesis in Hypnosis and the Healing Arts*. New York: W.W. Norton, 2002.

appetizing dishes that, we hope, will inspire readers to enjoy cooking up creative hypnotic encounters with the children and adolescents in their care.

William C. Wester, II, EdD, ABPP, ABPH
Laurence I. Sugarman MD, FAAP, ABMH

Acknowledgments

We have so many people to thank for their advice, encouragement, and help in making this book become a reality. We thank our parents, childhood teachers, and professional teachers who throughout the years have shared their wisdom and inspired us to use our imagination when working with children and their marvelous imaginations. Our families deserve high praise for their patience, endurance of our absences, and support as we overcame obstacles to our goal. We owe a sincere thanks to Shirley Soellner who formatted our personal chapters in accordance with the APA style format we selected, Bonnie Kaplan Brauer who assisted in editing and acting as a sounding board, and to the people at Crown House Publishing, especially Mark Tracten our managing editor, who has been most helpful and supportive. We are privileged to have been chosen by Crown House Publishing to publish this work.

Part I
Introduction to Hypnosis

Chapter One

Hypnosis with Children and Adolescents: A Contextual Framework

Laurence I. Sugarman, MD, FAAP, ABMH
William C. Wester, II, EdD, ABPP, ABPH

Hypnosis started when the first mother kissed it and made it better.
F. Bauman
Personal communication, September 21, 1996

He was 7 years old and the youngest of five children. He hated being the first in bed when so much happened in the evening just outside his bedroom door. He would sneak out, sit at the top of the stairs, and listen to his brother and sisters argue and laugh, his parents' stern voices, and hushed phone conversations. He wanted to miss nothing. Somehow, his mother would always know he had escaped his room, and send him scurrying back, yelling up the stairs, "You stay in that bed!" This repeated imprisonment fueled his resentment and his determination to undermine his mother's bedtime restrictions.

One evening, as he lay seething in his bed, he suddenly realized that his mother only forbade him to leave his bed, not his room. Inspiration struck! Lying under the covers, he gripped the mattress edges, mustered his concentration, squeezed his eyes shut with resolve, and willed his mattress to float carefully out his second floor bedroom window. He was aloft! He hovered rebelliously outside his parents' bedroom window, dashing away just before they spied him. He zoomed over the house in the cool night air, up over the rooftops. He sailed over his school and the backyard of his best friend Stuart's house. Over the trees and the park and his neighborhood he soared for hours and hours. As he tired, he began to descend. Breathing deeply, he landed back in his room just as he fell, peacefully, into sound sleep.

He woke in the morning refreshed, winning praise and extra cinnamon toast from his mother for staying in his bed after bedtime. Thereafter, he got away with it every night.

After a time he grew up, left home and became a man, husband, and father. He worked and traveled and worried. He did all those hard things that grownups do. And, even when he was much older, when his worries troubled him and he could not sleep, he would know to lie in his bed, a 7-year-old, tightly close his eyes, calm himself by floating through his neighborhoods, seeing his world from a different perspective, then make it back to his room just in time to fall, peacefully, into sound sleep.

His parents never found out.

What is hypnosis? What is different about hypnosis with children and adolescents? The fascinating, elusive answers to these questions are the subject of this text in general and this chapter in particular.

Since James Braid coined the term "neurypnosis" in 1843, ongoing debate has delayed consensus on a definition of this discipline (Braid, 1843). The 2003 American Psychological Association, Division of Psychological Hypnosis (Division 30) definition of hypnosis spawned a cacophony of criticism (Green, Barabasz, Barrett, & Montgomery, 2005–2006; Barabasz, 2005–2006; Woody & Sadler, 2005–2006; Yapko, 2005–2006; Spiegel & Greenleaf, 2005–2006; Heap, 2005–2006; Araoz, 2005–2006; Rossi, 2005–2006; Hammond, 2005–2006; McConkey, 2005–2006; Daniel, 2005–2006). Is hypnosis a natural state along a continuum of normal waking processes? Is it a socio-cognitive phenomenon manifested by role-enactment that is labeled hypnotic? Is hypnosis simply the "cultivation of imagination" (D. P. Kohen, personal communication, September 16, 1993), or is imagination less relevant to hypnotic processes than a sense of involuntary experience and subconscious activation? What are the important differences between reverie, self-hypnosis, and therapeutic hypnosis in a clinical setting? What is the validity of hypnotizability scales in clinical work? Is hypnotizability an innate trait or a self-limiting construct? Of the characteristics assigned to hypnotic experience or trance, which are most crucial: dissociation, suggestion, relaxation, absorption, or rapport? What is trance? What distinguishes hypnosis from the myriad of other mental states and human interactions that are not hypnotic (Lynn & Rhue, 1991)?

The essence of the debate is that, lacking some discrete, objective, exclusive device that measures when hypnosis has occurred, we define hypnosis from within our individual frames of reference. What is hypnosis? As Michael Heap put it, "I suspect the answer will remain: 'It depends what you mean by hypnosis'" (Heap, 2005–2006). It depends on context.

Because this book is about what hypnosis is with children, we adopt a broad definition that derives from the context of young lives. Experiencing the developmental ferment of infancy, childhood, and adolescence, young people are in the business of discovering how their minds and bodies are connected. Mother's first touch; the comfort of satisfied hunger; the repeated surprise of peek-a-boo; balancing on two legs, then two wheels; throwing a ball far; all of these events ultimately form, then reinforce, neural networks that structure subsequent memory and experience (Edelman, 2004). Emerging neuroscience research reveals that the blossoming, malleable neurohumoral pathways that join sensory input, memory, and physiological response at these deepest levels of a child's mind evolve into the frameworks of adaptation for the rest of our lives (Fitzgerald & Howard, 2003).

In childhood, the impetus for curiosity, novelty seeking, autonomy, and mastery are manifestations of this growing meshwork of psychophysiological reflexes. Imagination and dreams are the conscious representation of this subconscious psychophysiological development. Children live in the world of their imaginations, using their imaginative capacities to rehearse skills, cope with fears and challenges, and to set goals for themselves. These urges also drive creative social engagement, social learning, the senses of self and other, and the understanding of empathy (Hilgard, 1970; Olness, 1985).

We propose that hypnosis is about engaging these creative subconscious processes, with or without conscious awareness. This may occur in the reverie of a child's play (self- or auto-hypnosis) or in social interaction (heterohypnosis). The purpose of that hypnotic engagement is determined by its context. Stage hypnotists use hypnosis for the purpose of entertainment. Sales programs use hypnotic elements to sell a product. Acute trauma enacts deep subconscious processes with the same, though alienating, hypnotic rudiments. The spontaneous dissociation experienced by a sexually abused child typifies this naturally occurring trance (Kowatsch, 1991). When hypnotic elements are evoked in a clinical setting, supported by therapeutic rapport, with the intention of changing maladaptive, conditioned psychophysiological reflexes, we call that hypnotherapy. It has been noted that, "While all hypnosis is not therapy, all therapy is hypnosis" (James Maddox, personal communication, July 28, 1995).

If, at its simplest, therapeutic hypnosis is a type of human interaction that accesses and changes maladaptive subconscious psychophysiological reflexes, then it is no wonder that children, with virgin psychophysiological landscapes, are great adventurers, mapping new trails. If we can conceive of developmental tasks as psychophysiological imperatives that govern the formation of mind-body reflexes and behavioral response, then it is easy to imagine children in trance all the time and open to suggestion. It is not so much that children are "good at hypnosis"; more aptly, they live, full time, in the trance of intense psychophysiological development.

Doing Hypnosis with Children and Adolescents

Most professionals initially learn hypnotic technique as a series of discrete, ordered steps: (1) introduction, (2) induction into trance, (3) intensification, (4) therapeutic suggestions, (5) resumption of usual awareness ("de-hypnosis"), then, finally (6) ratification and reflection. Teleska and Roffman (2004)) have likened this to the "vessel" approach to hypnosis: the subject is dipped into the vessel full of hypnotic trance where some subconscious change occurs during immersion. Then the subject floats back up to the surface, is removed, and wiped off. This view of hypnotic interaction has some utility in that it provides a good model to build from and is often all that is necessary with many adults.

Medical students first learn to take a complete history and then perform a complete physical examination on every patient. For the purpose of training, they learn to follow the protocol of history, then examination in the same order, each time. Once they begin to interact with people in real clinical encounters, they learn that the history is unveiled in idiosyncratic layers as rapport with the patient grows. If they are paying attention, the students learn that how they respond to the patient will change both the symptoms and physical findings. They learn to revisit parts of the history and exam to discover their consistency and meaning. In time, they learn that there is never a complete history or physical examination, just an unfolding. Ultimately, they understand that the protocol for memorizing how to take a medical history and do a physical examination has little to do with actually interacting therapeutically with a patient. The protocol is just a way to begin to learn the skills.

With children and adolescents, whom we have identified as constantly being in the trance of psychophysiological change, the adult vessel metaphor seems to break down and typically the protocols do not work. The young person's tenacious and self-protective autonomy dictates the order and flow of the therapeutic encounter. The child who comes into the office entranced by the pain of appendicitis, his or her anxiety about receiving immunization injections, the induction of previous experiences with the therapist, or simply imagining the story that she read last night, does not require a formal hypnotic induction and may not cooperate with one. The therapist simply needs to join, with permission, in the flow of the trance. To the child entranced by the pain of a wound that requires sutures, the therapist can ask simply, "I wonder where you would rather be than here." When the child briefly averts his or her eyes as evidence of his or her subconscious search for that place, the therapist assists in the dissociation by saying, "Go ahead. Leave this hurt part here to heal up." Milton Erickson instructed, "Work primarily *with*, and not *on*, the *child*" [Italics added] (Erickson, 1958).

We find that hypnosis works best with children and adolescents when it is not done *to* them but *with* them. To do this well requires flexibility, creativity, and adaptability on the part of the therapist.

> I [LS] was conducting a small group practice experience at an intro- ductory workshop on pediatric hypnosis. After receiving my sup- portive, but critical feedback about the directive and authoritative tone of his suggestions to a subject, a young doctor stated, with some exasperation, "This is so hard because it is about giving up my con- trol over the patient!" I could not help but respond, gently, "No. It is about recognizing that you never had it in the first place."

Eye closure illustrates a common distinction between hypnosis with children and adults. Most children under 10 years of age fre- quently do hypnosis best with their eyes open and tell us so (Olness & Kohen, 1996). Since therapists have learned to equate eye closure with both the intensity of trance and validity of the hypnotic experience, they can be uncomfortable with this, even mistaking it for resistance or opposition. Some children, on the other hand, may equate eye closure with loss of control, having to go to sleep when they do not want to and not wanting to miss what is going on in the room while they use their hypnotic ability. As part of hypnotic induction, I [LS] ask children to do this experiment:

> "While you are [*imagining, letting those balloons raise your arm, relaxing, etc.*] find out if it is better with your eyes open or closed. Whatever is best for you and those eyes, let them stay that way because you know what is best." The child closes his eyes and either reopens them or leaves them closed. Whichever results, I say, "That's right." A 9-year- old boy told me, "I think it's good to keep my eyes open because it

helps to see colors better, because when I close my eyes all I see is black. I can see colors when I'm asleep but not when I'm awake." The child states, implicitly, his understanding that (1) he can imagine with his eyes open, using his surroundings for inspiration; (2) he uses different capacities during sleep; and (3) he knows that hypnosis is not sleep.

Similarly, young people may feel far more comfortable and engaged in hypnotic experience while not physically relaxed. Physical relaxation is certainly a compelling respite for most adults but is often too passive for children. "Relax" can be evocative of parental admonitions to "Calm down!" and "Be quiet!" It is far better to find out how the child will help himself or herself become most comfortable and able to have fun, rather than be relaxed.

In my [LS] consultation room, a 7-year-old boy with sleep disturbance, recurrent abdominal pain and divorcing parents happily imagined, and acted out, swinging back and forth on his favorite playground swing set. He moved vigorously back and forth on his chair while telling me he was going higher and higher. He abruptly stopped and looked side to side then sadly looked down. When I asked him what happened, he replied, staring at the floor, "There are two swings, next to each other. When I am on one I want to be on the other and if I switch I might fall off."

The vessel analogy of hypnosis also confines therapeutic work because it assumes a controlling and detached facilitator. Distinct from hypnotic elements of entertainment, sales, trauma, and story telling, hypnosis in therapy engages the young person's subconscious in a co-creative act in which the therapist is flexibly responsive to the subconscious clues, or ideodynamic signals of the subject. This responsivity is both a conscious and subconscious phenomenon within the therapist. This informs what we may call intuition, which Erickson and Rossi (1989) call an "unconscious response to [the patient's] minimal cues" (p. 18). Doing hypnotherapy and responding to intuition involves the recognition of the therapist's own trance, focused intently on the subject of therapy.

An 11-year-old boy with anxiety glanced at a glass ball on my [LS] bookshelf upon entering my office. This brief gesture led me to ask him if the rainy weather was ending outside. This, in turn, led to a discussion of weather, the rotation of the earth and, therapeutically, how we get a different perspective on our problems and how they change like the weather when we see them from far above.

The key to this approach to the patient is in understanding pacing and leading. *Pacing* is meeting the child or adolescent where he or she is and acknowledging that it is where he or she ought to be. *Leading* involves inviting, suggesting, offering a therapeutic direction for change. Pacing includes direct empathetic statements such as, "You look pretty frightened!" or "You sure are good at screaming!" Pacing can also be subtle, such as the affirmation of saying "that's right," or silence. Leading involves the language of possibilities. Hammond (1990) describes a variety of phrases that can be utilized to assist the child (or adult) with his or her journey and "assist you (the therapist) in internalizing this new way of speaking." Examples might include " ... and you will be surprised at ... ," "I wonder if you'll decide to ... ," or "One of the first things you can become aware of is ... ," and "It may be that you're already aware of ... " (pp. 40–41). Such phrases are subtle ways to help lead the child to discover more about himself or herself and his or her curious imagination.

Pacing and leading are best synchronized, by careful observation, focused attention, and listening for nonverbal and verbal cues, such as breathing patterns, body movements, and facial expressions. As we do this, perhaps in our own trance, we find ourselves going where the child needs to go. An example of pacing and leading towards therapeutic dissociation in an emergency setting with a child in pain can be as simple and powerful as, "I bet you would rather be someplace other than here right now. Go there while I help you with this."

While this text is brimming with clinical examples of hypnotic interaction with children and adolescents, these vignettes are not intended to be scripts or prescriptive types of imagery. They are illustrations of interactive, co-creative processes. They originate from the unique personalities of the therapist-child dyad at that moment in development. These singular examples exist to support the notion of hypnotic interaction as adaptive, flexible, and child-centered. This is essential because this responsive process reifies the therapist's faith that the child and adolescent are endowed with the internal resources to help themselves.

Locus of Control

> Healing consists in, and only in ... allowing, causing, or bringing to bear those things or forces for getting better (whatever they may be) that already exist in the patient. (Cassell, 1991/2004, p. 219)

It is certainly possible to do effective hypnotic work with children and adolescents in a directive, forceful, or authoritarian style. The early history of hypnosis records sparse, anecdotal reports of children, and little description of the technique used, but we can glean from accounts of the mesmerists that rigid, directive techniques were aimed at children and adolescents who were to remain passive or swoon in abreaction (Mesmer, 1779). This history and culture has no doubt informed and reinforced images of hypnosis from cartoons and fairy tales in which wizards, witches, and evil queens cast spells. Children have been coerced in the trance of repeated trauma to comply with authoritative commands.

It is also possible to prescribe imagery, and dictate solutions that involve metaphors the therapist finds poetic and elegant. Therapeutic stories can be comforting, familiar, and decrease alienation. Indeed, the therapeutic ritual of bedtime stories has soothed generations (Thomson, 2005). Kuttner's use of favorite stories with young children serves to support this strategy (Kuttner, 1988).

While a therapist may either successfully command a child to change a symptom in a hypnotic context or assist a child to find relief in a metaphorical story, both of these approaches are limited. They do not explicitly enlist the young person's innate resources. They fall short of the opportunity to invest in the young person's ability to discover his or her own stories, metaphors, and attributions of meaning. Both authoritarian, directive hypnosis and prescriptive imagery may potentially limit the young person's ability to help himself or herself.

Milton Erickson, whose sometimes subtle, very intuitive strategies signaled a shift in hypnotherapy, pioneered a more evocative, patient-centered approach to hypnotic interaction. His far-reaching influence on Bauman, Gardner, Olness, Kohen, and generations of child healthcare providers spawned a child-centered, creative focus on the use of therapeutic language, an emphasis on informal utilization of naturally occurring hypnotic states, and much more playful techniques. The critical contribution of these leaders in child hypnosis is their emphasis on employing hypnosis to invest in mastery and self-efficacy in children, moving beyond solution-focused therapy.

Locus of control studies focus on a young person's attribution of how internal or external factors affect him or her. This research demonstrates that innate coping skills and resilience are enhanced by an internalized locus of control (Culbert, Reaney, & Kohen, 1994). At the heart of a patient-centered, responsive hypnotic strategy is the faith on the part of the therapist that each youngster already has within him or her all of the resources to help himself or herself. This is the crux of Erickson's "Utilization Approach" in which the therapist uses whatever the patient brings to the encounter, recognizing it as essential and sufficient (Erickson & Rossi, 1992).

I [LS] was asked to help a frightened, uncooperative 7-year-old girl with chronic renal failure and extreme needle phobia. Asking what she would rather be doing than getting a "shot," she replied, "At home, playing with my kitties. When they scratch it doesn't hurt because they are just kittens." It was as if she was telling me, "Hey you, Doctor, use this metaphor. It will work!" It did, of course.

Helping children utilize their own capacities is particularly valuable when they have a chronic disease. Each medication, procedure, or removal from school for an appointment or hospitalization constitutes an implicit message that they cannot help themselves. The locus of control is externalized. More broadly, this loss of self-efficacy and alienation is an untoward effect of all allopathic therapy. Hypnosis can help children balance this loss of control but the use of prescriptive or authoritarian techniques constitutes yet another grown-up doing something manipulative to the child. A 14-year-old hospitalized for initial treatment of lymphoma explained, "Everyone keeps coming in and trying to teach me to calm down and relax. I already know how to do that, but they won't leave me alone!"

Roles of Parents

Milton Erickson said,

> You always point out to parents that the child has a tremendously important function for them. That they're really not going to get that full measure of satisfaction out of the child to which they are entitled unless the child is happy. (Haley, 1985, p. 86)

A major difference between hypnosis with adults and children is the presence and role of parents in the hypnotherapeutic process. A necessary developmental task of all children is to develop autonomy from their parents. The equivalent developmental task of all parents is to invest in their child's security, then let go. In a series of 505 hypnotherapeutic encounters with children, Kohen, Olness, Colwell, and Heimel (1984) found that negative outcomes were correlated with parental reminders and over-involvement. Parental nagging negated the autonomy necessary for success in self-regulation. The effect of family systems must be addressed before helping children help themselves.

Most parents have a positive attitude towards hypnosis with their children. They recognize, or can be helped to recognize, their own natural experiences with hypnosis. When hypnosis with the child is explained as an opportunity to invest in their child's vast creative ability to help themselves, parents generally are relieved that (1) they have a partner in helping their child and (2) that partner believes their child has the necessary resources and abilities to get better. This recognition on the part of the parents is enhanced when the therapist engages respectfully with the child in the parents' presence. When this parental acceptance is not the case, it ought to be construed as a warning that the parents are threatened in some way by their child's development.

Gardner (1974) carefully details strategies to help parents become allies in their child's hypnotherapy with three basic steps: (1) education, (2) observation, and (3) experience. Education involves explaining and noticing hypnosis in daily life, how this ability is enhanced with children, and how it may be utilized to help their child in this case. Once parents agree to allow the therapist to work with their child the parent can be reassured by observing their child using hypnosis. Generally, this is done after the child has learned self-hypnosis with the therapist, without the parents present, and has thereby developed a sense of comfort and competence on his or her own. Exceptions to this are explained below. During this observation, Gardner (1974) points out that it is important

> [T]o have the parent watch the therapist communicate with the child in hypnosis, requiring the child to give both nonverbal and verbal responses and then to transfer hypnotic rapport to the parents and have them also communicate verbally and nonverbally with the child. This exercise helps assure the parent that the child is in contact with his surroundings and in control of the hypnotic state as much as necessary." (p. 46)

Finally, Gardner recommends that parents can enhance their own understanding of the child's experience, exercise better self-control, and realize the individuality of hypnotic involvement by having their own brief trance experience with the therapist. After initial publication of these recommendations, Gardner decreased the frequency of having parents experience hypnosis intentionally. According to Olness and Kohen, "This change developed when it became clear that some parents—even in brief hypnosis—might use the opportunity to experience grief or other feeling … ," which could complicate the role of the therapist in relationship to the child (Olness & Kohen, 1996, p. 50).

In addition to Gardner's guidelines, we make it clear at the first visit that learning self-regulation is necessarily an exercise in autonomy, and therefore, a contract between the therapist and the child or adolescent, not the parent. If, for some reason, a parent feels that his or her son or daughter is not using or practicing the skills learned with the therapist, the parent may relay that concern to the therapist but not nag the child about it. We explain to the parent that this is a necessary part of helping the child help himself or herself.

Many clinicians record their initial hypnosis session and give the recording to child. This strategy serves a number of practical purposes. It extends rapport because the child brings the therapist's voice home. It reinforces the language, framing, and therapeutic suggestions with repetition. Knowing that their child has a tool to guide them can relieve parents of the need to become overinvolved in the process. The recording is not to be construed as the "right way to do hypnosis." Instead, it can be offered in a way that enhances therapeutic change and autonomy. This is illustrated in the following example:

> "I will make you a recording of what we do together today. That way you can choose to listen to it and remember how to use your self-hypnosis. The recording is like training wheels on a bicycle. They keep you in balance so you can learn what it feels like to be successful riding your bicycle. Of course, after you get good at it, you realize that they slow you down, so you take them off and go on without them. You will know when you don't need to use the recording anymore."

Some young people will make their own recordings, adding their own suggestions and music.

With preschool children and children facing life-threatening illness at any age, parental involvement is valuable and usually essential. In addition to reinforcing the primary attachment that is therapeutic in these situations, the heightened intimacy of hypnotic involvement with parent and child intensifies security and comfort. This is exquisitely exemplified in the "Candy Land" scene in Leora Kuttner's documentary video *No Fears, No Tears* (Kuttner, 1986). In this scene, a father gently and responsively engages his 7-year-old daughter who has leukemia in the guided imagery of visiting "Candy Land." Their co-creative process and his patient respect for her are evident in how he asks her about the details of the people she sees in "Candy Land." When we help parents become hypnotherapists in these settings, we are helping them help themselves as well as their children.

Caveats and Contraindications

We have presented hypnosis with children as an opportunity to help them utilize and strengthen their own subconscious resources in pursuit of health and adaptation. From the clinician's perspective, hypnotherapy is a skill set that can be integrated into a variety of clinical settings from the consultation room, to the examination room, the hospital bed, and the surgical suite. As such, it is always a helpful adjunctive therapy when it is used permissively and responsively. Dangers arise when hypnosis is used forcefully, as sole therapy, outside a therapeutic relationship or without a careful and repeated consideration of the patient's symptomology.

Clinicians integrating hypnosis into their care of children must first be careful and competent professionals within their areas of expertise (psychology, medicine, surgery, nursing, social work, counseling, etc.) considering a range of explanations for a given child's presenting problems. The temptation to make hypnosis a panacea must be tempered with careful diagnostic evaluation and re-evaluation. Olness and Libby (1987) reported that 20 percent of youngsters referred for hypnotherapy to a behavioral pediatric clinic had undiagnosed, organic etiologies for their presenting problems.

Clinicians must stay within their range of competency despite the range of problems for which hypnotherapy may be valuable. We may add hypnotic strategies to a problem that we also treat allopathically. For example, hypnosis has been shown to be a useful adjunct to asthma therapy (Kohen, 2000), and a primary physician trained in hypnosis may well employ hypnotherapy to help his or her young patients with asthma. While hypnosis is also helpful in the therapy of posttraumatic stress disorder (PTSD) in an abused child, the same primary care physician ought not to use hypnosis for that child unless he or she is specifically trained in treating posttraumatic stress disorder or forensic applications.

Olness and Kohen (1996) have outlined absolute contraindications to using hypnosis with children: risking physical endangerment, risking aggravation of emotional problems, hypnosis for fun or entertainment outside of a therapeutic relationship, and when more effective treatment is available. We would submit that these same principles apply for all forms of therapeutic interventions, including medications, surgery, manipulation, and non-hypnotic forms of psychotherapy.

We would add two relative contraindications. First, as discussed under the roles of parents, sometimes a symptom becomes a part of a family's ecology (e.g., a child's headache keeps mother and father from arguing). In this setting, attending to the family may be a primary intervention before or while helping the child. A second relative contraindication applies to situations in which the child has a long-term relationship with the clinician. Sometimes, based on the longevity of a relationship, the primary therapist is not the best therapist, despite his or her competency. In this setting a new relationship is best. A primary care physician, skilled in hypnosis and well known by the family, may not be the best therapist for the adolescent for whom he or she has cared since the child's birth. The teenager may benefit from and desire a fresh start with a new relationship.

The Psychobiology of Hypnosis with Children

One hundred and fifty years ago, writing about his study of hypnosis, James Braid (1865) coined the term "psychophysiology" and gave birth to the field, writing:

> The [hypnotic] phenomena are due entirely to this influence of
> dominant ideas over physical action, and point to the importance
> of combining the study of psychology with that of physiology, and
> vice versa. I believe the attempt made to study these two branches
> of science so much apart from each other, has been a great hin-
> drance to the successful study of either. (p. 369)

Over the last century investigators have started elucidating how
the brain and body influence each other. From the pathways of
stress mediated by the hypothalamic-pituitary-adrenal axis explicated by Hans Selye (1956/1976), to the brain body chemical
messengers researched by Candice Pert (1997), to the field of psychoneuroimmunology first explored by Robert Ader, David
Felten, and Nicholas Cohen (2001), these pioneers and their colleagues have begun to give Braid the answers to his questions of
how the mind influences the body.

In the clinical laboratory children have been shown to be able to
use hypnosis to elevate salivary immunoglobulin (Olness, Culbert,
& Uden, 1989), change blood flow (Clawson & Swade, 1975), alter
neutrophil adhesiveness (Hall, et al., 1992), change skin temperature, and conductance and other so-called "involuntary" psychophysiological reflexes (Lee & Olness, 1996; Dikel & Olness,
1980). These laboratory investigations have been utilized to study
how children can lower their frequency of respiratory infections
(Hewson-Bower & Drummond, 1996), exacerbations of asthma
(Kohen, 2000), frequencies of migraine headaches (Olness,
McDonald, & Uden, 1987), and chemotherapy-induced vomiting
(Jacknow, Tschann, Link, & Boyce, 1994). There is vast, unexplored
potential in prospective, controlled clinical trials of hypnosis with
children with a variety of common chronic conditions. Can children with a genetic predisposition to allergy, anxiety, hyperten-
sion, cancer, or other conditions, alter their risks by developing
skills in psychophysiological self-regulation?

Beneath this unexplored territory lies the exciting field of psychosocial genomics, explicated by Rossi. In *The Psychobiology of Gene
Expression* he investigates how social interaction, novel experiences, creativity and—necessarily—hypnosis affect gene expression in
the brain and, consequently, how these gene products regulate brain

growth, plasticity, and neural pathways (Rossi, 2002, pp. 188–252). In his prophetic monograph, "The Physiology of Fascination and the Critics Criticized," Braid (1865) postulates that hypnosis somehow activates the mind's ability to change conditioned, maladaptive psychophysiological reflexes. We are now beginning to understand the molecular and intercellular processes that activate nerves to grow new synaptic connections, reinforcing or changing memory and experience and, in turn, altering physiological reflexes throughout the body. Children and adolescents are fully engaged in this formative process, the trance of development, with profound implications for their neurobiological resilience into the future.

Erickson understood this was true in his work with adults. He utilized age regression frequently and increasingly. Rosen writes of Erickson's regression technique in his Foreword to Erickson and Rossi's *The February Man.*

> It became clear to me why Erickson tended to treat almost everyone *like a child*! ... In his later years, he seemed to be so enamored of corny jokes, childish puzzles, and games. I now feel he understood, probably from having learned it from working with adult patients in the hypnotically regressed state, *that it is precisely in this "child state" that we are most open to learning, most curious, and most able to change.* In order to intensify the patient's experience of regression, Erickson worked consistently to create a remarkably convincing illusion that he really was an older person talking to a young child. He had the "child" react and abreact to traumatic experiences and, through discussions, guided her through a reeducation process. As a result, *the "child" had new experiences to add to her memories*—positive experiences with a caring and understanding adult. These "corrective regression experiences," as I have called them, exerted a long-lasting effect on the patient, even after she returned to her "adult self." [Italics added] (Erickson and Rossi, 1989, p. vii)

Understanding hypnosis as stimulating change by engaging the patient's subconscious with novelty and creativity, we can understand Erickson's use of age regression as cultivating brain plasticity by uncovering the "inner child's" state of wonderment. When we work with children, no regression is required.

Conclusion

Our unifying thesis is that the therapeutic interpersonal process that we call hypnotic engagement or hypnotherapy with young people can serve to model respectful relationships, demonstrate confidence, and invest in a child's self-efficacy and mastery. Time and again, the authors of this text, along with so many of our colleagues who work with children in this way, have heard young people who have learned to prevent their migraines, control a habit, master the specter of anxiety, or undergo a feared medical procedure with equanimity, exclaim: "Now I know I can do this!" The evidence suggests that young people continue to generalize the skills learned in these contexts to other challenges in their lives (Kohen, Olness, Colwell, & Heimel, 1984). Ultimately we believe, and anticipate investigations will prove, that this powerful investment forms psychophysiological resilience.

An 8-year old girl presented to my [LS] office in ketoacidosis with new-onset diabetes. Knowing her previous fear of needles and recognizing the trance of the situation, I helped her discover how she could keep needles from bothering her by "turning down the pain switches" in her mind. I then sent her to the emergency department at the local hospital for stabilization, admission, and patient education. Her life was about to change. That evening, in the hospital, her mother expressed her gratitude that her daughter had learned this hypnotic "pain switch" technique, saying, "This is going to make things much easier. ..." Her daughter interrupted, "Especially since I am going to be a doctor when I grow up."

References

Ader, R., Felten, D. L., & Cohen, N. (2001). *Psychoneuroimmunology* (3rd ed.). New York: Academic Press.

Araoz, D. (2005–2006). Defining hypnosis. *American Journal of Clinical Hypnosis*, 48(2–3), 123–126.

Barabasz, A. (2005–2006). Wither spontaneous hypnosis: A critical issue for practitioners and researchers. *American Journal of Clinical Hypnosis*, 48(2–3), 91–97.

Braid, J. (1843). Neurypnology or the rationale of nervous sleep. In M. M. Tinterow, *Foundations of hypnosis from Mesmer to Freud* (pp. 269–368). Springfield, IL: Charles C. Thomas.

Braid, J. (1865). The physiology of fascination and the critics criticized. In M. M. Tinterow, *Foundations of hypnosis from Mesmer to Freud* (p. 369). Springfield, IL: Charles C. Thomas.

Cassell, E. J. (1991/2004). *The nature of suffering and the goals of medicine.* New York: Oxford University Press.

Clawson, T. A., & Swade, R. H. (1975). The hypnotic control of blood flow and pain: The cure of warts and the potential for the use of hypnosis in the treatment of cancer. *American Journal of Clinical Hypnosis*, 17, 160–169.

Culbert, T. P., Reaney, J. B., & Kohen, D. P. (1994). "Cyberphysiologic" strategies for children: The clinical hypnosis/biofeedback interface. *International Journal of Clinical and Experimental Hypnosis*, 42, 97–113.

Daniel, S. A. (2005–2006). The perspective of a teacher and clinician: The 2003 APA Division 30 definition of hypnosis. *American Journal of Clinical Hypnosis*, 48(2–3), 141–143.

Dikel, W., & Olness, K. (1980). Self-hypnosis, biofeedback, and voluntary peripheral temperature control in children. *Pediatrics*, 66, 335–340.

Edelman, G. M. (2004). *Wider than the sky: The phenomenal gift of consciousness.* New Haven: Yale University Press.

Erickson, M. H. (1958). Pediatric hypnotherapy. *American Journal of Clinical Hypnosis*, 1, 25–29.

Erickson, M. H., & Rossi, E. L. (1989). *The February man: Evolving consciousness and identity in hypnotherapy.* New York: Brunner/Mazel.

Erickson, M. H., & Rossi, E. L. (1992) *Hypnotherapy: An exploratory casebook.* New York: Irvington.

Fitzgerald, M., & Howard, R. (2003). The neurobiologic basis of pediatric pain. In *Pain in infants, children, and adolescents* (2nd ed., pp. 26–27). Philadelphia: Lippincott, Williams, and Wilkins.

Gardner, G. G. (1974). Parents: Obstacles or allies in child hypnotherapy? *American Journal of Clinical Hypnosis*, 17, 44–49.

Green, J., Barabasz, A., Barrett, D., & Montgomery, G. (2005–2006). The 2003 APA Division 30 definition of hypnosis. *American Journal of Clinical Hypnosis*, 48(2–3), 89–91.

Haley, J. (Ed.). (1985). *Conversations with Milton H. Erickson, M.D.: Volume III Changing children and families*. New York: Triangle Press.

Hall, H. R., Minnes, L., Tosi, M., & Olness, K. (1992). Voluntary modulation of neutrophil adhesiveness using a cyberphysiologic strategy. *International Journal of Neuroscience*, 63, 287.

Hammond, D. C. (1990). Formulating hypnotic and posthypnotic suggestions. In D. C. Hammond (Ed.), *Handbook of hypnotic suggestions and metaphors*. New York: W.W. Norton.

Hammond, D. C. (2005–6). An integrative, multi-factor conceptualization of hypnosis. *American Journal of Clinical Hypnosis*, 48(2–3), 131–135.

Heap, M. (2005-6) Defining hypnosis: The UK experience. *American Journal of Clinical Hypnosis*, 48(2–3), 117–122.

Hewson-Bower, B., & Drummond, P. D. (1996). Secretory immunoglobulin A increases during relaxation in children with and without recurrent upper respiratory tract infections. *Journal of Developmental and Behavioral Pediatrics*, 17(5), 311–316.

Hilgard, J. R. (1970). *Personality and hypnosis: A study of imaginative involvement*. Chicago: University of Chicago Press.

Jacknow, D. S., Tschann, J. M., Link, M. P., & Boyce, W. T. (1994). Hypnosis in the prevention of chemotherapy-related nausea and vomiting in children: A prospective study. *Journal of Developmental and Behavioral Pediatrics*, 15, 258–264.

Kohen, D. P. (2000). Hypnosis in the treatment of asthma. *The Integrative Medicine Consult*, 2(6), 61–62.

Kohen, D. P., Olness, K. N., Colwell, S., & Heimel A. (1984) The use of relaxation/mental imagery (self-hypnosis) in the management of 505 pediatric behavioral encounters. *Journal of Developmental and Behavioral Pediatrics*, 1, 21–25.

Kohen, D. P., Olness, K. N., Colwell, S. & Heimel, A. (1984). The use of relaxation/mental imagery (self-hypnosis) in the management of 505 pediatric behavioral encounters. *Journal of Developmental and Behavioral Pediatrics*, 1, 21–25.

Kowatsch, C. (1991). *The use of hypnosis in the treatment of multiple personality disorder.* [Videotape]. Cincinnati: BSCI Publications.

Kuttner, L. (Director, Co-producer). (1986). *No fears, no tears: children with cancer coping with pain.* Vancouver, B.C.: Canadian Cancer Society. [Videotape]. Available from Fanlight Productions, www.fanlight.com, 1-800-937-4113.

Kuttner, L. (1988). Favorite stories: A hypnotic pain reduction technique for children in acute pain. *American Journal of Clinical Hypnosis*, 30(4), 289–295.

Lee, L. H., & Olness, K. N. (1996). Effects of self-induced mental imagery on autonomic reactivity in children. *Journal of Developmental and Behavioral Pediatrics*, 17(5), 323–327.

Lynn, S. J., & Rhue, J. W. (1991). *Theories of hypnosis: Current models and perspectives.* New York: Guilford.

McConkey, K. M. (2005–2006). On finding the balanced path of hypnosis definition. *American Journal of Clinical Hypnosis*, 48(2–3), 137–139.

Mesmer, F. A. (1779). Neurypnology or The rationale of nervous sleep, London: Churchill. In M. M. Tinterow, *Foundations of hypnosis from Mesmer to Freud.* (1970). Springfield, IL: Charles C. Thomas.

Olness, K. (1985). Little people, images and child health. *American Journal of Clinical Hypnosis*, 27, 169–174.

Olness, K. & Kohen, D. P. (1996). *Hypnosis and hypnotherapy with children* (3rd ed.). New York: Guilford.

Olness, K., McDonald, J. T., & Uden, D. L. (1987). Comparison of self-hypnosis and propranolol in the treatment of juvenile classic migraine. *Pediatrics*, 79(4), 593–597.

Olness, K. N., Culbert, T. P., & Uden, D. (1989). Self-regulation of salivary immunoglobulin A by children. *Pediatrics*, 83, 66–71.

Olness, K. N., Libbey, P. (1987). Unrecognized biologic bases of behavioral symptoms in patients referred for hypnotherapy. *American Journal of Clinical Hypnosis*, 30, 1–8.

Pert, C. (1997). *Molecules of emotion: The science behind mind–body medicine*. New York: Touchstone.

Rossi, E. L. (2002). *The psychobiology of gene expression: Neuroscience and neurogenesis in hypnosis and the healing arts*. New York: W.W. Norton.

Rossi, E. L. (2006). Let's be honest with ourselves and transparent with the public. *American Journal of Clinical Hypnosis*, 48(2–3), 127–129.

Selye, H. (1956/1976). *The stress of life*. New York: McGraw-Hill.

Spiegel, H., & Greenleaf, M. (2005–2006) Commentary: Defining hypnosis. *American Journal of Clinical Hypnosis*, 48(2–3), 111–116.

Teleska, J., & Roffman, A. (2004). A continuum of hypnotic interactions: From formal hypnosis to hypnotic conversation. *American Journal of Clinical Hypnosis*, 47(2), 103–115.

Thomson, L. (2005). *Harry the Hypno-potamus*. Carmarthen, Wales, U.K.: Crown House.

Woody, E., & Sadler, P. (2005–2006). Some polite applause for the 2003 APA Division 30 definition of hypnosis. *American Journal of Clinical Hypnosis*, 48(2–3), 99–106.

Yapko, M. D. (2005–2006). Some comments regarding the Division 30 definition of hypnosis. *American Journal of Clinical Hypnosis*, 48(2–3), 107–110.

Chapter Two

Developmental Considerations: Hypnosis with Children

Leora Kuttner, PhD (RegPsyc)
Rosalind E. H. Catchpole, MA

Imagination is more important than knowledge. Knowledge is limited.
*Imagination encircles the world.**

Albert Einstein

For pediatric clinicians, it can be a creative and imaginative delight to use hypnosis with babies, toddlers, preschool, and school-aged children. Historically neglected, hypnosis has now increasingly been recognized as an effective tool for children of all ages— including the very young.

Just as there is profound change and development across childhood from birth to adolescence, so too, does the hypnotic phenomenon look markedly distinct at different developmental periods (Vandenberg, 2002). A hypnotic process in babies and toddlers is unique in that it is sensory- and motor-based and is often fleeting. For preschoolers in the age of unbridled imagination,

Note: This chapter was supported in part by a Social Sciences and Humanities Research Council Canada Graduate Scholarship Doctoral Scholarship and a Michael Smith Foundation for Health Research Senior Graduate Traineeship awarded to the second author.

*George Sylvester Viereck, "What Life Means to Einstein," *The Saturday Evening Post*, October 26, 1929.

hypnotic suggestions are integrated and externalized in play. This stands in contrast to the hypnotic presentation of the older child, adolescent, and adult, in which eye closure and physical relaxation are often (although not always) present. Children of about seven years and older are more willing to close their eyes, "go inside," and engage with their creative imagination in a structured hypnotic experience. With younger children, the hypnotic process is less structured and more action-oriented and present-centered.

In general, children are highly receptive to hypnotic suggestion and, when invited, will often easily engage with the play, creativity, and imagination inherent in the hypnotic experience (see videotapes by Kuttner, 1986; 1998). This is the easy part—the more challenging aspect for clinicians is to be able to move with the child appropriately for therapeutic benefit.

The successful use of hypnosis with youngsters requires careful attention not only to the particular clinical needs of the child, but also to the child's developmental level. This encompasses not only their chronological age, but also their cognitive, emotional, language, and behavioral development. Hypnosis with children is not a homogeneous phenomenon. Just as the use of puppets in hypnosis with a 17-year-old may be developmentally inappropriate, a 3-year-old will not be responsive to a lengthy verbal induction. Flexibility as a clinician is paramount. Being attuned to the child's whole being, his or her world, and the unique nature of his or her difficulty allows the clinician the best inroads into a child's inner life as a vehicle for therapeutic change.

Hypnosis can be used in many different ways with children, and can be combined with other therapeutic techniques. It can be used to engage a disengaged, fearful, or distrustful child (*see* the example of Jacob below), it can be used to transform the valence of emotional material—to make manageable the intolerable (LeBaron, 2003; *see* the case of Taylor), and it can be used to facilitate mastery (as with Samantha and Jeffrey, later in this chapter). The commonality between these uses is that hypnosis involves the *absorption* of the child into an *altered state of consciousness* in the service of creating a *therapeutic change* in *perception, emotion, behavior, or experience*.

This chapter will illustrate how to use hypnotic processes to engage with babies, toddlers, preschoolers, and school-aged children. We will outline how to address children's developmental needs and use appropriate hypnotic interventions in order to work productively with children and their parents.

Jacob

The following case of Jacob illustrates how to begin—to join with a child using hypnotic language.

Jacob, a bright, emotionally inhibited and regressed 5-year-old boy was referred for "extreme anxiety and non-cooperation with medical diagnostic procedures." He was clearly terrified at being in a hospital ward, and clung to his parents. I [LK] learned that he was gifted and had a passion for dinosaurs. I chose to engage with him via his intellectual strength and ignore, for the moment, the pressing medical needs.

The clinician's task in using hypnosis to engage a child in the process of therapeutic change is to take the child's theme and transform it into a therapeutic metaphor to promote change. Fluently, Jacob listed all the dinosaurs, using their Latin nomenclature, and described their characteristics in great detail. I chose to present the dinosaurs as a metaphor of courage and create an imaginative involvement in which he could become curious and challenged and his regressed emotional needs could be addressed.

Sitting on his hospital bed, I asked him if he wanted to hear an interesting story about how some dinosaurs discovered a new land. He nodded and with his eyes open I [LK] lowered my voice into intimate story mode:

> "Now, at first the dinosaurs were frightened—after all, they had never ever been away from their home. They wondered if they would ever find their way back. But there were also so many interesting new forms of life here: new flying creatures, new weird trees, new food … The dinosaurs began to feel slightly stronger. It was all so curious and new. They began to explore a little further away from their home base

and into this strange new territory, with these bigger trees and new life forms. They walked on their strong legs slowly...and carefully...and thoroughly...because they knew that if they watched, they could learn quickly about this strange place and then would know what was safe and where the dangers were and how to stay safe. Then they could take care of themselves properly, without having to be nervous and watchful all the time.

Now this was particularly true of Tyrannosaurus Rex. He was the bravest of them all, as you well know. Nod your head when you can see him exploring this strange new territory. [*Jacob nods his head, eyes still wide open.*] Good. Now, after he has had some sleep, he discovered that there were some very curious and interesting plants that he could eat. Nod your head again when you can see these plants: some will be in bright blue and purple, others may be green and red—you may even see ones that I haven't mentioned. [*Jacob is quiet, absorbed, with his eyes open and fixed on me.*] And then he discovered something that made him so happy—a big rock with knobbles on it that he could scratch his back on, because you know it's very hard for a dinosaur to scratch his own back."

In this example, hypnosis served two primary purposes. First, it promoted engaging with a frightened, distrustful child in a creative manner that interested him, and that accessed his competence. Second, it helped him to begin changing the emotional valence of the experience of being in hospital from something that was universally frightening to something manageable.

Imaginative Involvement as a Hypnotic Precursor

Classic hypnosis does not occur with young children. Instead, *imaginative involvement* is the preferred term, drawing attention to their differing behavioral responses compared to older children, adolescents, and adults. Imaginative involvement refers to a process in which a child is intensely absorbed in a "here-and-now" fantasy experience in which present reality is suspended in the interests of the current imaginative experience. It does not presuppose a dissociated ego state, or a profoundly relaxed physiological state with distinct altered state of consciousness, as occurs in the classic hypnotic state. Young children prefer not closing their eyes, as they associate this with going to sleep. Yet despite these differences, profound therapeutic changes can and do still occur. In a randomized controlled study of children aged 3 to 6, imaginative involvement was significantly more effective in relieving distress associated with a painful invasive procedure than either behavioral distraction or standard medical practice (Kuttner, Bowman & Teasdale, 1988).

In the early preschool years, the child has a more fluid sense of self and experiences blurred boundaries between reality and fantasy. A young child enters the imaginary world with eyes wide open. It is easy to miss the opportunity for therapeutic impact in these receptive light trance states, and it is easy to dismiss it as the child being "dreamy," "glazed," or "spaced out"—instead, this is a very receptive state. Direct suggestions are easily accepted and therapeutic change occurs simply and rapidly. From infancy onward, the young child learns most easily and effortlessly about the world through independent or interactive play. In fact, it is often only through play that the young child can be engaged in a hypnotic experience and sustained in that trance to shift distress or dysfunction.

Jeffrey

A kindergarten-aged child, Jeffrey, was referred to me [RC] for assistance in managing his emotions following a traumatic experience at school. He was a bright, intense boy who was highly creative and imaginative. He often drew his feelings and described them to me. On one occasion he became very distressed when discussing a "mad feeling"—becoming instantly absorbed in the experience that had led him to feel upset, and became overwhelmed by this distress in the session. I asked him to tell me what the feeling was like—how big it was ("as big as a house"), how it felt ("bumpy" and "swirling"), what color it was ("dark") and how long it lasted ("for four days"). He answered my questions intensely, wide-eyed, with a fixed gaze and a paucity of spontaneous movement—in an altered state. After a short

---

time, he spontaneously stated " … and then the feelings got as small as this piece of paper and then they grew into a tree and I chopped the tree down and threw it all the way to Africa." He later informed me that he meant to say that the feelings lasted "4 minutes" not "4 days."

This example illustrates the transformative power of imaginative involvement. This is not an example of formal hypnosis (as no direct hypnotic suggestions were made), but within a framework of safety and exploration, the child spontaneously used his own powerful imagination to transform his overwhelming feelings of distress into something he could process and then release. It also illustrates young children's fluid experience of time; young children are very susceptible to *time-distortion*. As Jeffrey creatively illustrated, 4 days of emotional distress became 4 minutes once he felt better. The cognitive processes with young children are often made up of loose associations and mixed with fantasy. As clinicians, we must not be sidetracked in attempting to rationally process what the child is speaking about—for to do so often stops the child's emotional work.

Changes in Clinical Hypnosis Across Development

Infants and Toddlers

Little attention has been paid to studying and developing the many forms of hypnotic processes informally practiced with infants and toddlers by parents worldwide. Despite a few excellent published reports on work with the preschool child (Olness, 1975; 1976; 1981) and reviews by Gardner (1977) and Kuttner (1988; 1991), there are few, if any, well-controlled research studies to expand our understanding of the hypnotic process with infants and toddlers. The work on hypnotic responsivity (Hilgard & Morgan, 1978; Morgan & Hilgard, 1979) suggests that the preschool child may not be as hypnotically responsive when compared with the older, school-aged child, and significantly there are no clinical scales to test hypnotic talent that go below 4 years of age. Does this indicate that hypnotic ability then starts at around

4 years of age? With a reliance on verbal suggestions as the therapeutic mode, this may be so. However, clinical experience indicates that short-term kinesthetic and sensory aspects of hypnosis occur with this age group.

Gardner (1977) reviews clinical evidence that supports the notion that infants and toddlers respond to parental repetitive soothing actions and can become entrained and entranced. She notes parents who report that playing soothing music, stroking a part of the child's body, or turning on a vacuum cleaner or electric shaver will quiet a fretting infant. It is clear that these phenomena are hypnosis in a primitive form. "The child under 6 is hypnotizable but not according to the sample practices commonly used with older children" (Morgan & Hilgard, 1979, p. 154). Hilgard & Morgan (1978) prefer the term "protohypnosis," in which "the very young child is better able to be distracted by listening to a story than by removing himself from the scene through his own fantasy" (p. 286). With a pre-verbal child, protohypnosis can be used for soothing and settling, but without the implied suggestions for change that are an integral part of the hypnotic process with older children.

Hypnotic sensory modality alters as a function of age, beginning with kinesthetic and auditory responsiveness and then later often developing visual facility (*see* Table 2:1). The younger child (birth to 2 years of age) understands the world through sensori-motor

Table 2.1: Changes in Hypnotic Technique with Advancing Development

Hypnotic Technique	
Less Advanced Development ⟵——————⟶	More Advanced Development
Shorter, Simpler Inductions	Longer, More Complex Inductions
More Intensity	More Subtlety
More Directive	More Indirect
More External Locus of Control	More Internal Locus of Control
More Kinesthetic	More Auditory
Repetitive Themes	Inventiveness
Use of Props	Use of Imagination without Props
Imitative, Familiar	Creative

Adapted from J. Reaney, Society for Developmental and Behavioral Pediatrics (SDBP) Workshop material, 1995.

experiences (Piaget, 1962). Hypnotic processes lend themselves to integration with other therapeutic strategies to facilitate effective change. Here, in the case of Taylor, hypnotic suggestion is combined with play therapy, behavioral rehearsal, and systemic intervention to transform intolerable needle procedures into a daily routine in which this toddler gains mastery.

Taylor

Taylor, a vigorous 20-month-old toddler, had just been diagnosed with Diabetes. As an only child, she and her parents were overwhelmed by the daily process of monitoring her blood sugar levels and administering regular insulin injections. Taylor picked up on their distress; she cried and struggled, and the daily routine became a battle ground. The Diabetes clinic referred the family to me [LK]. I showed Taylor how to blow bubbles, telling her to "blow her 'owies' away." She tasted the bubbles, caught and smacked the bubbles, while I continued with direct hypnotic suggestions: "This helps your body to feel happy and strong."

"Won't she associate the bubbles with the needle?" her worried mother inquired. "If she continues to have fun and feel empowered, then the bubbles will become stronger than her fear," was my reply. I invited the parents to buy her a Dolly who also happened to have Diabetes, so that Taylor could teach Dolly to sit on her Mom's lap for her needle and blow the "owies" out with her bubbles. Taylor engaged with this and the parents had a system in which they could organize themselves to test and administer Taylor's insulin.

At the next session the length to which Taylor had absorbed the new process became evident, when her father told how ritualized the process had become, with Taylor helping Dolly to have her needle followed by Taylor blowing bubbles during her insulin injection. In fact, he added, "All her toys have now got Diabetes!" They named all the toys and Dad asked, "And who else has Diabetes?" To our surprise this previously non-verbal toddler answered, "Me!"

Bretherton (1989) reviewed developmental evidence on the form and function of play across childhood, and reported that "for toddlers the boundary between reality and pretense tends to be diffuse ... especially when pretense is about highly charged emotional themes" (p. 390). As in the case above, the incorporation of hypnotic suggestion and play allows the difficult diagnosis to become integrated as a part of her sense of self.

In summary, hypnosis with babies and toddlers is:

- Not classic hypnosis—it is protohypnosis
- Sensory-based and/or motor-based (rhythmic, rocking, soothing)
- Repetitive, familiar, and predictable
- Simple, direct, minimally verbal
- Kinesthetic (such as a rapid regular rocking at a pace that approximates maternal heartbeat of 80 beats per minute)
- Auditory (such as songs, lullabies)

Preschoolers

Preschool children have short attention spans, are easily distracted, weave fluidly between fantasy and reality, and love magic and surprise. They are also unaccustomed to physical relaxation and often move and wriggle wide-eyed through an effective trance experience without interfering with its benefit. Cognitively, preschool children are concrete and literal in their communication and comprehension. Consequently, they benefit from the use of simple, clear, direct age-appropriate language. It helps to use their own words as a basis for hypnotic interventions. Preschool-aged children are spontaneous and tend to be less constrained by social rules or reality than are older children and adolescents. This requires that the clinician be highly flexible and follow the child as he or she moves in and out of a trance experience. Incorporating rituals or rhythms that capitalize on their non-verbal understanding as well as on the familiar soothing nature of rhythmic patterns, such as familiar songs or favorite stories is an excellent technique with preschool children.

In the "favorite stories" technique (Kuttner, 1988), the story becomes both the mode of induction and the substance of the trance. Hypnotic suggestions and reframing take place within the framework of the story line. This may include direct and indirect suggestions for increased comfort, coping, or decreasing pain.

Samantha

Prior to 5-year-old Samantha's feared bone marrow aspiration, our plan was to tell her favourite story of *Snow White and the Seven Dwarfs*. Just before the procedure she exclaimed, "I don't want that story! I want the story of Grandma Tildy and the Elephant!" Not knowing the story, I [LK] asked her to tell it. Sam provided the story complete with concrete details and sound effects. I then restated the plan: "Now how would it be if I were to tell you the story of Grandma Tildy and the Elephant while the bone marrow was getting done. I wouldn't be surprised if by the time we got to the end of the story the bone marrow was over and the band-aid was on. Wouldn't that be nice?" Sam nodded her head; a working contract plus hypnotic suggestion for outcome had been established. Anxiously holding her "kitty," she walked into the treatment room and climbed on the table. Informing the medical team of the plan, we began the story.

> "Grandma Tildy lived by herself, and was such a brave little lady, and one day there was a knock on the door ... (knock knock) ..."

Samantha's attention was fully absorbed by the story and dissociation from the procedure became evident. She was observed to wriggle when the sensation was discomforting, but her eyes were fixed and her concentration focused and unwavering. The intensity and excitement of the story was increased when the more painful sections of the medical procedures occurred, so that the hypnotic involvement remained more compelling than the pain.

Samantha was part of a research study, and as such gave quantitative indicators of her distress, pain, and anxiety. She initially gave one of the highest ratings of distress in the entire study, and rated both her pain and anxiety as 5/5. After first treatment with the hypnotic story,

---

her distress score was markedly lower. She rated her anxiety as 1/5 and her pain as 5/5, suggesting a split between her experience of pain and how much that pain bothered her. It seems as though the hypnotic story did not eradicate her sensation of pain, but rather transformed the meaning of the pain from frightening and upsetting to distant and manageable (adapted from Kuttner, 1988, pp. 293–294).

From infancy onward, the young child learns most easily and effortlessly about the world through independent or interactive *play*. It is often only through play that the young child can be engaged in a hypnotic experience and meaningfully sustained in that trance to bring about the needed change (Linden, 2003). Being present-centered, young children respond best to hypnotic interventions that utilize the "here-and-now experience" rather than relying on the child to "remove himself from the scene through his own fantasy or through reliving an earlier game or experience of his own" (Hilgard & Morgan, 1978, p. 286). Young children are easily able to become absorbed in fantasy—consider the prevalence of imaginary friends among this age group. Of interest, research finds that children with imaginary companions were more predisposed to engage in fantasy than those without, and, moreover, their fantasy was more vivid (Bouldin, 2006). The imaginary world is rich and accessible as a clinical tool with children of this age. Bretherton (1989) wrote, "As children become able to deal with highly charged events within the play-world, they also become more expert at deliberately blurring the map-territory distinction in such a way that real-world issues can be dealt with inside the playframe" (p. 391).

It is striking to observe children as young as 3 years of age who clearly demonstrate the ability to alter sensation, perception, and experience (Gardner, 1977; Kuttner, 1988; Olness, 1975, 1976, 1981; Olness & Gardner, 1988). Children this age can enter trance wide-eyed and maintain a trance during involved physical activity that is directly related to the trance (Olness & Gardner, 1988; Kuttner, 1988). Given the action-oriented nature of the preschool-aged child, and the distinctiveness of the child's hypnotic process, it is essential that the clinician adopt a highly flexible hypnotic style, allowing the child to move in and out of trance and remaining sensitive to the child's moment-by-moment responses. An active participation then develops between therapist and child such that the therapist paces the child, absorbing his or her attention in an informal child-centered manner.

Given the young child's relative ease in entering, leaving, and reentering a trance, it's often unnecessary to go through a lengthy induction with children under 6 years of age. It is often sufficient simply to say, "Now let's pretend," or "How about imagining ... and you can close your eyes, or keep them open ...."

Other simple and useful inductions for younger children include inviting the child to see his or her favorite cartoon on television, becoming a floppy Raggedy Ann doll or big strong oak tree, or taking on a pretend role of an astronaut or super hero.

Hilary

With the preschool child, parental dependency is still prevalent and normal. Often in the first few sessions, it is necessary and important to allow the parent to be present in the room since it enhances the young child's feelings of trust and safety. Sometimes, in therapeutically appropriate circumstances, the parent can be included in the hypnotherapeutic experience, such as in the case of 4-year-old Hilary, who had severe eczema that was marginally responsive to dermatological creams. Her referring dermatologist felt that anxiety may be playing a role in her condition. Her concerned, loving mother was involved in the hypnotic ritual. Before any medication was applied, her mother would pack a pink, cool cloud on Hilary's excoriated skin under her direction, until she felt its cool and pleasant effect. Below are some excerpts:

> **L. Kuttner [LK]**: So let's take this lovely soft cloud, scoop it up, and put it on the itchy parts so that it makes your skin feel so good, soft, smooth and very calm [*scooping up imaginary armfuls of cloud*]. What color is this?
>
> **Hilary**: [*With eyes wide open, staring*] It's pink.
>
> **LK**: Let's pack it on the parts of your skin that need to feel better. Show me where!

> *[Somewhat later.]*
>
> **LK**: Now I wouldn't be surprised that after having the lovely pink cloud, your skin will find it easier than ever before to take the good skin creams in, making the healing last even longer and keeping the redness and soreness away. Would you like Mom to put some pink cloud on?
>
> **Hilary**: Mum, here! [*pointing to her dry red elbows.*]
>
> **Mom**: Like this?
>
> **Hilary**: Yes, and there.
>
> **Mom**: [*Beginning to get into her stride.*] It's nice and cool like those strawberry yogurt sticks, making you feel good!
>
> In this example, by engaging Hilary's active imagination, mother and child were both participants in increasing the child's experience of comfort and healing.

In summary, hypnosis with preschool-aged children is:

- Action-based, allowing for movement
- Play-oriented and present centered
- Short, with engaging experiences
- Familiar, repetitive, using a "Let's pretend" or favourite story frame
- Involving parents as partners, when appropriate
- Flexible, humorous and playful
- Tailored to fit the child's presenting problem

School-aged Children

Research reveals that children at school age have a heightened capacity for hypnosis (Morgan & Hilgard, 1979) and evidence immediate autonomic changes (cardiac rate, skin temperature, galvanic skin response) when engaging in hypnosis (Lee & Olness,

1996; Lohaus, Klein-Heßling, Vögele, & Kuhn-Henninghausen, 2001). With increasing age (around 8 years and older) children are willing to close their eyes and their bodies visibly relax as they engage in the more classic forms of hypnosis. With their longer attention spans and better cooperation, they can use their inherent imagination (Vygotsky, 1990) for therapeutic benefit in trance. Relaxation is not as obvious as with adults, but it does occur and tends to be lighter. Breathing is often more regular, and facial expression more focused whether or not their eyes close. Morgan and Hilgard (1979) determined that between 8 and 12 years of age children reach the height of their hypnotic talent. Remembering that all hypnosis is self-hypnosis (that is, it is a child's own process) (Kohen, 1986a; 1986b; Zeltzer & LeBaron, 1982), it is important to inform school-aged children that this is their talent. With practice, children can learn to use hypnosis for themselves whenever and wherever needed. For example, Hawkins and Polemikos (2002) found that school-aged children who were experiencing sleep disturbance following a trauma benefited from learning and practicing self-hypnosis for sleep:

> Now, close your eyes as if you were just about to go to sleep so that you begin to feel all dreamy…you might notice how light you feel and perhaps even a tingling sensation as if you are sitting on a big fluffy ball of wool… And as you feel light, so you might notice that the cotton wool is like a fluffy white cloud…Would you like to go to a special or favorite and very safe outdoor place?…Then all you have to do is imagine your fluffy floating cloud is a magic cloud car. You can steer this car quite easily and fly it to your favorite place.… The more you practice, you might not even notice that you might not even wake up as you go to your special place…and there you will learn to sleep soundly all night long with enjoyable dreams. When you wake up in the morning you will feel wide awake and look forward to all the things that you have to do during the day. (p. 21)

With school-aged children, the trance experience becomes longer and more complex, and includes more suggestions and metaphor than with preschool-aged children (5 to 7 minutes is a good length). It always is more effective to use the child's own experiences, hobbies, or interests to make the experience relevant, attractive, and absorbing. Gathering this information from the child, parent, or nurse and using it in the trance experience improves cooperation and make hypnosis more successful.

Some common therapeutic problems that hypnosis is well suited to with this age group include: need for mastery; increased need for self-control; issues around self-efficacy and self-esteem; anxiety; and increased emotional comfort in social situations such as school and peer relations (Brown, Summers, Coffman, Riddell, & Poulsen, 1996; Culbert, Kajander, Kohen, & Reaney, 1996; Dobson, Bray, Kehle, Theodore, & Peck, 2005).

Sometimes, when a child is fearful, distrustful or not particularly wanting to come or be helped, hypnosis can be introduced more casually through a series of questions, the answers to which become material for a hypnotic experience:

- "If you were not here, what would you rather be doing?"
- "What do you love to do so that you don't even hear your Mom/Dad call you?"
- "Where's your favorite place where you can kind of enter another world and feel good or better than you do feel now?"
- "What helped in the past when you were worrying?"
- "Would it be okay if the (worry, pain, upset) didn't bother you? We can make that happen by going to that favourite place."

A wide range of inductions can be used with school-aged children (*see* Chapter Five). These include: eye fixation; coin drop technique; favourite-place imagery; learning and control metaphors; adventure imagery; superheroes and heroines; drawing; controls, wires, switches; video games; television or cartoon imagery. Ideomotor inductions are particularly intriguing to school-aged children and are easy to use in home practice. Creating an audiotape further supports the child's self-hypnosis, self-regulation, and independent practice at home.

Madeleine

Madeleine at 9½ has developed idiopathic leg pains, which were diagnosed as "growing pains." She found that nighttime was the worst time and falling asleep was consequently very hard. Planning together we developed a bedtime routine in which she'd find her "S" position, on her right side, curl up and start the series of "Ss": settle into the sheets, stop wriggled and stay still, soften her muscles and let them sink into the sheets…and then softly breath into her belly to help the sleepiness slip into her so that she could softly slip into dreams. We audiotaped the 5-minute session, and she religiously played it every night, learning to re-pattern herself.

Often when successfully engaged with an established hypnotic practice, children will integrate it into their way of coping and surprise you and their parents by adapting it to better suit their purpose—and in so doing truly make it their own!

Calum

Seven-year-old Calum had suffered from recurring and debilitating migraines since the age of three. Referred to me [LK] by his Pediatric Neurologist, Calum, with his supportive mom, eagerly learned how to turn down his pain switch in a focused hypnotic trance (Kuttner & Solomon, 2003). With practice, as Calum learned to trust himself and his capacities, he reduced his hypnotic trance of 7 minutes to 3 minutes. At a follow-up visit two months later Calum revealed that he'd become bored with the pain switch and spontaneously used another suggestion I'd made in passing. He took the notion of seeing a flickering candle and instead decided to become the wick of the candle. When in pain he would go inside himself, become the wick, and focus on melting all the wax [*the pain*] away and as it dripped down he would feel lighter and pain free.

In summary, hypnosis with school-aged children is:

- Focused and sustained easily for 5 to 10 minutes

- Natural, involving eye-closure and some relaxation
- Capable of creating dissociation from present reality to a preferred state or place
- Making use of their creative and hypnotic potential to alter emotional, physical, and behavioral issues
- Able to be independently practiced by the child at home or at school.

Resources

Brett, D. (1988). *Annie's Stories*. New York: Workman.

Fraiberg, S. (1987). *The Magic Years*. New York: Simon & Schuster.

Kuttner, L. (Director, Co-producer). (1986). *No Fears, No Tears: Children with Cancer Coping with Pain*. Vancouver, B.C.: Canadian Cancer Society. [Videotape]. Available from Fanlight Productions, www.fanlight.com, 1-800-937-4113.

Kuttner, L. (Producer). (1998). *No Fears, No Tears—13 Years Later*. [Videotape]. Available from C&W Bookstore, Children's & Women's Health Centre of BC, 4480 Oak Street, Rm. K2-126, Ambulatory Care Building, Vancouver, B.C. V6H 3V4, 1-800-331-1533, ext. 3, or http://bookstore.cw.bc.ca; also available from Fanlight Productions, www.fanlight.com, 1-800-937-4113.

References

Bouldin, P. (2006). An investigation of the fantasy predisposition and fantasy style of children with imaginary companions. *Journal of Genetic Psychology, 167*, 17–29.

Bretherton, I. (1989). Pretense: The form and function of make-believe play. *Developmental Review, 9*, 383–401.

Brown, G. W., Summers, D., Coffman, B., Riddell, R., & Poulsen, B. (1996). The use of hypnotherapy with school-age children: Five case studies. *Psychotherapy in Private Practice, 15*, 53–65.

Culbert, T. P., Kajander, R. L., Kohen, D. P., & Reaney, J. B. (1996). Hypnobehavioral approaches for school-age children with dysphagia and food aversion: A case series. *Developmental and Behavioral Pediatrics*, 17, 335–341.

Dobson, R. L., Bray, M. A., Kehle, T. J., Theodore, L. A., & Peck, H. L. (2005). Relaxation and guided imagery as an intervention for children with asthma: A replication. *Psychology in the Schools*, 42, 707–720.

Gardner, G. G. (1977). Hypnosis with infants and pre-school children. *American Journal of Clinical Hypnosis*, 19, 158–162.

Hawkins, P., & Polemikos, N. (2002). Hypnosis treatment of sleeping problems in children experiencing loss. *Contemporary Hypnosis*, 19, 18–24.

Hilgard, J. R., & Morgan, A. H. (1978). Treatment of anxiety and pain in childhood cancer through hypnosis. In F. H. Frankel & H. S. Zamansky (Eds.), *Hypnosis at its bicentennial: Selected papers*. New York: Plenum.

Kohen, D. P. (1986a). Applications of relaxation/mental imagery (self-hypnosis) in pediatric emergencies. *International Journal of Clinical & Experimental Hypnosis*, 34, 283–294.

Kohen, D. P. (1986b). Application of relaxation/mental imagery (self-hypnosis) to the management of asthma: Report of behavioural outcomes of a two-year prospective controlled study. *American Journal of Clinical Hypnosis*, 28, 196.

Kuttner, L. (Director, Co-producer). (1986). *No fears, no tears: Children with cancer coping with pain*. Vancouver, B.C.: Canadian Cancer Society. [Videotape]. (Available from Fanlight Productions, www.fanlight.com, 1-800-937-4113.)

Kuttner, L. (1988). Favorite stories: A hypnotic pain-reduction technique for children in acute pain. *American Journal of Clinical Hypnosis*, 30, 289–295.

Kuttner, L. (1991). Helpful strategies in working with pre-school children in pediatric practice. *Pediatric Annals*, 20, 120–127.

Kuttner, L. (Producer). (1998). *No fears, no tears—13 years later*. [Videotape]. (Available from C&W Bookstore, Children's & Women's Health Centre of BC, 4480 Oak Street, Rm. K2-126, Ambulatory Care

Building, Vancouver, B.C. V6H 3V4, 1-800-331-1533, ext. 3, or http://bookstore.cw.bc.ca; also available from Fanlight Productions, www.fanlight.com, 1-800-937-4113.)

Kuttner, L., Bowman, M., Teasdale, M. (1988). Psychological treatment of distress, pain and anxiety for young children with cancer. *Journal of Developmental and Behavioral Pediatrics*, 9, 374–381.

Kuttner, L., & Solomon, R. (2003). Hypnotherapy and imagery for managing children's pain. In N. L. Schechter, C. Berde, & M. Yaster (Eds.), *Pain in Infants, Children and Adolescents* (2nd ed.), (pp. 317–328). Philadelphia: Lippincott, Williams, & Wilkins.

LeBaron, S. (2003). The use of imagination in the treatment of children with pain and anxiety. *Australian Journal of Clinical Hypnotherapy & Hypnosis*, 24, 1–13.

Lee, L. H., & Olness, K. (1996). Effects of self-induced mental imagery on autonomic reactivity in children. *Journal of Developmental and Behavioral Pediatrics*, 17 (5):323-327.

Linden, J.H. (2003). Playful metaphors. *American Journal of Clinical Hypnosis*, 45, 245–250.

Lohaus, A., Klein-Heßling, J., Vögele, C., & Kuhn-Henninghausen, C. (2001). Physiological effects of relaxation training in children. *British Journal of Health Psychology*, 6, 197–206.

Morgan, A.H., & Hilgard, J.R. (1979). The Stanford hypnotic scale for children. *American Journal of Clinical Hypnosis*, 21, 78–85.

Olness, K. (1975). The use of self-hypnosis in the treatment of childhood nocturnal enuresis. *Clinical Pediatrics*, 14, 273.

Olness, K. (1976). Autohypnosis in functional megacolon in children. *American Journal of Clinical Hypnosis*, 19, 28–32.

Olness K. (1981). Hypnosis in pediatric practice. *Current Problems in Pediatrics*, 12, 1–47.

Olness, K., & Gardner, G.G. (1988). *Hypnosis and hypnotherapy with children* (2nd ed.). New York: Grune & Stratton.

Piaget, J. (1962). The stages of the intellectual development of the child. *Bulletin of the Menninger Clinic*, 26, 120–128.

Reaney, J. (1995) Workshop material. Society for Developmental and Behavioral Pediatrics (SDBP).

Smath, J. (1979). *But no elephants*. New York: Parents' Magazine Press.

Vandenberg, B. (2002). Hypnotic responsivity from a developmental perspective: Insights from young children. *International Journal of Clinical and Experimental Hypnosis*, 50, 229–247.

Viereck, G. S., "What Life Means to Einstein," *The Saturday Evening Post*, October 26, 1929.

Vygotsky, L.S. (1990). Imagination and creativity in childhood. *Soviet Psychology*, 28, 84–96. [Originally published in 1930].

Zeltzer, L., LeBaron, S. (1982). Hypnotic and non hypnotic techniques for the reduction of pain and anxiety during painful procedures in children and adolescents with cancer. *Behavioral Pediatrics*, 101, 1032–1035.

Chapter Three

Hypnosis with Adolescents and Developmental Aspects of Hypnosis with Adults

Julie H. Linden, PhD

Clinical Vignettes

Chronic Illness

Annie

Annie was 19 years old and struggling with cystic fibrosis. Her parents had made the first call to me and wanted help for her with managing her pulmonary treatments, her poor eating patterns, and her life-style choices. She was a conscientious college student who prided herself on good grades. When I met Annie I was very concerned about how thin she was. Annie did not see herself as having any problems except anxiety about getting her work done on time, and procrastination. Her perspective and its conflict with her parents laid the shaky foundation for her treatment. She accepted hypnosis as something that supported her independence, which eased her anxiety and helped her get her work done in a timely manner. When I broached the topic of her poor eating, she abruptly left treatment.

Trauma of War

Amina

I first met Amina when she was 15. She had left her war-torn country to study in the US and completed her high school, college, and graduate school in the States. At age 22 she married a compatriot from her home country. The marriage provided a respite and haven from the stress of adjusting to a new life, new culture, and new customs. She confided in me that she had been taught all kinds of self-hypnotic techniques for reducing her anxiety, and that none of them worked when she felt "that anxious." "So what do you do to cope?" I asked. "I sing at the top of my lungs. That is the only thing that works," she said. "Then keep singing," I told her. "Let's just make sure you have plenty of songs to sing when you need them."

Life under Duress

David

"I still remember the relaxation techniques you taught me" said, David, now 29. I had known David since he was 8 years old, and had helped him learn about his high anxiety, his ADHD, and his mood swings. "I know what I need to do to stop smoking, but I need to have someone walk through it with me. I can't do it alone." David had already reduced his smoking to four cigarettes a day by the time of our first session. With several hypnotic sessions, a target date for stopping, and a plan to get to that date, he quickly stopped all together, and remained smoke free six months later. "I know I should practice more to get to that very relaxed, Zen place, but I just don't have the time" he said. "I can't make myself do it."

Many hypnosis training courses teach that hypnosis can be used with any age group and any symptom. As the three vignettes illustrate, however, what we do and when we do it depends first and foremost on the acceptance of hypnosis by the subject (Murray-Jobsis, 1993). Adolescents as a group may be some of the more challenging clients or patients to work with because of the very developmental stage they are in. A look at adolescent development reminds us of some of the major tasks the adolescent faces in becoming an independent adult with his or her own set of values, beliefs, and life goals. Being mindful of these tasks can inform the process and outcome of our work.

This chapter will address the importance of understanding human development as it relates to, affects, and enhances our work with hypnosis clinically. A review of the literature on development and hypnosis underscores the theoretical notion that disturbance in personality is a result of a failure to progress along normal developmental stages (Baker, 1981; Brown & Froom, 1986; Murray-Jobsis, 1993; Winnicott, 1965). Hypnosis literature from Europe about a century ago, notably from the French schools of Nancy (where Hippolyte Bernheim practiced) and Salpêtrière (where Jean-Martin Charcot practiced), explored normal and abnormal human development with hypnosis and was "rediscovered" by trauma researchers during the more recent explosion of information on the origins of traumatic symptoms (van der Hart, Brown, & Turco, 1990). This early period of scientific exploration of hypnosis contributed to the psychoanalytical notion on the origins of personality disturbance.

There is general agreement that the path of development affects the outcome of the health of the personality. In this century, Baker (1981), Wolberg (1945/1964) and Murray-Jobsis (1993) (*see also* Scagnelli-Jobsis, 1982) are all pioneers in the use of hypnosis within the adult population to address symptomology that arose from hypothesized disturbances in developmental stages. Each applied principles of human development to hypnotic treatment, which, while lacking in rigorous empirical research, reported significant clinical success with the improvement of symptoms. Because of their work, we are invited to revisit the concept of developmental theories and their relationship to our hypnosis work.

Development and the Adolescent

Development refers to many areas of growth in humans usually divided into the traditional mind-body categories of physiological and psychological development. This convention is useful as a means to organize our understanding of human development as long as we recognize that each of these physiological changes has an effect on the psychological growth as well. The adolescent faces the challenges of a changing body and with this a self-conscious, often realistic, self-assessment of his or her body and related self-esteem issues. While causing its own set of conflicts for the adolescent it is doubtful that the identification process (figuring out one's identity) could move forward without this intense period of self-evaluation. New physical and emotional sensations mediated by changing hormones, a brain capable of more abstract reasoning and the task of becoming independent from his or her caregivers all collide in what many describe as a tumultuous period of change.

Physical Development

Physical development during adolescence is intrinsically tied to sexual development, since the transition the child's body goes through during a normal adolescence ends in a physically and procreatively ready individual. Sexual and physical development are so intertwined during this stage that puberty and adolescence are often used synonymously. However, adolescence refers to the period from puberty to adulthood, roughly the ages from 11–19, and includes psychological development as well as physical. Puberty, however, refers to the physiological changes of sexual maturity and other body development that take place during that time. No age range can accurately reflect any single individual's experience of adolescence, so these ages are simply a guide.

Any child's adolescence begins with the onset of puberty, which sometimes starts as early as age 8. Typically, adolescence is further divided into three parts. Early adolescence, ages 11–13, is the time when the teenager is experiencing increased capability in logical thinking and integrating bodily changes into his or her sense of identity. Mid-adolescence, ages 14–15, is a time of defining one's values and beliefs as distinct from those of the parents, of exploring the relationship to one's peers, to one's self and to the opposite sex, and taking increased responsibility for one's educational and vocational pursuits.

Late adolescence, from age 16 on, is successfully completed when there is a more stable sense of identity, when a balance exists between ones' aspirations, reality (abilities) and fantasies, and when the young person has an idea of the role he or she will hold/play in society, and how he or she will contribute to the world at large. Each culture has its own tenets that define this period of growth and some developmental psychologists have expressed concern that western culture has extended adolescence well into the twenties. Such statements are very much influenced by the particular set of criteria used to define this period of growth, and usually have more to do with the societal goals (Macoby & Jacklin, 1974) than physical development. I am reminded of the time I asked a colleague for advice about my 20-year-old son's confusion of what he wanted to do when he grew up, and my colleague, then age 50, said, "Well, that's normal—I still don't know what I want to do when I grow up."

Psychological Development

Psychological development of adolescents is complex and its description made more difficult because of a lack of empirical research. However, several theories have been formulated that describe various aspects of human development including emotional, sexual, cognitive, social, and moral development and help us to better understand adolescents. These theories suggest sequential patterns of development, and each one estimates the ages at which particular developmental characteristics can be seen. These theories offer great benefits in our being able to explain to parents what to expect and why in their changing child's behavior (Galinsky, 1987). In addition these theories inform us as to what is "normal" development thus providing some criteria with which to compare our clients.

A rich understanding of development will lead to more effective interventions when using hypnosis, especially with approaches that foster dissociation and regression, such as ego state therapy (Watkins & Watkins, 1997) or age-regression techniques. The "age" of an ego state or the age to which a person regresses is often indicative of the very developmental task the person may be stuck on. For example, Jill, age 35, spontaneously regressed in her hypnotic trance to her first grade class where the teacher would not allow her to leave the room to use the bathroom. At age 6 she could not hold her urine any longer and wet the chair, and in remembering this episode understood the origins of her embarrassment about public speaking and was able to resolve that fear.

Conversely, the presenting symptoms for which hypnosis may be useful often indicate the "age" at which an event occurred that was stressful or traumatizing. For example, Janet had worries about going anywhere and being unable to find a bathroom. I suspected that her bathrooming issues might be rooted in toilet training experiences. Now 45, she wanted to complete her college education but her fear had her paralyzed. She remembered bedwetting incidents during which her mother took the mattress outside to dry, which embarrassed Janet. Before the age of 5 she had made a pact with herself to never be far from a toilet. Once this child's secret agreement was made conscious, and she could use her more adult understanding that toilets could be found or improvised anywhere, she moved forward and completed college and graduate studies.

Freud (1962/2000) proposed a theory of *psychosexual* development. He understood the interplay of mind and body when he titled his theory and, while some specific content of his theory has been disputed, the relationship between the psyche and soma remains a major contribution of his work. Eric Erikson (1950) formulated a theory of psychosocial development and his eight stages, each focused on the resolution of a social crisis, have continued to frame our thinking about social growth and development. Erikson defined this stage as the adolescent struggle of identity versus role confusion. Piaget (Inhelder & Piaget, 1958; Puloski, 1980; Piaget, 1983) is known for his theory on cognitive development elucidating the distinct stages that occur cognitively over the course of childhood development. Moral theories on development include Kohlberg's work (Kohlberg, Levine & Hewer, 1983) and Gilligan's (1982) that expanded on the gender differences in moral thinking. Brazelton and Greenspan (2000) offer a more practical model that addresses the basic needs of children for healthy development. This is only a partial list of the many theories that abound on development and is reviewed to highlight the importance of developmental theories on all forms of psychotherapy.

Utilizing Knowledge of Development

In Chapter Two, Kuttner reviewed child development in some detail. It is my opinion that the utilization of hypnosis is enhanced when we understand the developmental stage of the person with whom we are working. Applying what we know of psychological and physical development to work with adults will help to clarify not only the current developmental stage of the client/patient but the symptoms may also provide the clues for the stage of development at the time at which a symptom began. In addition, knowledge of what the stage of development is will help us match our suggestions to the client's hypnotic age.

One of the few standards taught about development and hypnosis is that hypnotic performance peaks between the ages of 8 and 11 (Hilgard & Le Baron, 1984; Olness & Kohen, 1996). As has been eloquently discussed by Sugarman and Teleska in Chapter Four, hypnotic performance does not equal hypnotic ability. Finding the "trance in the encounter" is our task and children do this far more easily than adolescents or adults. One major reason for this has to do with the changes brought by our physical and cognitive development. The child lacks many of the self-reflective self-conscious thoughts that inhibit adolescents and adults. The adolescent and adult have a critical mind that is "on" more than the child's. It is hypothesized that by the time of adolescence both an observing ego and participating ego are present and the observing ego is a critical observer with qualities similar to those proposed in the superego (Hilgard & Hilgard 1975). The observing ego may be more left-brained, more logical, analytical, and more cautious. It is like a set of brakes on the more primitive fantasies and imagination of the child.

Children's fantasies are often an extension of their everyday experiences. As a child, while driving through the southwest, Mary remembered seeing buffalo ranging on the prairie. She was trapped in the car with bickering parents and squished between her arguing siblings. She "rode" the buffaloes and lost herself in the experience of feeling the air on her face, and the freedom her cowgirl persona provided. No one had to tell her how to do this; it came naturally. Adults often need to be reminded to daydream. They can be awkward and shy about using their imagination, after years of being told to stay focused in reality. Adolescents are somewhere between their childhood natural ability to "imaginate" (as 7-year-old Susie called it) and the more reality-oriented adults they are becoming. Their fantasies are about their peers, and often about wished for sexual encounters with those peers. Because peer influences are so powerful for the adolescent they can be utilized in many hypnotic encounters. Fourteen-year-old Ian wasn't sure that he could decrease his anxiety with relaxation training and other hypnotic techniques, but when he pictured the movie screen and saw his friend anxious about a test, he knew just what his friend needed to hear. He didn't like that his friend looked so "uncool" when he was anxious. Giving his friend advice with the hypnotic projective technique ultimately eased Ian's own anxiety.

When I work with adults I have to ask fairly specific questions in the interviewing process to learn about their interests, hobbies, and activities that they enjoy. Unlike children where imagination seems ever present, the adult has not only learned well the difference between fantasy and reality, he or she also seems to have learned that fantasizing is "bad"; it is what children do (and what adolescent wants to be seen as childlike?). In my experience, both adolescents and adults respond well to learning that their creative energy is enhanced when they practice using their imaginations. An exception to this is in the presence of more severe pathology such as chronic PTSD, Dissociative Identity Disorder, or severe attachment disorders. In such cases, the imagination has become restricted because it is feared it will lead to unwanted memories and feelings. These cases require a very judicious use of imaginative techniques and, of course, expertise in the disorder being treated.

Adolescents and adults who spontaneously give vivid details to their inner imaginings while in trance usually have experienced what they describe as a "deeper" hypnotic, more regressed trance. "Wow! That was so cool," said Joey, "I haven't felt that relaxed since my mom used to sing to me at bedtime when we would snuggle with Snowball (the pet dog)." In my experience with utilizing the "descending the staircase" technique, people often find themselves on the stairs from a childhood home and can describe in elaborate detail the colors, material, and placement of those stairs. This "deep" or "regressed" state may indicate some emotionally laden material is connected with the visual or sensory memory.

It is almost as if when imagination begins to be used again the floodgates to the past open up (Linden, 1997). This phenomenon is one of the reasons that hypnosis training emphasizes the increase in transference between the client and clinician. All too often, it is not about transference, but simply about the increase in access to repressed or buried imaginings. This is, clinically, an advantage of hypnosis, for as noted in the chapter on trauma and hypnosis (Chapter Seven), access to affect that has been dissociated is the road to resolution of distressing symptoms.

It is well established that children who were traumatized as youngsters, with type II complicated trauma, have had lots of practice with dissociating (being in spontaneous trance) (Gil, 1998; Cardeña, 2000). When in hypnosis as adults they behave more like children do. These children in grown-up bodies are capable of a great deal of "trance logic," crossing logical and sensory boundaries quite easily. The adult, who is capable of producing a negative or positive hallucination, or of altering the smell of ammonia to the smell of a rose, may do this by regressing to an earlier developmental stage in hypnosis, when these abilities were natural. Perhaps our hypnotic virtuosos, the highly hypnotizable, are more facile at accessing those childhood experiences.

A characteristic of children's thinking is its concreteness. In addition to our need to speak about things that are familiar to children—things that relate to their limited experiences—we also need to choose language, often much simpler than our adult vocabulary, and to be aware that children understand this language in concrete ways. For example, the pediatrician who talks with a child about "pokes" or "pinches" instead of immunizations is adapting his or her adult vocabulary to the child's and choosing words to which the child can relate his or her experiences. With adolescents and adults who become regressed in the trance state, sensitivity to this concept can enhance the work we do. In fact, a regressed adult subject will look confused with adult verbiage or concepts, and may even come out of trance in order to respond to a question posed during hypnosis. A related issue occurs when some of the fixed ideas that remain in the unconscious are in a specific language, often child-like concrete language. During hypnotic work, reevaluation of old dictums from parents that affect adult functioning, or removal of these fixed ideas that might relate to anxious or phobic behavior, depends on identifying the specific language. An example of this involved an adult who had been traumatized in her early development, at age 3, by parents who fought verbally. One particular fight escalated to a physical encounter that involved the father hitting the mother on the leg. The mother, aghast, cried, "You hit me in the shin!" My client, as a child, had no idea what a shin was, and understood it must be very bad because of the distress of her mother's cries. In trance she was able to be relieved of the intense affect related to this memory when I explained to the child ego state what a shin was.

In some cases where the person's native language is different from the language in which they are being hypnotized, there may be positive or negative consequences to the treatment. For example, trance depth may be less and the experience less intense emotionally, which may or may not be helpful. Language is personal and while the full discussion of this topic is outside the intent of this chapter, attention to the native/non-native language of the person being treated is important.

The previous example of child's language laid down (think of a concrete foundation to a building) in a stressful or traumatic scenario is a reminder that trauma researchers have once again put development in the forefront (Garbarino, Kostelny & Dubrow, 1991). When PTSD researchers (Bonanno, 2004) asked why some people were so resilient and others remained symptomatic following the same kinds of trauma, they were led to developmental considerations. Predisposing factors to the formation of PTSD responses to trauma include among other things: the age of the developmental phase of the person at the time of the trauma, personality, previous exposure to trauma and genetic predispositions (van der Kolk, 1987), all of which are developmental considerations (Eccles, Midgley, Wigfield, Buchanan, Reuman, Flanagan, & Iver, 1993).

Sometimes our work with past experiences, old traumas, is indirect. It involves the environmental or contextual factors that contributed to the creation of a personality style or disorder. In this arena, knowledge of development can lead to more accurate diagnosis, since the behaviors we are addressing may identify the age at which the individual was stressed or traumatized rather than any particular traumatic experience. For example, the person with Borderline or Narcissistic Personality Disorder suggests that investigation of the quality of early attachments (Murray-Jobsis, 1993), when these patterns begin, would be worthwhile. The person with a discrete phobia, such as fear of elevators or airplanes, may have had anxiety begin to develop later, maybe between the ages of 6–10, while working on separation from parental figures and still in need of support and outside comforting. The ability to identify a developmental time frame for the origins of current symptoms will help to direct the choice of hypnotic intervention. Symptoms related to disruptions or disturbances in early attachment may benefit, for example, from renurturing techniques, whereas symptoms related to anxiety in the workplace may benefit from future-oriented rehearsal techniques of adult competencies.

While the choice of which intervention or technique to utilize is also related to the subject's preference, the clinician's knowledge of the timeframe (chronological and developmental age) of symptom development will enhance the outcome. A 70-year-old client who wanted help with a long history of anxiety and was assessed to have had significant disturbances in early attachment, did best when she imagined herself on the lap of her grandmother in a rocking chair, while practicing relaxation or breathing techniques. When she pictured herself alone, her anxiety always increased. This kind of subtle shift in the imagined suggestion, informed by the developmental knowledge of the client, is representative of the importance of knowing our client's developmental history.

This concept of a child's need for comfort is, in my experience, equally important in our work with adults. If the adult is in a regressed state, he or she is often confused and overwhelmed and appreciates comfort and support. Ego-strengthening principles work well with adolescents and adults. We are taught to praise and to congratulate the accomplishments of our subjects hypnotically (and I would add, therapeutically) for a reason. The support and comfort that warmth and nurturance provide to an adolescent or adult can increase the effectiveness of our clinical work partly because it mimics good parenting, and partly because it is ego strengthening. When the adult is in a child ego state, the clinician accepts the need for dependence and provides a safe holding environment while encouraging the movement towards independence and individuation. The adolescent ego state, at a different development stage, may require the clinician to encourage autonomy and to tolerate, even encourage, the rejection and rebellion necessary for separation and individuation without abandoning the adolescent ego state.

We can often capture our clients' attention when we add surprise, an element of novelty, fun, and creative play to our hypnotic interventions. Rossi (2002) theorizes that novelty may be essential to neurodevelopmental change in our hypnotic work. Adolescents are intrigued when an adult is fun, humorous, and creative. They are often convinced that most adults are just supervising, boring authorities in their lives. To be otherwise may ignite cooperation and motivate them to change. Anbar (2001) has developed an automatic typing technique in which he uses two keyboards on a computer to do hypnotic work, combining a familiar medium for teens and a sound knowledge of adolescent development. In this technique, the teen can communicate (typing rather than speaking) private thoughts while exploring contributing factors to symptoms. The novelty of the doctor approaching the teen in this way engages them hypnotically and produces health-promoting results.

Thus far the importance of understanding normal developmental stages with regard to our hypnotic work with adolescents and adults has been explicated and emphasized. Age regression, ego state therapy, and ego-strengthening hypnotic techniques are just a few examples of how knowledge of development improves our therapy in hypnosis. There are a range of hypnotic techniques that can be used to enhance development whether at the level of modifying behavior, uncovering the roots of symptoms, renurturing to improve personality development, or just reinforcing healthy aspects of the developed individual (Halas, 2000). Many of these techniques are extensions of psychotherapeutic practice such as hypnotic dreaming or reframing of the meaning of an event.

In a hypnosis workshop in which the theme was hypnosis and human development over a lifetime, students explored the words used to connote aging and images that could be paired with those words to create a more positive association with the aging process. One of my colleagues shared a metaphor that he utilized with medical students that aptly captured the theme of development:

> "When we are in our twenties, we choose our careers. When we are in our thirties, we become established in these careers. In our forties, we take our long strides, and when we reach our fifties we reflect for a while and blend in all the things we've been putting aside—as if we are stirring cookie dough and then scrape into the mix the dough still on the sides of the bowl. In our sixties, we stop striving and let whatever is there within us simply bubble up from the dough." He admitted not being sure of what to do in the seventies, and was told, "That is when you eat the cookie" (P. Bloom, Personal communication, July 23, 2006).

This metaphor is a reminder that development is an active, not a static, process.

A few final words on work with adolescents and adults and some caveats to remember. Adolescents have parents, and for all of their strident efforts to exclude them in the process of individuation, our work with adolescents is enhanced when we think of them as part of the family system.

Tony

One teenager, Tony, 15 years old, whom I saw for some preparation for surgery, would fight with his chauffeuring mother on the way to the session, slam the car door (I could hear it), and storm out of her presence saying he didn't need to see any doctor for any help. He would enter my office, work hard with self-hypnotic techniques, never revealing any discomfort with the idea of being in session. He repeated this before each session. His mother, unaware of what he did during the sessions, called after just two sessions to ask if it was worth the fight to keep him coming. "Yes," I told her. "Whatever he is saying to you doesn't match his behavior with me, so I think we can assume his behavior with you is about asserting himself and not about what he is getting from the work we are doing. If you can keep up the great job you are doing getting him here, I think he will benefit from our work together." His surgery went well, and he later asked for more hypnotic work for other issues he wanted to address. So, it is useful to think in terms of the family system and the adolescent as part of it, being mindful of the needs of each person in the system and preventing unnecessary sabotage by any member.

Adults, no matter how they are acting, are adults. What I mean by this is that even in regressed or abreactive states, the person with whom you are working has all of the stored resources accumulated over his or her lifetime. Unlike the child whose resources are few and as yet undeveloped, the adult has many more resources. Even with the most severe disturbances of personality development, one can appeal to some adult resources in ways one cannot with a child. Treating the adult with adult expectations while working with childlike parts of the personality, conveys the important message (and perhaps suggestion) that the person is capable of adult behavior and expected to act responsibly in and out of the therapist's office, regardless of what she or he experienced inside the office. To treat the adult as a child will, conversely, elicit more childlike behaviors.

This chapter outlines the importance of considering developmental stages of growth in our hypnotic work with adolescents and adults. Key models of human emotional, sexual, cognitive, social, and moral development highlight the complexity of human development. The interface of hypnosis with human development has been explored. Each example is illustrative of some aspect of thinking in developmental terms while working hypnotically. This chapter demonstrates that developmentally appropriate hypnotic strategies allow us to engage children of differing ages, even those residing in grown-up bodies, to further promote their health and well-being.

References

Anbar, R. (2001). Automatic word processing: A new forum for hypnotic expression. *American Journal of Clinical Hypnosis*, 44, 27–36.

Baker, E. (1981). An hypnotherapeutic approach to enhance object relatedness in psychotic patients. *International Journal of Clinical and Experimental Hypnosis*, 29, 136–147.

Bingham, M. & Stryker, S. (1995). *Things will be different for my daughter*. New York: Penguin Books.

Bonanno, G. (2004). Loss, trauma, and human resilience. *American Psychologist*, 59, 1, 20–28.

Brazelton, T. B. & Greenspan, S. (2000). *The irreducible needs of children*. Cambridge, MA: Perseus.

Brown, D. (1985) Hypnosis as an adjunct to the psychotherapy of the severely disturbed patient: An affective development approach. *International Journal of Clinical & Experimental Hypnosis*, 33(4):281–301.

Brown, D. & Fromm, E. (1986). *Hypnotherapy and hypnoanalysis*. Hillsdale, NJ: Erlbaum.

Cardeña, E. (2000). Hypnosis in the treatment of trauma. *The International Journal of Clinical and Experimental Hypnosis*, 48, 2, 225–238.

Eccles, J., Midgley, C., Wigfield, A., Buchanan, C., Reuman. D., Flanagan, C., & Iver, D. (1993). Development during adolescence: The impact of stage-environment fit on young adolescents' experiences in school and in families. *American Psychologist*, 48(2), 90–101.

Erikson, E.H. (1950). *Childhood and society.* New York: Norton.

Freud, S. (1962/2000) *Three essays on the theory of sexuality.* Translated, edited, and revised by James Strachey. New York: Basic Books.

Galinsky, E. (1987). *The six stages of parenthood.* New York: Addison-Wesley.

Garbarino, J., Kostleny, K., & Dubrow, N. (1991). *No place to be a child.* San Francisco: Jossey-Bass.

Gil, E. (1998). *Play therapy for severe psychological trauma.* [Videotape and manual]. New York: Guilford.

Gilligan, C. (1982). *In a different voice.* Cambridge: Harvard University Press.

Halas, M. (2000). Hypnosis for the many faces of menopause: Enhancing normal development and treating trauma-related disruptions. In Hornyak, L. & Green, J. (Eds.). *Healing from within: The use of hypnosis in women's health care.* Washington, D.C.: American Psychological Association.

Harper, G. (1999). A developmentally sensitive approach to clinical hypnosis for chronically and terminally ill adolescents. *American Journal of Clinical Hypnosis*, 42:1 July, 50–60.

Hilgard, E. & Hilgard, J. (1975). *Hypnosis in the relief of pain.* Los Altos, CA: Kaufmann.

Hilgard, J. & LeBaron, S. (1984). *Hypnotherapy of pain in children with cancer.* Los Altos, CA: Kaufmann.

Inhelder, B., & Piaget, J. (1958). *The growth of logical thinking from childhood to adolescence.* New York: Basic Books.

Kohlberg, L., Levine, C., & Hewer, A. (1983). *Moral stages: A current formulation and a response to critics.* New York: Karger.

Linden, J. (1997, June). *Transitions: Adolescents, war and hypnosis.* Paper presented at 14th International Congress of Hypnosis, a joint meeting between ISH, ASCH, and SCEH. San Diego, CA.

Macoby, E., & Jacklin, C. (1974). *The psychology of sex differences.* Stanford, CA: Stanford University Press.

Miller, P. (1983). *Theories of developmental psychology.* San Francisco: W.H. Freeman.

Murray-Jobsis, J. (1993). The borderline patient and the psychotic patient. In Rhue, J., Lynn, S. & Kirsch, I. (Eds.), *Handbook of clinical hypnosis.* Washington, D.C.: American Psychological Association.

Olness, K. & Kohen, D. P. (1996). *Hypnosis and hypnotherapy with children* (3rd. ed.) New York: Guilford Press.

Piaget, J. (1983). Piaget's theory. In P. Mussen (Ed.), *Handbook of child psychology* (4th ed). Vol. 1. New York: Wiley.

Pipher, M. (1994). *Reviving Ophelia: Saving the selves of adolescent girls.* New York: Balantine Books.

Pulaski, M. (1980). *Understanding Piaget: An introduction to childrens' cognitive development.* New York: Harper & Row.

Putnam, F. W. (1997). *Dissociation in children and adolescents: A developmental perspective.* New York: Guilford Press.

Rossi, E. (2002). *The psychobiology of gene expression.* New York: Wiley.

Scagnelli-Jobsis, J. (1982). Hypnosis with psychotic patients: A review of the literature and presentation of a theoretical framework. *American Journal of Clinical Hypnosis, 25,* 33–45.

van der Hart, O., Brown, P., & Turco, R. (1990). Hypnotherapy for traumatic grief: Janetian and modern approaches integrated. *American Journal of Clinical Hypnosis, 32,* 4, 263–269.

van der kolk, B. (1987). *Psychological trauma.* Washington, D.C.: American Psychiatric Press.

Wall, V. (1991). Developmental considerations in the use of hypnosis with children. In Wester, W. & O'Grady, D. (Eds.), *Clinical hypnosis with children,* (pp. 3–18). New York: Brunner/Mazel.

Watkins, J., & Watkins, H. (1997). *Ego states: Theory and therapy.* New York: W.W. Norton.

Wester, W., & O'Grady, D. (Eds.) (1991). *Clinical hypnosis with children.* New York: Brunner/Mazel.

Winnicott, D. (1965). *The maturational processes and the facilitating environment.* Madison, CT: International University Press.

Wolberg, L. R. (1945). *Hypnoanalysis.* New York: Grune & Stratton.

Wolberg, L. R. (1964). *Hypnoanalysis* (2nd ed.). New York: Grune & Stratton.

Chapter Four

Hypnotic Abilities

John A. Teleska, MEd
Laurence I. Sugarman, MD, FAAP, ABMH

a·bil·i·ty (ə-bĭl′ə-tē) n., pl. –ties. 1. The quality of being able to do something: mental, physical. ... 2. A natural or acquired skill or talent.[1]

Whatever I say it is ... will distract me from recognizing and utilizing the many possibilities that are.[2]
Milton H. Erickson, when asked
to define unconscious processes

In this chapter, we look at the phenomenology of hypnosis in an effort to tease out (1) what we mean by "hypnotic ability," (2) how we learn to engage it in therapy, and (3) whether it can be measured in a clinically useful way. To do this, we first discuss hypnotic abilities by building on the notion of subconscious (psychophysiological) reflexes introduced in Chapter One. This expansive but inclusive framework stretches beyond traditional notions of hypnotic phenomena and has important implications for working with children and adolescents. Next, we consider what helps us utilize these broadly defined capacities in therapy; that is, what are the postures and responses of the clinician that facilitate hypnotic engagement? Finally, we narrow our focus to the problem of attempting to gauge hypnotic ability in the midst of a dynamic process that we call hypnosis.

---

[1] W. Morris. (Ed.). (1981). *The American Heritage Dictionary of the English Language.* Boston: Houghton Mifflin. (p. 3).
[2] S. Gilligan. (1987). *Therapeutic Trances: The Cooperation Principle in Ericksonian Hypnotherapy.* New York: Brunner/Mazel.

Abilities: Conscious, Subconscious, and Hypnotic

Conscious Abilities

Sitting in his sixth grade classroom, Christopher listens intently to his teacher as she talks to the class about the ancient Egyptians. He decides to raise his hand and ask a question. Upon receiving the teacher's response, he decides to nod his head "Yes" to signal his satisfaction with the answer. He is consciously deciding to make those movements and aware that he has made them. In this case, raising his hand and nodding his head are *conscious abilities*.

Subconscious Abilities

While giving his report about King Tut, in his excitement about the "Boy Pharaoh" and, without thinking about it, Christopher's arms and hands move in support of what he says verbally. Someone raises his or her hand with a question. Christopher acknowledges the person and, without thinking about it, he raises his eyebrows and tilts his head towards him or her. He or she begins to talk, and, again without thinking about it, Christopher begins slowing nodding his head as he realizes it is a good question. He is not consciously managing his arm and hand movements, facial gestures, and head nodding, but they are not random movements. They are coherent expressions of his experience and responses. In this case, his body language is a *subconscious ability*.

Uniquely Coordinated Subconscious Abilities

Christopher's experiences illustrate the fact that everybody has subconscious abilities. In addition to body language, we intelligently and responsively accomplish digestion, respiration, walking, and hand-eye coordination all without conscious management. We are able to access memories relevant to what is being read, to experience interest or disinterest in parts of a conversation, construct mental images where relevant and inspect them, fill in gaps in a discourse, and plan a response—all of which are managed by what Lakoff and Johnson (1999) refer to as the "cognitive unconscious" (pp. 10–11). Depending on many variables—developmental stage, the social ecology in which one grew up, the nature of the significant relationships of one's life, to name a few—these subconscious competencies are varied and uniquely coordinated within each of us.

Subconscious Abilities and Psychophysiological Reflexes

We are using a slight, but important, shift of semantics here with this focal term "abilities." One might consider accessing relevant memory, walking, reading, and body language as subconscious or psychophysiological "reflexes" (*see* Chapter One). An *ability* implies a talent, potential or enacted, to do something, usually good, with the implication that it is acquired. A *reflex* is a more generic, reactive, mechanical process that can be adaptive or maladaptive. The reason for this shift of meaning is that *psychophysiological reflexes can be utilized as talents for therapeutic benefit in hypnosis*. Both reflexes and abilities are mutable. They can be trained. The reader is urged to keep in mind, as in Chapter One, that regardless of which term is used, both abilities and reflexes are behavioral manifestations of real neural and neurohumoral interconnections within the child's and adolescent's mind. The plasticity of these intercellular interactions is exercised in hypnosis (Rossi, 2002).

Subconscious Abilities and their Uses Change with Maturation

Consider how the subconscious abilities associated with imagination develop as we grow up. For our purposes, we define *imagination* as the ability (both conscious and subconscious) to create sensorial experiences "in the mind" without, at the time, requiring a corresponding "real" source of sensorial stimulation. Our imaginings can involve sight, sound, movement, skin sensation, smell, taste, and combinations of these. A child's experience may blur the distinction between what we call "real" and "imagined." Many children spontaneously enact playing with an invisible (to adults) companion or conversing with Teddy Bear. As we mature, our ability to imagine does not weaken; rather, we use it in different contexts, and typically learn to hold the distinction between real and imagined more tightly than when we were younger. We use our imagination to explore our sexuality (by fantasizing), to imagine what life choices might yield pleasing outcomes, to choose a new vacation destination, to plan a project, to plan for retirement, or, as clinicians, to think about how to precede therapeutically with a patient.

Ask a youngster to imagine watching his or her favorite TV program; many children can do it and report on the program in detail. Many adults cannot. Ask a young adult what he or she imagines he or she wants for himself or herself in the future, in work, in relationship: most can respond, and at greater length than would a child. Ask an older adult, dealing with issues of physical decline, to recount pleasant events in which he or she felt good. He or she often can remember a lot in a way that reminds him or her *now* about feeling more comfortable. At any age, we cope by escaping and separating ourselves from pain and discomfort, either by consciously evoking our imagination or, less consciously, by dissociating from perceived threats. As with any ability, how imagination can be accessed and engaged depends on linking it with relevant contexts in the person's life.

Hypnotic Abilities

Using the methods of hypnotic induction, a clinician suggests to me that, without any conscious effort on my part, the more one of my arms lifts off my lap the more I will go into a trance. As my arm gradually levitates, I am not consciously aware of making it happen. My subconscious ability to move my arm has been engaged in the context of a hypnotic interaction. It is useful to consider any natural or acquired ability accessed and engaged in the context of hypnotic interaction as a hypnotic ability. So, in this case, the lifting of my arm is a hypnotic ability.

We define a *hypnotic interaction* in clinical settings as an encounter that (1) is intentional, (2) is informed and organized by the premises and elements of hypnosis, and (3) accesses and engages the patient's innate abilities for his benefit. It follows that hypnotherapy occurs on a continuum from formal hypnosis to "hypnotic conversation" (Teleska & Roffman, 2004). In formal hypnosis, hypnotic elements might be structured as are those critiqued by Sugarman (*see* Chapter One). Roffman (*see* Chapter Thirteen) offers a looser framing that includes hypnotic interaction occurring outside of formally defined trance.

Implications

The implications of this conceptualization of hypnotic ability are significant. There are no abilities that exist uniquely in the hypnotic domain. The hypnotic phenomena commonly described in the literature—arm levitation, ideodynamic signaling, analgesia, anesthesia, dissociation, amnesia—are based on natural or acquired subconscious abilities that have been accessed and engaged in the context of a hypnotic interaction. Table 4.1 clarifies this: in each row, the left column describes a subconscious ability and the right column describes the hypnotic ability that results from utilizing that subconscious ability in a hypnotic context.

This framing of hypnotic abilities also suggests that there are many paths to a therapeutic goal. Because people have different structures of subconscious abilities, different clinician/patient dyads will entail different hypnotic interactions to generate similar hypnotherapeutic results. For example, in Table 4.1, row 4, pain control is not always and only accomplished by utilizing the patient's subconscious ability to selectively not notice certain sensations. People have unique subconscious abilities and require different hypnotic approaches to accomplish pain control. Erickson & Rossi (1979) describe 11 hypnotic approaches to the engagement of the patients' potential abilities to facilitate pain control, including direct suggestion, amnesia, hypnotic analgesia, hypnotic substitution of sensation, hypnotic displacement of pain, hypnotic reinterpretation of the pain experience, dissociation, and time distortion (pp. 97–192). The clinician's proclivities—his or her expectations, past successes and failures, and what he or she is able to notice and engage within the patient—also shape the hypnotic interaction.

Table 4.1: Examples of Subconscious Abilities Used as the Basis for Hypnotic Abilities

Subconscious ability (i.e., not consciously managed) …	… that which, when engaged in the context of hypnotic interaction, might be the basis for…
1. Body language consisting of arm and hand motions, facial gestures, head movements—each of which is expressive of part of the person's internal experience	Arm levitation; Ideomotor signaling
2. Waking fantasy, dreaming, lucid dreaming	Guided imagery; Positive hallucination (sensing something that others do not)
3. Selectively noticing what is assessed as important either in the domain of physical things (e.g., watching the snake on the trail while not paying much attention to the surrounding greenery or not noticing the chairs or people around you while engaged in watching a movie), or information (e.g., quite naturally attending to the ideas in this book that interest you and are useful to you)	"Going into trance"; the focused, selective attention that can occur in trance; Negative hallucination (not sensing something that others do)
4. Selectively *not* noticing certain sensations (e.g., the feel of one's shoes, or the feel of one's glasses resting on the ears and the bridge of the nose, or the drone of a neighbor's lawn mower)	Possible pain control, analgesia, anesthesia; Negative hallucination (not sensing something that others do)
5. Forgetting (e.g., someone's name, or where you put the keys, or your glasses)	Amnesia
6. Our natural response to trauma: When overwhelmed by one's experience, setting aside the part of ourselves that is overwhelmed, so that we can stay as functional as possible (e.g., the soldier setting aside fear while in the battlefield)	Dissociation: the ability to behave and respond as if we are divisible into parts (e.g., conscious, and subconscious, as in, "You can let the part of you that knows when your bladder is full wake you up just enough get out of bed and go to the bathroom and come back to bed")
7. Withstanding the disappointment or anger of the other when you are not as they want, need, or expect you to be	No simple name or description; nonetheless, a useful ability to engage as individuals become more of who they are that may be different from those around them

Essentially, within this broad context, the hypnotic process is determined by the combined abilities of the dyad.

Another implication of this framing is that most hypnotic talents do not have names. Hypnotic abilities—or phenomena—that have been given names in the literature typically satisfy the following conditions: (1) they are easy to describe (e.g., arm levitation, amnesia), (2) a significant portion of the population studied can access the requisite subconscious assets that form the basis for the named hypnotic ability, and (3) a significant number of clinicians and researchers have learned to use hypnotic interaction to generate the named hypnotic phenomenon. Each child possesses far more abilities and resources than we recognize. The bottom row in Table 4.1 describes an example of what could be considered a subconscious ability that has no common name when engaged in hypnotic interaction: Withstanding the disappointment or anger of the other when you are not as they want, need, or expect you to be. Evoking this ability in a hypnotic interaction might be useful to an adolescent in the process of appropriately individuating from his or her parents or siblings.

As a result of the interplay of natural human development and our personal histories, each of us has our own types of abilities, conscious and subconscious. We have abilities that no one has thought to name. Milton Erickson's genius was expressed in the creativity with which he accessed and engaged the unique capacities of each of his patients on behalf of promoting their health and well-being (Haley, 1986). The hypnotherapist need not think of his or her work as confined to engaging a standard set of hypnotic abilities— that some people are good at and some not. Rather, it is the hypnotherapist's charge to study and to collaborate with each patient to create a hypnotic interaction that accesses and engages that patient's unique and innate talents.

Engaging Subconscious Abilities in Therapy

Hypnosis does not exist. What exists is the interaction between a given context and the aptitude of the subject to respond to that context.
H. Bernheim (1916)

69

Matthew

At 14-year-old Matthew's first visit to seek help for controlling his chronic, debilitating migraine headaches, I [LS] asked him to track how his head felt on an analog scale of his own choosing. He chose a scale from zero to 10, with 10 being the worst. I labeled 10 as "unimaginably horrible, like if your head exploded!" and zero as "normal." This was my usual strategy, designed to have the adolescent "own" the scale's creation but to keep it inclusive of his experience. Matthew also learned a simple relaxation and dissociation technique with which to experiment at home.

Two weeks later Matthew returned with his record of self-monitoring. He was pleased to report that his experimenting with self-hypnosis was beginning to help him. I was puzzled as I reviewed his written notes. In black ink, he had recorded numbers from zero to 6. In red ink, he had recorded numbers from negative-1 to negative-4. When I asked, "What's this?" Matthew, smiling, explained that *I* had labeled the scale from 10, "unimaginably horrible" to zero, for "normal."

"So, what are these other numbers?" I asked.

He replied, "You said zero was normal. Normal isn't the best you can feel. I want to go for negative numbers."

Not only did Matthew master his migraines, he went on to college to major in both psychology and graphic design.

What types of attitudes and skills contribute to a clinician engaging a young person's subconscious reflexes as talents in therapy? In this section, we suggest a variety of ways that the therapist can develop those resources within themselves. Chief among them is to read and study the breadth of clinical experience offered in the literature at the end of this chapter.

Recognize that Change Belongs to the Person Changing

The subconscious ability by which a child learns to gain relief from chronic migraines belongs to the child. In a clinical setting, the hypnotic engagement of those abilities is a co-creation of the patient and clinician. This is illustrated in the clinical vignette, above. Not only is it critical for the clinician to recognize that the patient "owns" his or her trance, but it is also important that the child or adolescent know it. Sometimes, in the midst of rapport, the patient misattributes the source of his or her own resources. What if Matthew had claimed, incorrectly, that the *therapist* had told him about "better than normal?" Then that attribution becomes an avenue to explore in service of resolving his migraines.

Explore Your Own Subconscious Abilities

One cannot fully recognize the "trance of the encounter" without becoming familiar with how it feels to consciously explore subconscious talents. This can best be done by (1) learning, with the help of a trained mentor or colleague if needed, to go into trance; (2) experimenting with engaging your own subconscious abilities to answer a troubling question or make a choice; (3) practicing using all of your senses to observe your own experiences so that you can engage with the child's and adolescent's multisensory experiences.

Discover and Engage the Patient's Motivation

Is the child seeing you because he has a problem, the parents think they have a problem, the child thinks the parents have a problem, the parents think the child has a problem, or some combination of all of these? If a child still sucks his or her thumb to irk his parents, then the solution to thumb sucking will have to include the motivation to irk parents. In such a case, Erickson (Haley, 1986) prescribed 20 minutes of loud, slurping thumb sucking every evening while the parents read the newspaper (p. 196). The child quickly lost interest in thumb sucking. For a child suffering from migraines, or embarrassed by bedwetting, or scared of needles, or in pain, there will be a motivation to learn self-regulation in a way that will afford relief. The more the child (or an adult, for that matter) experiences interacting with you as on behalf of what motivates them, the more he or she will include your influence in generating a therapeutic outcome. To illustrate this, Paul Lounsbury (personal communication, May 21, 1999) tells this story of a patient he worked with over the span of 10 years.

> Alice began to have diarrhea when she was 11. Nothing stopped the diarrhea, and she was beginning to lose weight. It turned out that her mother and father were in the habit of taking the family for long drives over the weekend, during which they would usually have a screaming argument with each other. Alice's diarrhea prevented her from going on these unpleasant family outings. I told Alice that was a pretty good solution for her, except that her body wasn't holding onto the food long enough for her to get sufficiently nourished. She agreed to receive some help to improve her "already-pretty-good" solution. Without specifying the symptom, I suggested that she could replace the diarrhea with a better problem that did not threaten her well-being but still prevented her from going on the family trips when she did not want to. She stopped the diarrhea and developed migraines, but mostly on weekends. Often the family wouldn't take Alice on these trips because of the *threat* of her getting a migraine. She didn't always get them when she stayed home. As Alice became older, I worked with Alice's growing abilities to have more options for setting boundaries about what she would and would not do without having to use migraines.

Lounsbury's recognition of Alice's motivation for having a symptom (separating herself from her parents' arguing) created the opportunity for Alice to choose a healthier solution. Implicit in the therapist's acceptance of Alice's motivation and his concern that diarrhea was unhealthy is his respect for Alice's self-worth and ability to help herself.

Promote Positive Expectancy—Clinician and Patient

The expectation that you, as clinician, hold for a therapeutic inter-action affects both you and the child or adolescent in your care. Language choices can promote positive expectancy (*see* Appendix at the end of this chapter, and the many examples in Hammond, 1990). These semantics are important, but only if they are an authentic expression of the therapist's confidence. Without this attitude, semantics are just a shell without the nut.

What promotes the clinician's development of authentic positive expectancy? Erickson's answer to the question, "How do you know what to do?" reveals his expectations of himself, his patients, their interaction, and the therapeutic outcome:

> "I don't know. ... I don't know what I'm going to do. I don't know what I'm going to say. ... All I know is that I trust my unconscious to shelve into my conscious what is appropriate. ... And I don't know how the clients are going to respond. ... All I know is that they *will*. ... I don't know why. ... I don't know when. ... All I know is that they'll respond in an appropriate fashion, in a way that best suits them as an individual. And I become so intrigued with wondering exactly *how* their unconscious will choose to respond. And so I comfortably wait for their response, knowing that when it occurs I can accept and utilize it."
>
> He paused, his eyes twinkling. "Now I know that sounds ridicu-lous ... *BUT IT WORKS!!*" (Gilligan, 1987, p. 83)

Fundamental to Erickson's authenticity was his sincere delight in discovering something to wonder about in each patient. For the busy clinician, the essence of this attitude is looking forward to discovering how this unique child will learn to help himself or herself.

Hypnotic Ability Can Violate Our Current Understanding of Physiology

In her teaching, Kay Thompson offered many examples of hypnosis and hypnotic abilities that violate current notions of physiology. For instance, when she tells her patients to stop bleeding she says, "… Why do people stop bleeding? Because I tell them to. Nobody ever told them before" (Kane & Olness, 2004, p. 316).

One can think of it this way: abilities—out-of-awareness hypnotic abilities—are sometimes engaged by presupposing they might exist. Children are told they can exhale out the discomfort of an injection by blowing out, making a pinwheel turn. And they do (Sugarman, 1997/2006). Ewin (1983) found that suggestions of being "cool and comfortable" during the first two hours after sustaining a burn engaged patients' hypnotic ability to reduce the depth of their tissue injury. Before reading such a study, we may not have had reason to expect human ability included such phenomenon.

The precursors of such studies were clinicians' anecdotal experiences with patients that led them to hypothesize and then design investigations. There are many clinicians doing this sort of work who do not research it. They quietly function as healers collaborating with their patients to generate therapeutic outcomes. Studies and reports of these anecdotal experiences are valuable to read because they evoke what might be possible in our own clinical practices. Thompson offers this:

> [T]hose people who work in surgical situations and who work with pain patients assume that pain relief, if it's utilizing hypnosis, must follow the [*known*] neurological pathways. That is not a valid assumption…you have to be aware that hypnosis violates some of the physiological and neurological kinds of expectations. That's all right. That's what hypnosis is so good for.

> Once you … set aside your assumption that you know how the world works, then it opens a great many things to you as a person, in order to believe in the things that other people can do. … (Kane & Olness, 2004, p. 323)

As the clinician's view of hypnotic abilities broadens, so too does the clinician's awareness of the patient's resources available in therapy. This contributes to the clinician's positive expectancy.

Ryan

Ten-year-old Ryan had severe asthma. He learned to reduce his frequent inhaler use when he started guitar lessons. The more he practiced the guitar, the fewer asthma symptoms he experienced. He could even control the asthma by playing his guitar in his mind. Over a period of five years Ryan became proficient at the guitar and was able to stop using all but occasional medications for asthma. The consulting pulmonologist concluded that he had outgrown his asthma. Ryan claimed that he "outplayed" the asthma, adding, "Maybe how I imagine it works is really how it works."

Build Rapport

The Michael Jordan Metaphor
Kids are so good at using their subconscious capabilities for whatever interests them that attempting to influence their process is like playing a pick-up game of basketball with Michael Jordan, arguably the best professional player of his generation. He is so much more talented and experienced than you are that you will not even touch the ball unless he lets you. You have to give him a reason to let you. That reason starts with *rapport*.

Rapport occurs when the patient recognizes himself or herself in the clinician's responses to him or her. From the clinician's perspective, rapport cannot be assumed to exist simply because we care, are altruistic, mean well, and are approachable. It is evidenced in the minimal cues of the patient in response to our own: the open posture, the slow nod of the head, the softening of facial expression, the eye contact. These pieces of data can be identified and written in the record of the encounter. They are the platform upon which rapport is built.

From the patient's point of view, rapport is getting the message that "Somebody out there knows I am here." This is exemplified in a rudimentary way in the following vignette.

April

Our friend Nancy and 6-month-old daughter, April, came to visit. Nancy and my wife sat in chairs and talked with each other; April lay on her back on the floor. I [JT] sat at April's feet and watched her. Her eyes darted about, and she made sounds, some of them loud and piercing. She sporadically moved her arms and legs, opening and closing her hands, moving her head from side to side. Some movements looked deliberate in that the turn of the head seemed coordinated with where April chose to focus her gaze. For a few minutes, I made sounds and facial gestures in an attempt to engage April. Her attention would rest on me momentarily and then continue hopping around. I stopped doing anything in particular to engage April, and just watched her. I found the opening and closings of her hands and her finger movements held *my* attention. I held my hand up and mimicked her right hand motion as best I could. She immediately watched my hand—and to my surprise, kept watching it, *as long as I mimicked her motions*. If I stopped moving my hand, but continued to hold it up, within seconds, April's gaze would drift. When I returned to mimicking her hand motions, her gaze would come back to my hand. If I ignored her hand motions, and moved my hand as I chose, she lost interest. *She most attended to my hand motions when I mimicked her hand motions.*

While April's hand movements were not intentional in the way that an adult is capable of intentional hand movements, her level of awareness of her hand motions was sufficient so that she responded with attention when my hand motions mimicked hers.

This is the same sort of human responsivity that is at play when we, as clinicians, notice and respond to our patients in a way that engages *both* of us in a therapeutic interaction. When we react intentionally to behavior that the child executes without conscious management, we are including in the conversation that from which subconscious behavior arises. Those subconscious responses can be word choices, metaphor choices, eye blinks, body language, attitudes, voice changes, pauses in speech, posture changes—any observable behavior of which the child may be unaware. As we relate to more and more of the child's behavior, we nurture and encourage more and more of his or her subconscious resources.

In a clinical setting, this "feeding back" of subconsciously derived behavior contributes to an unfolding of patient's deeper assets, making them available. "Rapport is deepened when you are vulnerable and somebody meets you there" (Nancy Winston and Paul Lounsbury, personal communication, April 29, 2006). For example, building rapport with a young drug addict who has lied to his parents, his teachers, and police officers is *not* accomplished by indicating that you intend to treat him as trustworthy. Rapport is built by letting him know you don't trust him to do what he says. He knows he is not trustworthy, and he knows you are seeing part of who he knows himself to be.

Rabbits and Tunnels: The Child Owns the Meaning

Pediatrician Judson Reaney tells this story about a patient in his care:

> An 11-year-old boy was learning to keep his bed dry. He imagined that he had a racetrack between his bladder and his brain with race cars carrying the message, "Gotta go" up to his brain. He decided that a second car would race back to tell his bladder what to do. He became dry in a single session of hypnosis. After two months of keeping his bed dry, he called the office because he was wetting the bed again. He explained, "There are rabbits crossing the road, and the cars have to slow down or hit them, so I don't get the message in time."
>
> Rather than wondering about the figurative meaning of this development, I assumed that he had the answer and so, expressing my faith in his ability, I asked him, "Gee, what are you going to do about that?"

The boy responded, "I'm going to build fences along the track with tunnels under the road for the rabbits."

He kept the bed dry after that. (Judson Reaney, personal communication, 2006)

Dr. Reaney, an experienced clinician and hypnotherapist, still does not know or need to know what those rabbits represented to that boy. Might the rabbits have held deep symbolic significance? Perhaps, but all that was needed for this child was Dr. Reaney's support and faith that the child's understanding was sufficient within itself to resolve his own problem. Perhaps that is why he came back. I shared Dr. Reaney's clinical vignette with a 10-year-old girl who had just learned to have a dry bed 29 out of 30 days.

I asked her, "What do you think the rabbits are?"

Without hesitation, she replied, "They're his doubts. And the tunnels are how he is not going to let them get in the way."

Resistance—What is Being Left Out?

What is being left out? How will the patient bring it into the interaction? If the child has an objection to a suggestion, find out more about the objection and then refine the suggestion to include what had been left out. Assist the entire patient to "Yes." It is helpful to replace the word "resistant" with "self-protective."

In the following vignette, the adolescent's apathy to the clinician's suggestions could be interpreted as resistance. The clinician did not explore what was left out. Despite this, the hypnotic interaction may have influenced the therapeutic outcome. The clinician's framing of hypnosis ("… might find some relief in self-hypnosis") was broad enough to allow the young woman to help herself.

Lisa

Seventeen-year-old Lisa had a severe, continuous headache for a month after being thrown from a horse. She was an accomplished equestrian and always wore a helmet when she rode. A thorough evaluation after the accident had revealed no brain injury, and the neurologist could not explain the ongoing pain but recommended amitryptaline (a tricyclic antidepressant often used for chronic pain), which Lisa refused. Curiously, she had had a similar headache associated with an unexplained, passing illness one year ago. Her primary care physician, trained in hypnosis, suggested she might find some relief in self-hypnosis and she agreed, but with indifference. She participated passively in an exercise in relaxation and imagery in which she chose to be riding a powerful horse away from a mountainous headache that drifted into the distance. After this experience she agreed that she "might be a little better." The next day the doctor called to inquire about her progress and her mother answered saying, "She doesn't want to talk with you and thinks that hypnosis is stupid." The following day, Lisa tearfully revealed to her mother that she had been raped one year ago. She had never told anyone, until now. Her headache resolved as she worked with a therapist to process her trauma.

Hypnotizability Scales as a Measure of Hypnotic Ability

Researchers need measures to build correlations so they hypothesize about a group of individuals. Several generations of hypnotizability scales now exist (Council, 2002), some of which are dedicated to measuring the hypnotic responsivity of young people. Using these scales, researchers are accumulating a growing list of correlates. For example, young subjects assessed using hypnotizability scales as "high hypnotizables" are found to be significantly better than "low hypnotizables" at using (the researcher's version of what they call) hypnosis for ability to respond positively to instruction to relax (Sebastiani, Simoni, Gemingnani,

Ghelarducci, & Santarcangelo, 2005), control pain, and negatively hallucinate (Raz, Fan, & Posner, 2005).

These scales are presented and discussed in Olness and Kohen (1996) and Plotnick and O'Grady (1991). There is a long-running debate in the realm of hypnosis about whether such instruments should be routinely part of clinical work. There are those who vigorously promote such integration to discriminate which patients will most benefit from hypnosis from those who will not (Plotnick & O'Grady, 1991). In reality, the majority of clinicians do not use these scales (Cohen, 1989) for a variety of reasons. These include (1) the belief that low scores create negative expectancy, (2) poor predictability of clinical outcome (especially with children), and (3) the formality of imposing a rigid structure on the encounter.

As clinicians working with patients, we find these scales, their measurements, and their correlates interesting and suggestive of domains in which to use hypnosis with our patients. In the clinical realm, however, these instruments can be limiting constructs. If we think of hypnosis as utilizing and developing myriad unnamed subconscious abilities in each individual, then these scales cannot measure more than a narrow swatch of the rich landscape in which hypnosis operates. For example, if a given child performs well on the scaled tasks (e.g., arm levitation, hallucination, post-hypnotic suggestion) he or she is deemed "hypnotizable." If those same tasks are prescribed and elicited as "hypnotic phenomena" in the therapeutic encounter and linked, by the therapist's suggestions, to a positive outcome that is subsequently achieved, then, as a prescriptive strategy, the hypnotizability scale predicted the outcome. Because the scale's demands were used by the subject to meet the goals, the scale is self-validating.

The instrument becomes limiting when the presumption is made that these tasks represent the *whole of the subject's capacity for subconscious change* using hypnosis. For example, the Stanford Hypnotic Clinical Scale for Children (Morgan & Hilgard, 1978/1979) assigns lower scores to younger children who do not relax physically. If relaxation is believed to be a correlate of hypnotizability, (i.e., to predict cooperation and positive outcome in hypnotherapy) then the therapist would *correctly* conclude that doing hypnosis using relaxation would be less effective for a child who scores low on this item. But the therapist, generalizing this correlation, may further decide *incorrectly* that using hypnosis *at all* would be less effective for this child. Olness and Kohen (1996) liken this assumption to "tying a child's hands behind his or her back and then concluding he or she is not mature enough to tie his or her own shoes" (p. 25). It may be more apt to claim it is like assuming that a 4-year-old who has not learned to tie her shoes cannot learn to do so.

Actually there is little evidence of such limitation. We are aware of no clinical studies with children in which low scores on such scales predicted negative outcome. This is primarily because most children score high. These high scores likely reflect not only the facility of children's imaginations but also their ability to develop rapport and adapt to the implied performance expectations inherent in the evaluation. These factors may be as important, if not more predictive, of ability to utilize subconscious resources for therapeutic change.

Given that children are hypnotically talented—in the business of developing subconscious psychophysiological self-regulation—perhaps it is not hypnotizability we need to measure but predictors of the types of personality characteristics, affective styles, and learning profiles that will help us more efficiently determine the strategies to apply to a given child for a given problem. As well, it would be interesting to identify those qualities that make a therapist a good match for a given child. In other words, can a scale predict the specificity of a strategy? Kohen and Olness (1996) note that an ideal scale for children would "… at least in part be (1) brief (e.g., 5 to 15 minutes long), (2) interesting and absorbing, (3) developmentally sensitive and specific, (4) learning style sensitive and specific, (5) multisensory and discriminating between senses, (6) free of cultural bias, and (7) predictive" (Daniel P. Kohen, personal communication, February 28, 2000; Kohen & Olness, 1996). One could argue that the practical application of such a broadly inclusive scale would involve such a co-creative dynamic between evaluator and child that it would itself be a hypnotic encounter.

Andre Weitzenhoffer, co-developer of the Stanford Hypnotic Susceptibility Scales, Forms A and B (Weitzenhoffer & Hilgard, 1959) and other measurement tools, had this to say about the role of measuring hypnotic ability in practice (Weitzenhoffer, 2002):

> This is not a well-recognized fact, but it has never been independently, empirically or theoretically shown that (a) hypnosis has or should have depth or degrees, and (b) that suggestibility is or should be a measure of this depth or degree. (p. 212)

> [T]he majority of available hypnosis scales cannot directly tell us anything regarding the presence of hypnosis, its extent, or the subject's capacity to develop it. Anything said in these regards is a pure guess, although possibly an educated one. (p. 213)

> How useful is it to know, for instance, that a patient can do an age regression when all one needs to do is to produce an analgesia? Generally, not greatly. For this reason, in my own practice … I do essentially no pretesting of suggestibility. My advice is not to spend the time on testing, which can be better spent doing something more constructive. (p. 217)

Clinicians function in different contexts than researchers, and, more importantly, clinical patients function in a different context than do experimental subjects. Assigning a specific set of behaviors/responses as "The-Hypnotic-Phenomenon-To-Use-As-Metrics-Of-Hypnotic-Ability" serves primarily to measure the extent of the intersection of the measurer's preconceived (and perhaps rigid) notions of what constitutes hypnotic ability with the patient's naturally evolved subconscious talents and competences. Working on a problem that matters to them, clinical patients are differently motivated to be available to hypnotic engagement than is a person taking a hypnotic susceptibility test. Kay Thompson (Kane & Olness, 2004), a gifted clinician and teacher of hypnotic engagement, said:

> I refuse to restrict myself and the patient to their ability to learn based on some artificial criteria determined by somebody, when the individuals who established those criteria really didn't have any motivation to go into trance. (p. 15)

We suggest the clinician is better served by studying the unique coordination of abilities, subconscious and otherwise, that each young person already *has* in order to help him or her do what he or she *can*, rather than what he or she *cannot*.

Resources

Journals

American Journal of Clinical Hypnosis

Australian Journal of Clinical and Experimental Hypnosis

Contemporary Hypnosis

The International Journal of Clinical and Experimental Hypnosis

Journal of Personality and Social Psychology Imagination, Cognition, and Personality

Books

Erickson, M. H., & Rossi, E. L. (1996). *Hypnotherapy: An Exploratory Casebook*. New York: Irvington. [*Among the Erickson/Rossi books this is the one to start with; it is thorough and articulate.*]

Haley, J. (1986). *Uncommon Therapy*. New York: W.W. Norton. [*This book contains Haley's articulate description of Erickson's psychiatric techniques as gleaned from a series of transcribed conversations with Erickson (see next listing)*].

Haley, J. (Ed.). (1985). *Conversations with Milton H. Erickson Vols. I-III*. New York: Triangle Press, distributed by W.W. Norton. [*This book contains conversations between three very good therapists (Erickson, Haley, and Weakland) about specific cases. Gregory Bateson occasionally joins in.*]

Hammond, C. (Ed.). (1990). *Handbook of Hypnotic Suggestions and Metaphors*. Des Plaines, Iowa: American Society for Clinical Hypnosis. [*This book contains an extensive collection of trance suggestion for thousands of situations. It is a standard reference for hypnotherapists.*]

Kane, S., & Olness, K. (Eds.). (2004). *The Art of Therapeutic Communication: The Collected Works of Kay F. Thompson*. Carmarthen, Wales, U.K.: Crown House. [*The collected works of a gifted healer and teacher.*]

Moerman, D. (2002). *Meaning, Medicine and the "Placebo Effect."* New York: Cambridge University Press. [*This book discusses the importance of the meaning people make and its effect on their health and healing.*]

Rosen, S. (Ed.). (1991). *My Voice Will Go with You: The Teaching Tales of Milton H. Erickson*. New York: W.W. Norton.

Rossi, E. L., & Cheek, D. B. (1988). *Mind-Body Therapy: Methods of Ideodynamic Healing in Hypnosis*. New York: W.W. Norton. [*Ideodynamic means unconscious motor control. Cheek, a colleague of Erickson's, made creative use of hypnosis in his many years as an obstetrician. Rossi collected the scattered papers and made a book. This book contains great material far beyond the borders of OB-GYN.*]

Rossi, E., Erickson-Klein, R. & Rossi, K., Editors. (2006) CD. *The Neuroscience Editions. Volume 1: Healing in Hypnosis; Volume 2: Life Reframing in Hypnosis; Volume 3: Mind-Body Communication in Hypnosis; Volume 4: Creative Choice in Hypnosis. Version 1*. Phoenix, AZ: The Milton H. Erickson Foundation Press. [*These four volumes on CD contain transcripts of some of Erickson's seminars, workshops, and lectures. Although out of print, you may still find some of the book versions.*]

Short, D., designer. (2002) CD. *Milton H. Erickson, M.D.: Complete Works*. Phoenix, AZ. The Milton H. Erickson Foundation Press. [*This CD contains an indexed and searchable collection of all of Erickson's published papers.*]

Zeig, J. (Ed.). (1980). *A Teaching Seminar with Milton H. Erickson*. New York: Brunner/Mazel.

References

Bernheim, H. (1916). *De la suggestión* [About Suggestion]. Paris: Albin Michel.

Cohen, S. (1989). Clinical uses of hypnotizability. *American Journal of Clinical Hypnosis, 32*, 4–9.

Council, J. (2002). A historical overview of hypnotizability assessment. *American Journal of Clinical Hypnosis*, 44(3–4), 199–208.

Erickson, M. H., & Rossi, E. (1979). *Hypnotherapy: An exploratory casebook*. New York: Irvington.

Ewin, D. (1983). Emergency room hypnosis for the burned patient. *American Journal of Clinical Hypnosis*, 26(1), 5–8.

Haley, J. (1986). *Uncommon therapy*. New York: W.W. Norton.

Hammond, C. (Ed.). (1990). *Handbook of hypnotic suggestions and metaphors*. Des Plaines, Iowa: American Society for Clinical Hypnosis.

Gilligan, S. (1987). *Therapeutic trances: The cooperation principle in Ericksonian hypnotherapy*. New York: Brunner/Mazel.

Kane, S., & Olness, K. (Eds.). (2004). *The art of therapeutic communication: The collected works of Kay F. Thompson*. Carmarthen, Wales, U.K.: Crown House.

Kohen, D. P., & Olness, K. N. (1996). Self-regulation therapy: Helping children to help themselves. *Ambulatory Child Health: The Journal of General and Community Pediatrics*, 2, 43–58.

Lakoff, G., & Johnson, M. (1999). *Philosophy in the flesh: The embodied mind and its challenge to western thought*. New York: Basic Books.

Morgan, A., & Hilgard, J. (1978–1979). The Stanford hypnotic clinical scale for children. *American Journal of Clinical Hypnosis*, 21, 78–85.

Morris, W. (Ed.). (1981). *The American heritage dictionary of the English language*. Boston: Houghton Mifflin.

Olness, K. N., & Kohen, D. P. (1996). Norms of hypnotizability in children. In *Hypnosis and hypnotherapy with children* (pp. 18–32). New York: Guilford Press.

Plotnick, A. B., & O'Grady, D. J. (1991). Hypnotic responsiveness in children. In W. C. Wester & D. J. O'Grady (Eds.), *Clinical hypnosis with children* (pp. 19–33). New York: Brunner/Mazel.

Raz, A., Fan J., & Posner, M. I. (2005, July 15). Hypnotic suggestion reduces conflict in the human brain. *Proceedings of the National Academy of Sciences*, 102(28), 9978–9983.

Rossi, E. L. (2002). Psychosocial genomics and the healing arts. In *The psychobiology of gene expression: Neuroscience and neurogenesis in hypnosis and the healing arts* (pp. 188–252). New York: W.W. Norton.

Sebastiani, L., Simoni, A., Gemingnani, A., Ghelarducci, B., & Santarcangelo E. L. (2005). Relaxation as a cognitive task. *Archives Italiennes de Biologie*, 143(1), 1–12.

Sugarman, L. I. (Producer) (1997/2006). *Hypnosis in pediatric practice: Imaginative medicine in action*. [DVD and Learning Guide]. Carmarthen, Wales, U.K.: Crown House.

Teleska, J., & Roffman, A. (2004). A continuum of hypnotic interactions: From formal hypnosis to hypnotic conversation. *American Journal of Clinical Hypnosis*, 47(2), 103–115.

Weitzenhoffer, A. M., & Hilgard, E. R. (1959). *Stanford hypnotic susceptibility scales, forms A & B*. Palo Alto, CA: Consulting Psychologists Press.

Weitzenhoffer, A. M. (2002). Scales, scales, and more scales. *American Journal of Clinical Hypnosis*, 44(3–4), 209–219.

Appendix: Therapeutic Language

In the highly charged, sensitive arena of our clinical encounters with children, adolescents and their parents, words take on more power, conveying meaning, both positive and negative, beyond usual awareness. Language is more than the words. It is the *when*, and the *how*, and the *why* of what we say that brings therapy to the relationship. In order to maximize the therapy in the use of language, consider the following concepts and examples.

Patient Centered

Use the young person's own words, once elicited, to describe symptoms:

- "I am *most* interested in how [*symptom*] feels to *you*" (e.g., not to your parents).

Avoid controlling, authoritarian language:

- Replace "I want you to ..." and "You should ..." with "You can choose ...," "You may, when you are ready ...," or "When you decide ..."

Do not let symptoms or problems "just go away." Something the child did made it better:

- "I wonder what you do to make it better," and "How did you do that?"

Empowering

Express an implicit authoritative belief in the child's efficacy and mastery:

- "What do you do when *you make* that [*symptom*] feel better?"

Avoid, at all costs, the verb "try." It implies failure. We do not "try" to do what we know we can; only what we doubt we can.

- Replace "try" with *"Do your best."*

Reframing

Descriptions of problems provide a new way to look at them, re-address them, and change them. Description leads to control.

- Allow dissociation: *"the* [not *your*] headache."

Use the young person's words to reframe symptoms. Avoid charged words like "pain" and "hurt."

- Replace "pain" and "hurt" with "That *tight feeling* in your chest," or "The *banging* above your eye you called a headache."

Provide an alternative version:

- "I notice that sometimes the bed is not wet. So, I wonder how *you keep the bed dry."*

Promoting Positive Change

Use "when" for desired behaviors and outcomes:

- *"When* you are feeling better" and *"When* you practice your relaxation exercises."

Use "if" for undesired outcomes that may occur:

- *"If* you have another problem with asthma."

Use the past tense for past problems:

- "Those headaches you *had."* "When your asthma *bothered* you."

If the young person asks why you use past tense for what he or she believes is a present problem, explain that he or she came to you for help and you intend to help, but you can not tell the future. You do believe *the symptom experience will be different* because it is always changing.

Add the word "yet" to statements of self-doubt:

- "You say you don't know how, *yet.*"

Ego-Strengthening

Refer to the child's or adolescent's past experience of growth and development of new capabilities, such as learning to walk, talk, control his or her bowel and bladder, overcome fears of going to the doctor, and getting injections . This is all evidence of capability for growth and change.

- "You already know how to do it"; "You are *right*"; "You are the boss of your body."

Empathizing

Explore common ground in understanding feeling and experience:

- "I wonder how this [*problem*] feels to you." "That must have really bothered you when …" [*Note the past tense*]. "You have worked really hard at this haven't you?" Sometimes silence is the best empathy, followed by, "It's hard, isn't it?"

Avoid the word "but"; it is oppositional. Replace "but" with "and," siding with the patient:

- "I know you don't like having this problem, *and* you can change it."

And when they say, "I don't know," add the word "yet."

- "I don't know, *yet*."

Challenge:

- "I know, and part of you does."

Shrug, and wait. Silence is a great motivator.

Do not ask questions for which "I don't know" is a possible answer. Instead ask:

- "I wonder what you *imagine* ..." "What do you *think might* be the reason...?" This allows you to follow-up with, "I didn't ask if you *know*. I don't *know* either. I asked you what you *think/imagine*."

Be bold and reframe the relationship:

- "Well I don't know. I'm just the doctor. *You're* the patient."

What About Parents?

Avoid talking to parents as if the child was not in the room:

- "I am going to talk with your mother now. You don't have to listen, of course. But let me know, when I am all done, if you think she gets anything wrong."

If a parent answers for the child, refocus:

- "Well, that's how *your mother* would answer my question. What do *you* think?"

Chapter Five

Induction and Intensification Techniques

William C. Wester, II, EdD, ABPP, ABPH

Children are wonderful to work with because of their very creative and active imaginations. When they are experiencing a problem, children generally want assistance and look forward to learning a variety of skills that will help them resolve it. Most children have heard about hypnosis and, like adults, children need to learn about it.

The therapist must take time to introduce the hypnotic process to the child and parent(s). This preparation can start even before the first session by sending the parent(s) a copy of a brochure entitled, "Questions and Answers about Clinical Hypnosis" (Wester, 1982/2002). This brochure was first published in 1982, and revised in 2006. It contains a definition and brief history of hypnosis, information on professional training for therapists, myths and misconceptions about hypnosis, and other information typically discussed during the initial interview. When you first interview the child and parent(s), the therapist must allow time to develop rapport and answer any questions the child or parent(s) may have.

When the child arrives for the first session, the therapist can provide the parent(s) and child with additional reading material about hypnosis. An excellent resource to have available is *My Doctor Does Hypnosis* (Elkins, 1997). This short book is of great value, especially for the younger child. The story is about a girl who goes to a therapist who uses hypnosis to liberate her from her hurt feelings. She learns how to do self-hypnosis by relaxing and utilizing her imagination to help herself feel better. Finally, she learns that other people also use hypnosis to help themselves feel better.

I hope that your referrals come from colleagues who have already set the stage for hypnotic treatment based on their knowledge of hypnosis and your reputation. If you are asked to see a child in the hospital, make sure the staff, nursing staff, and any other professionals know why you are there and what you are trying to accomplish. You do not want to do really good hypnotic work only to have what you've done undermined by some inappropriate negative statement such as, "I don't believe in this stuff."

There are many other factors that the therapist can evaluate prior to hypnotic treatment. Crasilneck and Hall (1985) identified seven questions to consider during the initial intake interview:*

1. Why has the child come for treatment at this time?
2. Who sent/referred the child?
3. Is the child sufficiently motivated to give up the symptom(s)?
4. Is the symptom being used to manipulate others?
5. Is the symptom organic or psychogenic?
6. What is the child's degree of impulsivity and what is the child's level of frustration?
7. What is the child's general personality or history?

Even though you do a thorough evaluation, there are a variety of factors that can go wrong, such as parental pressure, shyness, hyperactivity, lack of attentiveness, and general defensiveness. Remember that these factors may be the child's way of telling you something. Find ways to deal with these barriers. For example, if a child sits in my chair covering his or her face with his or her hands and will not speak, I simply say, "That's okay, you don't have to talk —I guess you don't want to see the magic marble." At this point the child always lifts at least one hand to look and rapport begins. A simple magic trick follows and the child gets to keep the marble.

---

* Copyright (1991) from *Clinical Hypnosis with Children* by W. Wester & D. O'Grady. Reproduced by permission of Routledge/Taylor and Francis Group, LLC.

Induction Techniques

The hypnotic treatment outcome will be greatly enhanced if the therapist builds rapport and carefully assesses the child. The next step, based on all of the pre-hypnotic information obtained, is to select a suitable induction technique that takes into account the child's chronological age, intelligence, and emotional/maturity level. Table 5.1 is an excellent way to illustrate this point (Wall, 1991).

Olness and Kohen (1996) divide induction techniques into visual imagery, auditory imagery, movement imagery, storytelling, ideo-motor, progressive relaxation, eye fixation, distraction, and uti-lization (the use of videotapes, audiotapes, or the telephone). I offer the following induction techniques to provide the reader with a variety of induction techniques and specific verbalizations.

Clinical Vignette

Butterflies

S.P.

The vignette is that of a 12-year-old boy, S.P., who presented with sep-aration anxiety. He described his anxiety as "butterflies in his stom-ach" and was unable to spend the night at a friend's home. This is the second session, and he states that he has gotten better but still cannot fully spend the night at a friend's house without having butterflies, even though this feeling is less intense than it was before. There was a strong family history of anxiety disorders. The therapist uses a learning model and combines several induction techniques, which also act as an intensification technique, with a great deal of reinforce-ment and reframing. S.P. sits in a recliner and props his feet up.

W. Wester [WW]: Just close your eyes and keep your eyes closed as I talk with you [*direct approach used only because I knew this child and the fact that he was 12 years old*]. Look at the next few minutes as a very special time that you have set aside for yourself. This is a

Table 5.1: Developmental Stages and Hypnotic Interventions

Age, Years	Jean Piaget	Erik Erikson	Linguistic Research	Hypnotic Interventions
0	0-2 years Sensorimotor thought	0-1 year Stage I Trust vs. mistrust	0-2 years Not investigated	Rocking, patting, stroking, repetitious auditory input such as singing or rhyming, visual distraction with toys or presentation of familiar toy to hold
1				
2				
3	2-7 years Preoperational thought	1-3 years Stage II Autonomy vs. shame and doubt	2-6/7 years Metaphors possible if tied to perceptual stimuli (visual) "Because" relationships understood	Use of visual/movement stimulation while giving language input, e.g., talk through a puppet
4				Use of "because" causality in stories
5				Story telling
6	Includes intuitive thought in 5-7 year-old	3-5 years Stage III Initiative vs. guilt	"If" relationships developing, more complex perceptual metaphors possible	Stories with "because" and "if" possible at 6-7 years
7	7 years to puberty	6 years to puberty Stage IV	Increasing capacity to use internal representations of acts and activities	Eye-closure techniques more comfortable (over age 5)
8				
9				
10	Concrete Operational thought	Industry vs. inferiority	Use child's area of knowledge Concrete thinking observed	Arm rigidity: e.g. oak tree Eye fixation (on hand, coin, wall, spot) Arm lowering
11			Ability to recognize and use voice intonation to interpret meaning	Special/favorite places Listening to music
12				Favorite physical activities or sports Magic carpet Cloud car
13	Adolescence	Adolescence Stage V Identity vs. identity confusion	Egocentrism may be a function of increased cognitive awareness and the new ability to think about oneself relative to peers and to think about thinking	Adult induction methods Naturalistic/permissive methods allowing for patient control while setting internal boundaries: e.g., safe room or space Favorite sport
14				
15				
16				
17	Formal Operational thought		Inductive and hypothetico-deductive reasoning increases into early 20s	Use of physically based inductions Use of more abstract, less consciously aware metaphor
18				
19				
20	Not investigated	Three adult stages	Not reported here	

time to just really relax, a time to let go of tension and tightness in your body, and most importantly a time to learn. Just like the way you learn in school, you can learn something that can be very helpful to you in some very special ways [*begins to establish the learning model*]. As you listen to my voice and with each breath you take you can begin, that's right, to let yourself relax more thoroughly, more comfortable, and a little more deeply. As you do that you can feel the chair supporting your body [*supportive suggestion*]. You can feel so comfortable and relaxed now. You can feel the arms of the chair beneath your hands and fingers. You can feel your feet propped up with the foot rest and it just feels so good to get so comfortable and so relaxed [*reinforces general relaxation since the presenting problem was anxiety*].

You have already learned during our first session [*reinforces learning model*] that you have a very special talent [*reinforces skill building*] and can utilize your mind in a very special way to help yourself [*reinforces self-hypnosis*]. See yourself in your mind, for a moment, at home. See yourself sitting in front of your TV set [*TV induction*]. Just take a moment to get settled. You can have a soft drink with you if you like, but just see yourself where you would normally sit and the TV is in front of you and you have the remote so that you can turn the TV on and off, make the sound go higher or lower, and even allow the TV to stop at any point just like an instant replay of a sports game [*reinforces control*]. As soon as you see yourself sitting right there and watching TV, real comfortable and relaxed, just let me know by moving this finger or any finger [*I touch his right index finger—permission to touch a finger, hand, or arm was obtained from the parents and the child during the first visit*]. That's fine.

Turn the TV on for a moment to a sports channel. You like soccer, so just turn it on to one of your soccer games. It's fun to be home and watching yourself on TV playing soccer. See yourself right there [*enhancing imagery*] just so comfortable and relaxed and enjoying that soccer game. As soon as the channel is turned on to your soccer game, once again, just let me know by moving your finger [*pause—the finger slowly rises*]. That's fine. For just a moment tell me what's happening right now with the soccer game.

SP: I'm just about ready to kick a penalty shot at the end of the game.

WW: Go ahead and see yourself kicking that shot and tell me what happens.

SP: It went in!

WW: Boy, is that a good feeling. Just relax now so comfortably and so deeply. See yourself right there still watching TV but turn the channel. You have control over the remote. Turn the channel until you see yourself on the TV at one of your friends' home. Pick any friend you wish. See yourself at their home and you're going to spend the night. Just see yourself right there, perhaps just you and your friend, or there may be a couple of other people there as well. Just see yourself playing a game, maybe playing with the computer, or whatever you would like to do [*permissive choice*]. You now know that you are going to spend the night. Just tell me what kind of feeling you have knowing that you are going to spend the night.

SP: I feel a little nervous but confident that I will be able to spend the night.

WW: Let's see what you [*reinforces his responsibility and self-hypnosis*] can do to further help that feeling of confidence. Notice how much fun you are having being at your friend's house. That very special part of your mind knows that you will be able to spend the night at your friend's house. Just see yourself as you watch yourself on that TV feeling really good and really comfortable. See yourself feeling more and more confident and seeing those butterfly feelings, almost like a real butterfly, gently flying away. As you relax further you can become even more comfortable and more and more confident. That very special part of your mind can be so helpful to you. The next time you're asked to spend an overnight at a friend's house, you will find that your level of confidence will become stronger and stronger each time you are asked to do that [*post-hypnotic suggestion*]. You are going to feel more and more comfortable and relaxed and look forward to the fun you can have being with your friends. Because of what you have learned there will be little or no worry and that butterfly feeling will become less and less. You will be able to sense and feel that butterfly feeling leaving as the butterfly flies off into the distance. See yourself on that TV now with that high degree of confidence and all the butterflies have left. You are having fun and feeling real good. Tell me how you're feeling right now about spending the night.

SP: I think can spend the night now and won't have butterflies anymore.

WW: That's great! [*I repeat his statement.*] That very special TV you have in your mind—just lock that thought in and it will be part of you now. Even from the very first moment that you hear about an opportunity to stay at someone's home you will feel confident because you now know that you can really do it and those butterfly feelings will just fly away. [*I could have ended the session at this point but I felt that reframing of the butterflies would be helpful. I got up and moved to the child's side to use an arm levitation to significantly reframe the butterfly feelings.*]

I am going to come around to your other side so you can experience something interesting about hypnosis and relaxation. You are really doing great [*positive reinforcement*]. I am going to move this arm and hand and just let it float like this. [*I lift his arm up, gently bouncing it to achieve arm catalepsy and then slowly remove my hand and fingers allowing the child's hand to float.*] Very nice—just feel how the hand and arm feels as it floats. It can float there all by itself. That's right. As you feel that, just remember that feeling as I slowly let your arm and hand back down to rest on the arm of the chair. Just relax now even more deeply and completely. That floating feeling is going to remind you of a light feeling and gentleness and the way in which the butterfly flies. It can just gently and easily fly away.

It's interesting that butterflies can stay up in the air and just float. Butterflies don't harm anyone. They are a very gentle, very calm kind of insect. So in the future, in addition to your high confidence, your mind will also remember that feeling you had in your arm and hand and that will remind you that the butterflies can just fly away, just float away as you feel more comfortable and relaxed. And now turn that channel once again back to that soccer game and as soon as you see it just let me know by moving your finger. That's great. Tell me one more thing that is happening right now during that soccer game.

SP: We are just about ready to kick off.

WW: That's super. You have learned some very interesting things today. Once you learn something, just like when you learned how to ride a bike, you don't forget it, and in fact, you get better and better at it. The first time you got up on a bike it might have been a little clumsy, but as you practiced it, you became a super-biker [*truism*]. By using hypnosis and skills you have learned, you will continue to feel more comfortable and confident and look forward to having a lot of fun staying over at a friend's house [*reinforcement of learning a new skill yet permissive in terms of how quickly*]. Turn that TV and soccer game off knowing that's yours to use at any time you wish. And now in your own mind count from 1 to 4, and when you reach 4 your eyes will open and you will be completely alert and feel really good, comfortable, and refreshed. Very good! How do you feel?

SP: I was really relaxed, and it was like I was floating and not sitting in the chair. When you lifted my arm up it was just like it was staying there by itself and floating. I liked it a lot. I was real relaxed and I felt comfortable. I could picture the TV and the practice field clearly.

WW: How do you feel now?

SP: I feel fine—I feel good.

Relaxation

Use the relaxation techniques you have learned from reading and workshops, and use them with a child but alter the techniques so that the relaxation is age appropriate. Always remember that children will do what they need or want to do. In the above vignette I use comfort and supportive statements, and I reinforce the more progressive relaxation procedure used in the first session.

In the first session, after doing a clinical intake interview with S.P. and his mother, I excused his mother and had him sit in my recliner and prop his feet up. I simply asked him to close his eyes (he could have kept his eyes open) and listen to my voice. The following was also recorded on an audio tape so that S.P. could practice his relaxation in preparation for the second session (reinforces self-hypnosis).

> **WW**: Just relax now and focus on your breathing. We all breathe but we don't think about it very much. Just be aware of air coming in and out of your body each time you take a breath. That's right. Allow your breathing to further help you to relax and then at the same time notice how all the muscles in your scalp have started to relax and become smooth. That is a great feeling. Use your creative mind now and imagine a liquid-like relaxation flowing from your scalp down into the muscles of your forehead, around your eyes, cheeks, mouth, and chin. Let that wonderful feeling continue to flow down through the muscles in your neck, shoulders, arms, and hands. Sometimes the hands feel heavy or light and that is okay [*because this is so common it reinforces something changing*]. The relaxation flows down now into the muscles in your back and chest. As that feeling comes DOWN [*emphasis on "DOWN" automatically intensifies relaxation*] through your waist and DOWN through your hips, just feel supported by the chair and relaxing deeper and deeper. From the hips now down into the legs, ankles, and feet. The entire body now, from the top of your head to the tip of your toes, relaxed and comfortable. That's such a nice feeling you can relax even more deeply as I count backwards from 7 to zero. [*I slowly count from 7 to zero interspersing additional suggestions of total relaxation.*]

Allow the transition from a relaxation technique to a deepening technique to flow smoothly. Keep all inductions simple, and as you observe the relaxation behaviors, move forward, if needed, to further intensify the response. Graduate students learning about hypnosis frequently go on and on with relaxation suggestions while losing great therapeutic time. You can tell when your patient is ready to move forward.

The teddy bear technique is frequently used with young children whereby each finger represents one of the three teddy bears. You start with the child holding three fingers up on the arm of the chair. As each teddy bear gets tired and sleepy, it slowly comes back down to rest on the arm of the chair. By the time the third teddy bear is down you should have been able to bring about eye closure and a good level of relaxation. Once again, eye closure is not necessary, and you can just begin therapeutically interacting with the child because he or she has become engaged with the teddy bears.

Imagery

In the above vignette, I used sports imagery because soccer was a big part of this young man's life. It was easy to go from visual TV imagery to movement imagery as described by Olness & Kohen (1996). They nicely differentiate the visual (multisensory) imagery techniques, such as a favorite place or TV, from the movement imagery techniques, such as a sports activity or flying blanket.

It is absolutely necessary to interact with the child who is experiencing hypnosis. This will not interfere with his or her level of experience. Children have marvelous imaginations and have no trouble using their creativity to see something in their mind, especially if it is a fun, learning experience. I will sometimes start with a procedure I use in the forensic hypnosis arena as a way to put the child at ease and get into how imagery works. For example, I will say, "Just close your eyes and take yourself in your mind to your house and, with your eyes closed, just count the number of windows in your house." You can just see his or her little head bobbing as he or she goes from room to room counting windows.

The standard in the field is imagery of a favorite place or TV. I like to add "special place" as I begin with my induction:

> "Use your creative mind to think of a very favorite or special place you have been or would like to go. Allow yourself to be right there seeing and feeling everything that is so special. As you enjoy that favorite or special place I am going to be talking to that special part of your mind we have talked about."

The TV technique is perhaps as popular as the favorite place. It is easy to use and almost all children, even those coming from lower disadvantaged groups, have a TV or have seen a TV. Make the experience as real as possible with sounds, remotes, colors, and any other sensory processes to make the experience as real as possible. Another example of a TV or theater approach is to say,

> "Just see in your mind a TV screen [*or see yourself in the front row of a theater*] and as soon as you have that image, let me know by moving one of your fingers. You are in control of all of the dials and now turn the TV on [*have the image appear on the screen*] and turn the dial to your favorite program. As soon as you see your program, let me know by moving your finger once again."

Ideomotor approaches are good, but not necessary. You can simply have the child tell you what is happening. "Just relax and enjoy your program. Watch it carefully now because I am going to ask you what is happening at different times. You can relax deeper and deeper as you continue to enjoy your program (or show)." Additional deepening, relaxation, and treatment suggestions can be interspersed at this time (Wester, 1991).

For movement imagery, I use the "magic carpet" instead of a flying blanket. It really makes no difference, but I come from a background of using magic with kids to build rapport, and the "magic carpet" fits with my approach.

> "See yourself at a family picnic and ask mom or dad if, for just a few minutes, you can go over to the grassy area by yourself. When you get there you will find a fairly large piece of carpet on the grass. Let's call it a magic carpet. Go ahead and sit on the carpet and notice what happens. The carpet does whatever you think and want to do. It is very safe. For example, as you think up, it goes up a few inches, and as you think right, it turns right. Remember the carpet is totally safe. Go ahead and go up higher so you can see your family at the picnic. It's fun to see what they are cooking. You can do whatever you wish for a few minutes and then land your carpet. You have been in control of that carpet and have learned how to use your special creative mind in this way. If your mind can help you control the carpet, just imagine how helpful this will be when you need to control other things." [*use suggestions consistent with therapeutic strategies*]

The Fluffy Technique

Some therapists use the concept of a teddy bear (described above) or rag doll. Once again, Olness and Kohen (1996) describe a variety of ideomotor techniques including, hand levitation, finger lowering, arm rigidity, or the mighty oak tree. The Fluffy technique is basically a relaxation procedure whereby "Fluffy the dog" models a variety of behaviors, and the child repeats these behaviors. For a long time I used a Raggedy Ann or Raggedy Andy doll, until I found the most wonderful white, fluffy, stuffed dog. Younger children quickly respond when I bring out Fluffy. I hold Fluffy in my lap and begin to flop the ears, legs, head, and then hold Fluffy in the middle and flop the whole dog. While interacting with the child, I ask the child if he or she likes Fluffy and would like to have Fluffy teach him or her some things that will help him or her with his or her problem (whatever the presenting problem might be). The "yes" set is established, and I begin by asking the child if he or she can make his or her arm floppy just like Fluffy can make his front leg floppy. I repeat this for the head and other legs, and at the same time, I ask the child to close his or her eyes and become just as floppy as Fluffy. I add other relaxation and attending suggestions as I follow therapeutic strategies.

Eye Fixation

It is my belief that eye fixation techniques with adults are unnecessary because the primary goal is to bring about eye closure. It is so much easier to say to the patient, "Just sit back and relax, prop your feet up, and close your eyes." Adults also tend to associate eye fixation with some of the myths and misconceptions about hypnosis, especially if a pendulum is used. An exception might be the use of an eye fixation technique, such as a coin resting on the cupped fingers with an elevated arm, with a reluctant patient, or with a patient who asks you to use some type of pendulum.

On the other hand, the use of eye fixation techniques with children and young adolescents can be an excellent approach. Remember that children do not come to hypnosis with all of the adult myths and misconceptions. I typically use a coin and have the child raise his or her arm to an above eye level position. He or she holds the coin facing down between his or her thumb and first two fingers. The arm of course gets heavy and suggestions can be directed toward the heavy feeling and associated with losing his or her grip on the coin at the same time.

> "As your arm gets heavier and heavier, in just a moment, you will notice that the coin begins to slip from your fingers and when that happens your eyes will close and your arm will come back to rest on the chair (or bed if the child is in a hospital). I will put my hand beneath your hand to catch the coin as that happens." [*suggestive that it will happen*]

The coin can also become a "magic coin" and used for needle sticks, self-hypnosis, or other procedures. When a hospital staff member comes in to give a shot (referred to as a needle stick) it is fun to watch the child say, "Just a moment—I need to use my 'magic coin' to rub the spot where you are going to give me the needle stick to make that area numb." Another interesting eye fixation technique is to have the child draw a happy face on his or her thumb with a magic marker. Once again, the arm is elevated above eye level with the happy face facing the child as the therapist begins the induction.

Arm Levitation

In Chapter Ten, a vignette describes the balloon technique I used in treating a 12-year-old boy experiencing panic attacks. What is nice about this technique is that the therapist has so many options, and as long as the therapist is patient, the arm will move in an upward direction. Sometimes it takes more than one balloon, or suggestions need to be made about being able to slide a piece of paper between the hand and the arm of the chair. All movement can be reinforced, and children find this experience to be interesting and fun. The therapist can be just as creative as the child when using this procedure. For example, one child was really interested in pulleys. The therapist had the child explain what type of pulley would be needed to pull the arm up off of the chair. Then the therapist used imagery following the child's prompt with suggestions for deeper relaxation.

You can also use reverse arm levitation with the arm starting off in the elevated position. Have the child just close his or her eyes and imagine something heavy on the back of the hand that makes the arm and hand want to move downward (remind them that the object will not hurt them and the arm and hand will come down slowly). Children will be very creative with this and imagine anything heavy from a book to a rock.

Distraction Techniques (Rapid Inductions)

Some situations require a rapid induction that is best accomplished by distraction. I clearly remember a young girl who came to the emergency room for treatment of a laceration of the hand. She had been playing tag with her brother and slipped, and her hand went through a window pane. The baby sitter wrapped her hand immediately with a sterile bandage and drove her to the emergency room. I just happened to be walking past the ER with the Chief of Psychiatry. The ER staff called upon him to help with this hysterical child who was very frightened, especially since her mother wasn't with her. He turned to me and asked me to do whatever I could to help this child.

I hesitated for a moment (I was on staff at this hospital), put on a pair of sterile gloves, and approached the frightened child. I said,

> **WW:** "I'm Dr. Wester [*as I straightened out her arm*] and you know that is the prettiest blue blood I have ever seen." She looked at me with a puzzled look, immediately calmed down some, and said, "That's not blue it's red." I replied, "I know blue from red and I think it's blue. If you let the other doctors and nurses look at it we can see if it is really blue or red, but you know you can really help them if you first close your eyes and find the very special place in your mind where all the wires to the body connect and find the wire to your right hand. [*The child closed her eyes and the staff began removing the bandage.*] As soon as you find that wire to your right hand just let me know. [*The child responded that she*

had found the wire as the staff cleaned the wound.] Every wire has a switch, and you can use your powerful mind to turn off the switch to your right hand for just a moment. When you do that you will not feel any discomfort as the doctor fixes your hand—just pressure. And then in just a few minutes you can turn the switch back on and open your eyes, and we can check again to see if the blood was really blue or red" [*The doctor uses several stitches to close the wound*].

I continue talking to the child and then say to her,

WW: "You can turn the switch to your right hand back on now and you will be surprised how good it feels. Let's see now—you were right, the blood is really red [*as I point to the gauze*]. You did a great job helping the doctors learn a new way to help you, just as if you were a real teacher. Your parent(s) will be so proud."

In a similar situation, a young boy came to the ER having a severe "asthma attack." Once again I happened to be in the ER working with a trauma patient and was asked to help. I asked permission of the parent, put my arm around the young boy's shoulder and said,

WW: "That's one of the best wheezing episodes [*immediately reframing the episode*] I have ever seen. [*I began to synchronize my breathing with the child.*] Do you think you can make it worse? [*The child looked at me with a very strange expression.*] Well, you really don't have to make it worse, but notice as I slow down my breathing that you're breathing and wheezing also slows down and becomes better. That's right, just relax now and feel great that you have just learned a new way to help yourself. In the future, if you ever have another wheezing episode, you can use that very special part of your mind you have just used to help yourself. You can just close your eyes and see in your mind a favorite place or see a special switch that you have to turn down the wheezing." [*I gave the child and the parent a further explanation of what I had done*]

One might argue that hypnosis was not really used in the above cases. Hypnosis involves suggestion, modeling, and rapport and does not have to involve a formal induction. These children responded to a variety of suggestions in a rather busy and loud environment. Their motivation was obvious, and we had everything to gain by using the child's wonderful creative capacity.

Intensification Techniques

Intensification techniques (deepening) need to be discussed whether we are treating adults or children. Most therapists, who are less experienced with hypnosis, get overly concerned with the depth of a trance state and take extra measures to try and assure themselves, more than the patient, that the patient is now in a deep trance-like state. Going down in an elevator, walking down a flight of stairs, and a variety of counting techniques are typically used to deepen hypnosis. There is no question that there are levels of trance characterized by certain observable behaviors. In a light state of hypnosis, we are likely to see such things as eyelid catalepsy, relaxation, limb catalepsy, and even glove anesthesia. In a medium state of hypnosis, we are likely to see such things as partial amnesia, simple posthypnotic suggestions, simple hallucinations, and an increased detached feeling. Finally, in a deep state of hypnosis, we are likely to see such things as total amnesia, surgical anesthesia, eye open trances, age regression, and positive and negative visual and auditory hallucinations.

Hammond (1987) describes the following procedures to enhance the depth of the hypnotic state:*

1. *Fractionation.* The child is alerted and re-hypnotized several times.
2. *Downward movement.* The child sees himself or herself walking down a set of stairs or moving down an escalator.
3. *Interspersing the child's motivation and needs.* "And you are relaxing deeper and deeper because you...."

---

* Copyright (1991) from *Clinical Hypnosis with Children* by W. Wester & D. O'Grady. Reproduced by permission of Routledge/Taylor and Francis Group, LLC.

4. *Contingent suggestions.* "With every sound of my voice, you can drift deeper and deeper....," or "With every breath you take, your level of relaxation increases more and more."
5. *Breathing and counting.* Counting backwards from 10 to 1 with interspersed suggestions, or focusing on breathing with deepening suggestions.

Because most of what we do as therapists is done within a light to medium trance state, we do not have to put a great deal of emphasis on depth of trance. Remember that all hypnosis is self-hypnosis. We each have the ability to engage in trance if we want to, if we cooperate, and just allow it to happen. Trance is whatever the patient says it is. They go where they need to go. We generally expect those undergoing surgery or other significant procedures with hypnosis to be highly hypnotizable, but again the patient will do what he or she needs to do. For example, one of my childbirth patients was delivering her third child under hypnosis and all of a sudden the birth was compromised. A quick decision was made to do a cesarean section. I explained this to my patient and transferred the glove anesthesia we had practiced to my hand. The doctor told me where he was going to make the incision and as I ran my fingers across that area I used suggestions of this area being numb and insensitive. This was tested with ideomotor movement, and the doctor made the cut and delivered a healthy baby. We are trained how to test for depth of trance before proceeding with certain procedures.

Children really do not care or ask about depth of hypnosis. Intensification of the hypnotic experience is a much better term for us to use as we work with children. They are challenged to learn new things, to use their creative mind to help themselves, and to have fun with their new skill. Experienced therapists simply make decisions about the necessary depth of trance as they proceed with treatment and adjust their technique/approach/strategy as necessary. Induction and intensification techniques are kept simple and selected based on a variety of variables such as chronological age, intelligence, personality, and level of emotional maturity. The narrative at the beginning of this chapter demonstrates pyramiding of techniques that then becomes an intensification technique.

Conclusion

Throughout this book a variety of other induction and intensification techniques will be included in the chapter vignettes. My graduate students are instructed that inductions are usually easy and it is what we do then that really counts. In the case of children, and adults, we must remember that this is their experience. It is true that all hypnosis becomes self-hypnosis with the eventual goal of allowing the child to manage his or her problem with his or her newly developed skills. Keep your inductions simple, learn to go with the flow, and follow the child's lead. Have fun helping the child master this new skill, and use your creative mind in the same way that you are asking the child to use his or her creative mind.

References

Crasilneck, H. B., & Hall, J. A. (1985). *Clinical hypnosis: Principles and applications* (2nd ed.). New York: Grune & Stratton.

Elkins, G. R. (1997). *My doctor does hypnosis*. Chicago: American Society of Clinical Hypnosis Press.

Hammond, C. (1987). Induction and deepening techniques. In W. C. Wester (Ed.), *Clinical hypnosis: A case management approach*. Cincinnati, OH: BSCI Publications.

Olness, K., & Kohen, D. P. (1996). *Hypnosis and hypnotherapy with children* (3rd ed.). New York: Guilford Press.

Wall, V. (1991). Developmental considerations in the use of hypnosis with children. In W. Wester & D. O'Grady (Eds.), *Clinical hypnosis with children*. New York: Brunner/Mazel.

Wester, W. C. (1991). *Clinical hypnosis: A multidisciplinary approach*. Cincinnati, OH: BSCI Publications.

Wester, W. C. (2002). *Questions and answers about clinical hypnosis*. Columbus, OH: Ohio Psychology Publications.

Chapter Six

Ethical Considerations with Children and Hypnosis

Thomas W. Wall, PhD, ABPP, ABPH

Psychologists are committed to increasing scientific and professional knowledge of behavior and people's understanding of themselves and others and to use such knowledge to improve the condition of individuals, organizations, and society. Psychologists respect and protect civil and human rights and the central importance of freedom of inquiry... They strive to help the public in developing informed judgments and choices concerning human behavior.

Ethical Principles of Psychologists and Code of Conduct
American Psychological Association (APA), 2002[1]

The above statement is not limited to psychologists. It applies to any healthcare professional involved in the delivery of services whether medical, dental, or psychological; it applies to all patients of all ages including pediatric populations and is independent of the procedure, therapeutic technique, or theoretical orientation.

The evolution of hypnosis as a legitimate treatment modality has greatly expanded in the last 50 years in healthcare delivery. This includes an increasing emphasis in the hypnosis literature on treatment approaches to pediatric populations and research in an effort to unravel the mystery of hypnosis and the neurobiology of the hypnotic experience. Olness and Gardner (1981) have noted the history of hypnosis and its application to the problems of children. Their collaboration resulted in the first comprehensive text in this area entitled *Hypnosis and Hypnotherapy With Children* published in 1981. A second edition by the same authors was published in 1988. Wester and O'Grady (1991) published an edited

---

[1] For actual code go to:www.apa.org/ethics/code2002.html

volume, *Clinical Hypnosis with Children,* followed by the third edition of *Hypnosis and Hypnotherapy With Children* by Olness and Kohen published in 1996. These books contain chapters on the application of hypnosis to specific pediatric problems, developmental considerations, correlates of childhood hypnotic responsiveness, and various induction techniques to name a few. They do not reference the explication and/or application of professional ethics within this population, which makes the central topic of this chapter on ethical considerations with children of vital importance.

A literature review reveals the scant attention this topic has received. Virtually no citations were found that directly address professional ethics in the practice of hypnotherapy with children. In the psychotherapy literature, Grisso and Vierling (1978) discuss a minor's right to treatment from a developmental perspective. Koocher (1976) notes the "fact that children in psychotherapy need to have their rights protected simply does not occur to most practitioners." Bersoff (1995) examines the issue of children being allowed to exercise the right to consent to psychological treatment. Hambleton (2002), Scheflin (1997), Adrian (1996), and McConkey (1995) have all written articles that address ethics within a hypnotic context, but focus on adult issues.

In the forensic application of hypnosis, several references review the many key issues in that setting. Sheehan and McConkey (1993), Coons (1988), Relinger and Stern (1983) and Orne (1979) are representative of the literature in this important area. T. W. Wall (1991) noted that recognition and application of ethical principles and professional standards in the use of hypnosis contribute to the legitimacy and acceptance of hypnosis in healthcare. He notes, "The professional and ethical use of hypnosis is through acceptance and adherence to ethical practices of professional conduct in our clinical work, our teaching, and the promotion of hypnosis" and this includes the application of ethical principles in the use of hypnosis with children.

Given the paucity of literature in the area of professional ethics and hypnosis, the 2002 Ethics Code of the American Psychological Association and the 2000 Code of Conduct of American Society of

Clinical Hypnosis (ASCH)[2] will serve as a guide in applying certain ethical principles to hypnosis with children. It is important to remember that children are not small adults and their understanding of therapeutic procedures, hypnosis, the treatment setting, and their rights will require special attention. The various applicable ethical standards and codes of conduct may have to be modified somewhat in the treatment setting to account for the child's developmental level.

By necessity parents will be required to participate in the application of many ethical and treatment decisions depending upon the age of the child. Pope and Vasquez (1991) have noted that that the ethical responsibilities of psychotherapists (and any other healthcare provider) are founded upon the recognition that therapy/ treatment involves three important variables: trust, power, and caring. Nowhere do these variables require more sensitivity in their application than with children. In the development of the therapeutic relationship and maintenance of the therapeutic alliance, these three variables are woven into both the application of treatment decisions and the ethical standards guiding the appropriate behavior of healthcare providers.

Professional ethics becomes the norm of conduct that forms the basis of our shared identity as healthcare professionals. Thus, professional ethics represent three basic tasks. First, professional ethics involves acknowledging the reality and importance of the person whose life is affected by our professional actions. Second, professional ethics involves a thorough understanding of the nature of the professional relationship, its boundaries, and our professional interventions. And third, professional ethics involves our affirming that we are accountable for our professional actions. The 2002 APA Ethics Code and the 2000 Code of Conduct by ASCH embrace each of these principles. The 2002 APA Ethics Code separates aspirational principles (General Principles) from enforceable standards (Code of Conduct). The aspirational principles encourage psychologists to perform their professional skill at the highest level. The Code of Conduct includes standards under which psychologists may be disciplined. The ASCH Code of

---

[2] For actual code go to: http://asch.net/forms/conduct-rev.pdf

Conduct emphasizes principles and standards without distinguishing between the two. Both Codes are based on the general standard that psychologists or other healthcare providers should follow: what a "reasonable psychologist/healthcare provider" would do in the performance of their professional obligations. These codes are similar to the codes of other professional healthcare organizations that require their members to maintain membership by practicing within a prescribed code of professional conduct.

Briefly, the aspirational General Principles suggest a value orientation in which psychologists strive to do good by promoting the welfare of others and strive to do no harm. Moreover, they recognize their responsibility to obtain and maintain high standards of competence in their own work. Psychologists maintain integrity in all psychological activities, which involves honesty and accuracy in communication in the practice of psychology. Psychologists strive to provide all people with fair and equitable access to treatment. The final principle calls for psychologists to "respect the dignity and worth of all people, and the rights of individuals to privacy, confidentiality, and self-determination." Fisher (2003) notes that psychologists are aware and attentive to the circumstances of individuals who may have limited capacity for autonomous decision making (such as children) and take extra precautions to safeguard these individuals' rights and welfare. While the APA standards are for psychologists, the ASCH Code of Conduct pertains to any professional discipline consistent with membership in that organization.

Competence

Using these principles as guidelines, a number of issues emerge that have particular relevance to children in hypnotherapy or any other procedure that involves the use of hypnosis or hypnotic procedures. Maintaining high standards of competence means providing services to populations, children for example, only in those areas within the boundaries of competence based on one's "education, training, supervised experience, consultation, study or professional experience" as specified in both Codes of Conduct. Work with children requires that the clinician have formal training in pediatrics, child psychology, pediatric dentistry, or have taken sufficient postgraduate training and supervision with children in one's respective professional discipline and area of expertise before using hypnosis. It also assumes appropriate training and certification in the use of hypnosis in general and its application to children before applying this approach to a pediatric population. Competence also requires an appreciation for developmental considerations in the use of hypnosis with children (Wall, V., 1991). Further, competence means the provider of services is both familiar with and maintains his or her professional and scientific knowledge. This means being familiar with the current and relevant scientific and professional literature in one's professional discipline, keeping abreast of the hypnosis literature, and being aware of the implications for children.

The 2002 APA Code of Ethics, and in particular the 2000 ASCH Code of Conduct, note that psychologists' and other healthcare professionals' work is based upon established scientific and professional knowledge of the discipline and hypnosis. The ASCH Code of Conduct directly addresses this issue by defining a members' expertise through professional education, training, licensure, and relevant experience. Further, members recognize and are respectful of limitations to their expertise. No professional field is without its "fringe treatments" and dubiously trained practitioners. In psychology, and especially in hypnosis, this amplifies the importance of adequate training and grounding one's work firmly in established scientific and professional knowledge.

In this regard, it is helpful to appreciate what are called "deterioration effects." Specifically these are linked primarily to three therapist-controlled variables. The first is a mismatch of the treatment method; that is, the provider fails to provide an adequate treatment method or persists in using an inappropriate treatment method despite its inadequacy. The second is the provider's persistence in using a technique that worsens, rather than improves, the patient's condition. The third is the expression and/or engagement of the provider's countertransference reaction in the form of attitudes or biases that can negatively influence the relationship or treatment. It is important to emphasize that competent healthcare professionals need to undertake an ongoing effort to maintain their competency and be aware of these possible influences.

Clinical Example

A 10-year-old boy is referred to a psychologist for treatment with hypnosis for thumb-sucking. Unless the psychologist has specific training in hypnosis in general, hypnosis with children, and a background in child psychology, an appropriate referral should be made. The principle of staying in one's area of competence applies here. At the time of the initial referral, it is important to set these limits. For example, the healthcare provider might say, "I have considerable training using hypnosis with adults and very little training with children. I would be glad to work with you to find someone trained in hypnosis with children for your son. It is important to both your son and me that I stay in the areas for which I am trained."

Clinical Example:

An 8-year-old girl is referred to a child therapist for hypnosis to treat enuresis. The healthcare professional has taken one course in using hypnosis with children and learned that hypnosis is appropriate for treating bedwetting. For the non-medical provider, the first treatment decision involves a self-assessment regarding the question of whether this particular case of enuresis is in one's area of competence. The clinician needs to rule out any medical conditions as to the cause of the enuresis. Once it is determined that there is no medical condition, the next ethical decision could be both a boundary and/or competence issue if the possible cause of the enuresis could be in an area requiring specific training and professional experience as in the treatment of child abuse.

Supervision

For those healthcare providers who have experience working with children and desire to include the application of hypnosis into their future treatment plans, supervision needs to be addressed. There are clinicians who have considerable pediatric experience and little, if any, training in hypnosis. Training is available through continuing education offerings by the American Society of Clinical Hypnosis or the Society of Clinical and Experimental Hypnosis (SCEH). The Society of Developmental and Behavioral Pediatrics (SDBP) has offered a workshop on hypnosis with children and adolescents at introductory, intermediate, and advanced levels as part of its annual meeting every year since 1987. University graduate psychology programs and medical training centers may offer advanced training in both hypnosis and its application in a pediatric context.

In addition to advanced training, the clinician interested in expanding his or her competence might engage a colleague for supervision who is trained both to work with children and has considerable experience with hypnosis and children. In a supervisory relationship there are three people: the patient, the supervisee, and the supervisor. Pope and Vasquez (1991) have offered that the supervisor has an ethical obligation to insure that the tasks of supervision, roles within supervision, and the responsibilities of each are clear. Since the supervisor is ultimately responsible, ethically and legally, for the services provided by the supervisee, the supervisor shares the responsibility for the welfare of the patient. A supervisor must be well trained to treat children in his or her own discipline and have his or her own advanced training and experience using hypnosis with children. In addition, as Stoltenberg and Delworth (1987) have stated, "it is vital that the supervisor be well trained, knowledgeable, and skilled in the practice of clinical supervision." In a supervisory relationship the supervisor has the responsibility to continually assess the adequacy of the treatment offered as well as the professional development of the supervisee. It is the responsibility of the supervisee to engage in informed consent with the patient. In fact, in some states laws or regulations may specify the legal obligation of supervisees to disclose their status.

Informed Consent

Competency of the Patient

Koocher, Norcross, and Hill (1998) have defined *informed consent* as "the patient's voluntary agreement to accept treatment based on an awareness of the nature of his or her disease, the material risks and benefits of the proposed treatment, the alternative treatments and risks, and the choice of no treatment at all." Informed consent (Stromberg, et al., 1988) involves four elements. The first is *competency of the patient*, that is, the patient is capable of understanding the issues within informed consent. To meet this criteria the clinician must have done an adequate assessment, have a correct diagnosis, and developed an appropriate treatment plan. Fisher (2003) noted that adults not legally competent and most children under the age of 18 do not have the right to provide independent consent to receive psychological services, yet this varies from state to state. For example, in the state of Washington the age of consent is 13.

For children who are legally incapable of giving informed consent, the clinician must obtain permission from a legally authorized person. There are instances in which permission for treatment from a parent or guardian of children under 18 is not required or possible. This would be the case for an emancipated minor, a legal term conferred on a person who may not have attained the age of legal competency as defined by state law. He or she may be entitled to receive treatment and participate in informed consent as if he or she has the appropriate legal status by virtue of assuming adult responsibilities. Examples of this would include being self-supporting and/or married. Sometimes the term "mature minor" is used to denote someone who is not an adult as defined by state law, but according to state law is entitled to be treated as an adult for certain purposes. These might include treatment for psychological problems, treatment for drug abuse, or treatment for venereal disease.

In all instances with children and adolescents it is important that the clinician communicate the elements of informed consent in a language that can be readily understood. That is, for children who may or may not be considered legally capable of giving informed consent, the clinician should provide an appropriate explanation, seek the child's permission to proceed, consider the child's preferences and best interests, and obtain appropriate permission from a legally authorized person. Knapp and VanderCreek (2003) have noted that when consent by a legally authorized person is not permitted or required by law, the clinician must take appropriate steps to protect the child's rights and welfare.

Disclosure of Information

The second element of informed consent involves *disclosure of material information;* meaning the patient must be given relevant information. This requires a sensitivity to communicate appropriately given the age of the child and with language that satisfies the third criterion, which is that the child can understand what is proposed regarding treatment and treatment decisions.

Understanding by the Patient

The third is element is *understanding by the patient,* which involves knowing what the provider of service is proposing and why. This could include a fuller explanation to the parents or guardian and an age-appropriate discussion with the child. This is done in "layman's terms," thus avoiding the use of jargon and providing the necessary information within the capacity of the person to understand. Given that the effectiveness of any treatment is dependent on the establishment of a therapeutic alliance with the development of trust and safety, there is much to recommend explaining what is to occur in treatment and having the child become involved in decisions that will contribute to the therapy itself and the therapeutic outcome.

Voluntary Consent

The last element of informed consent is *voluntary consent,* which means the patient must be allowed to make decisions without coercion. The doctrine of informed consent is a legal concept relating to the right of the individual to be "free of coercion and unwanted interference." This means that the consent to participate in any treatment must be voluntary and so documented. The principle was clearly stated in 1914 by U.S. Supreme Court Justice Benjamin Cardoza who argued that every human being of adult years and sound mind has the right to determine what will be done with their body. This meant that the patient, rather than the doctor, has the right to decide whether to undertake a particular treatment or not. Sometimes this is referred to as the "right of self-determination." For the patient and/or his or her parent or guardian to make the decision to participate in treatment, it must be meaningful based on an adequate range of information provided by the clinician proposing the course of treatment and must be *voluntary*. Inherent in this is the interpretation that failure to disclose the proposed course of treatment, the consequences of a treatment procedure, and especially the risks and possible side effects could be seen as a dereliction of professional duty and possible grounds for negligence.

Documentation of Informed Consent

It is important that informed consent be documented. In many states it is a requirement that an office policy statement be given to the patient and/or their parent or legal guardian. Among other things, this policy statement might contain information regarding the background and training of the clinician, emergency procedures, freedom of choice to participate in treatment, the right to withdraw consent at any time, the limits of confidentiality, the fee structure and the possible use of collection, and any other possible entries that would add to the professional qualifications of the clinician and his or her office procedures. There is considerable case law supporting the use of collection as a breach of confidentiality unless specified in the office policy statement.

In addition, informed consent should be documented in terms of the diagnosis and proposed course of treatment, alternative treatments if applicable, as well as some assessment that the patient understands what is being proposed and gives his or her permission to participate. The main legal test that informed consent was given is based on evidence in the form of documentation. That is, there is evidence in the record that informed consent was rationally given with a good faith effort to present the issues accurately so they could be understood, evidence that choice was given, and evidence that there was an appreciation of the nature of the situation of the child through an appropriate assessment. This might include as evidence a document signed by the child depending on his or her age and/or his or her guardian that he or she accepts both the office policies and the elements of informed consent as outlined above. Meeting the requirement of obtaining informed consent before a course of treatment confers the status of the patient as autonomous and capable of deciding what is in his or her best interest.

Informed consent is a process of decision making with an emphasis on communication and clarification and it needs to be an ongoing process as the decisions and directions of treatment may be altered from the basis of the original assessment, diagnosis, or through the course of treatment. Informed consent, then, is a process of information gathering, communication of intended procedures, the elucidation of any contingencies, and agreement by the patient and/or his or her parent or guardian to the proposed procedures that encourages the patient's autonomy.

There are several questions to help the clinician assess whether consent was informed:

1. Does the child and/or parent or guardian understand the qualifications and status of the treatment provider?
2. Does the child understand the purpose of the initial session?
3. Does the child understand the proposed treatment, implications of treatment, and possible alternatives?
4. Does the child understand his or her access to the therapist?
5. Does the child understand the issues of confidentiality depending on his or her age and the exceptions to confidentiality?

Confidentiality

Lakin (1991) has observed that a communication is judged to be confidential if it is not intended to be disclosed to a third person other than those reasonably involved in the treatment procedures, which might include family members and/or a legally designated guardian. He notes the general rule is that the patient, not the doctor, has the privilege to disclose, or to prevent anyone from disclosing any communications between the clinician and the patient that are made for purposes involving the treatment. In the case of a child, disclosure of healthcare information is legally dependent on the age of the child and the respective state laws that govern when the child is legally dependent/independent.

The clinician has the responsibility to safeguard the confidential information obtained in the course of treatment. This means the practitioner shall disclose confidential information to others, including family members, only with the informed consent of the patient with certain exceptions. As previously noted, the exceptions usually involve the age of the child and his or her legal status. At the beginning of a professional relationship, to the extent the person can understand, the clinician shall inform the child and the parent or legal guardian of the limit the law imposes on the right of confidentiality with respect to their communications with the healthcare professional. This means the clinician has the responsibility to clarify any limits of confidentiality between a minor child and his or her parents or legal guardians at the onset of proposed services. It is recommended that the clinician discuss this fully in advance, especially with a legally dependent child, including that the clinician will always act in the best interests of the child in deciding whether to disclose confidential information to the legal guardians without the minor child's consent. In working with children and adolescents this becomes a very important issue in the establishment of trust, the development of a good therapeutic alliance, and the condition of safety. If disclosure of private patient information and openness to the treatment are to develop, the limits of confidentiality must be agreed upon in advance before consent can be given.

Healthcare providers who deliver services in an organizational context, such as a hospital setting, mental health center, child guidance clinic, or other entity, need to be especially careful to utilize informed consent. This requires that consent be given before treatment begins, as in a private context, but must also include the relationship of the provider to the organization and the nature of the relationship the provider will have with the child and the parents or legal guardian. This should include delineation of the services provided and the information obtained, who will have access to the information, and the limits of confidentiality.

Mandatory Reporting of Child Abuse

Another important exception to confidentiality is the mandatory reporting of child abuse or suspected abuse. Kalichman (1999) noted, "Child abuse is one of the great social maladies of our time." Moreover, he noted that in 1997, there were over 3 million children reported as victims of child maltreatment in the United States, representing more than a 40% increase since 1988. Only about 40% of all cases of child abuse are reported based on examination of community-based studies of reported child abuse.

Healthcare professionals are mandated under specific conditions defined by law to report child abuse and failure to do so can have serious legal consequences. Kalichman and Craig (1991) have reported that surveys of practicing psychologists show that 31% believe reporting has adverse consequences for their patients and their treatment. The primary argument against reporting is the belief that it can have destructive consequences to their services. This argument puts the clinician and possibly the child at risk and violates mandatory reporting laws—if the concerned clinician is unsure how or when to proceed, he or she is advised to seek a consultation with child protective services.

As Kalichman (1991) has noted, the problem of mandatory reporting laws is their application in mental health service settings without regard to the nature of these services. The particular settings and the relationships within which suspected child abuse is observed in "mental health service settings are qualitatively different from those of emergency medicine and pediatrics, the original targets of mandatory reporting legislation." Whether using hypnosis or engaged in any other professional endeavor with children, as mandated reporters of child abuse we need to view the welfare of children and their families with the greatest consideration when deciding to report suspected child abuse. The manner in which reporting occurs, if deemed appropriate, requires thoughtful consideration for the situation, previous reporting experiences and consultations, and the circumstances of the specific family.

While it is beyond the scope of this chapter to discuss the issues of "recovered memories" or any other disclosures through the use of hypnosis, the reader is cautioned to be familiar with the forensic literature and the use of hypnosis as well as the research on the veracity of memory and the differences between implicit and explicit memory. No assumptions should be made about the historical accuracy of recall with or without hypnosis. Whether a memory is accurate or not, it should be considered as part of a person's narrative memory and treated as such in therapy.

The remaining mandated reporting situations relate to dangerousness to self or other and abuse of a vulnerable adult. The former sometimes becomes known to the clinician working with children or adolescents in a treatment setting. All states have mandatory reporting laws and the respective laws of the state in which one practices bind the healthcare professional. Child protection statutes pertaining to the definition of a child's dependence vary from state to state. It is the healthcare professional's responsibility to know their local statutes in this regard. Informed consent is a decision-making process regarding treatment and as well as guiding those decisions that could arise in the course of treatment that might involve the necessity of mandatory reporting.

In summary regarding informed consent, Nagy (2006) has offered the following guidelines for hypnosis and the informed consent process:

1.   Address the patient's/parents' preconceptions, questions, and fears about hypnosis.

2. Explain the potential benefits and risks in engaging in hypnosis.
3. Describe how hypnosis can contribute to therapy as an adjunct.
4. Provide a general indication of how therapy and hypnosis will proceed.

While this list is not exhaustive, it will vary by context and be up to the clinician how to address each area with the parents and the child or adolescent according to age and developmental capacity to understand the elements of informed consent.

Boundaries

Clinical Example

You have been using hypnosis with a 12-year-old girl to improve her mastery/competence and to reduce her anxiety in school. In the course of treatment, you determine she has been neglected/mistreated both physically and emotionally. At the end of the session, the girl asks for a hug before leaving the appointment. Independent of the gender of either the child or therapist, the question needs to be asked: How will physical contact independent of its intent be interpreted by the child? In order to provide the child safety and nurturance the therapist might say, "You and I both know that sometimes when people have hugged or touched you in the past, it was not safe." If the clinician knows the mother is safe, then the clinician could proceed by saying, "Let's have your mother come in and show her how I can give you a safe hug." With the mother now present, the therapist might say to the child, "Go ahead and close your eyes and picture us in my office with your mom sitting here and we stand up and I meet you in the middle of the room and we have a hug. And you know that you are safe and we are friends." This is done so that mother sees the boundary set and the child experiences the safety and nurturance of the therapist and the appropriate interpretation of the hug is made at home.

Clinical Example:

Another type of boundary decision involves the extent of treatment and whether it is appropriate for the developmental level of the child. In the earlier enuresis example, the clinician might determine that the best practice, depending on the age of the child, is to treat the enuresis only since the child may not be "ready" to engage in treatment of more difficult psychological issues. In such cases, the therapist might use the hypnotic experience to resolve the presenting symptom and improve a general sense of mastery and competence. This is an example of a developmentally set boundary. The therapist may stay in contact with the child or family until there is a developmental readiness to deal with possible underlying causes.

All codes of ethics share the common value of taking reasonable steps to avoid doing harm. An area that concerns all professionals involves possible exploitation of the treatment relationship. One source of this involves boundary violations, which can be physical and possibly suggest some intrusion into the physical space of the patient. The 8-year-old daughter of a former patient was discussing the meaning of a boundary with her mother. The girl's conclusion was to define a boundary as "a fence made of no's."

Gutheil and Gabbard (1993; 1998 have written extensively regarding boundaries in clinical practice. They make a distinction between a boundary violation and a boundary crossing. They note that one's professional role, time, place and space, gifts, clothing, and physical touch are all potential boundaries. It is important to remain in one's professional role, thus maintaining the professional distinction. Sometimes children respond to the clinician as a parental figure, creating the possibility of transference elements. Time is part of the therapeutic frame that serves as a boundary, defining limits and providing structure. Children's capacities to focus or engage in hypnotherapy over time may vary with age and development.

Treatment usually takes place in the practitioner's office, treatment room, or playroom. The boundary of the area where treatment occurs can include a hospital room or any place that is associated in the child's mind as a place of safety and where he or she can feel secure. Sometimes in an effort to establish rapport and a therapeutic relationship with children or adolescents, the clinician may take them on a walk or engage in some other activity important to the development of their relationship. Gifts can be an especially sensitive area with children. Often the child will make something to give to his or her healthcare provider or the clinician might give something to the child that has meaning within the context of the treatment.

Gutheil and Gabbard (1993) acknowledge that clothing represents a social boundary that needs to be appropriate for the situation and could represent a boundary violation with possible destructive consequences if the clothing is sexual or seductive in nature. Sometimes language is seen as a boundary with children. As mentioned earlier, language needs to be appropriate to the treatment, the child's developmental level, and presented in understandable terms.

Perhaps most important is the physical boundary. The therapeutic relationship like any other relationship is always subject to the risk of exploitation. A violation in any of the three aforementioned values—trust, caring, and power—contributes to the vulnerability of the professional relationship. This requires extra sensitivity in working with children especially in the area of physical contact. Sometimes appropriate touch conveys caring and yet its application needs to be assessed as to the meaning it conveys. Two questions serve as a useful guide for the variables outlined by Gutheil and Gabbard (1993) in screening for risk of harm and/or exploitation: What am I attempting to teach my patients by what I say and/or do? And what are my patients learning? If, through our self-supervisory capacity, we are continuously aware and assess our answers to these two questions the risks to the treatment will be greatly minimized.

Children and Hypnosis

Clinical Example:

A father brought his 3-year-old daughter to treatment because they had been in an auto accident; neither had been seriously hurt. The man in the other car, however, had been thrown from his vehicle and landed on the windshield of the father's car. The child developed sleeping difficulties, high levels of anxiety, and kept referring to the image of a "bloody man." The presenting problems were the anxiety and nightmares associated with the trauma of the accident. Hypnosis had been recommended to the family by the pediatrician as an appropriate intervention.

During the first treatment session the clinician asked the girl to tell her something she liked to do and a special place she liked to go. She chose Disneyland as a favorite place and especially Snow White's Wishing Well just outside the Magic Castle. This was used because it had importance for the child and contained both auditory and visual images appropriate for a child this young. The "hypnotic induction" involved asking the child with eyes open or closed, to go to the wishing well and listen to Snow White and the seven dwarfs singing. She was given the suggestion that when she went home and was feeling worried, she could visit Snow White and the seven dwarfs in her imagination or pretend world. During the next visit the therapist and girl visited Snow White and the seven dwarfs and the therapist asked the girl to see "the man over there." The child asked, "What man?" The therapist indicated, "The one over there." The child said, "Oh, I see him." The therapist said, "He looks fine now," and the girl agreed as they both looked at the wishing well.

During the third session, the therapist had the child return to the image of Snow White and the seven dwarfs at the wishing well and asked about any recurring nightmares. The child opened her eyes, put her hands on her hips, and said, "You silly, you know he's fine." The child controlled the pace and child and therapist were equals in the treatment.

Koocher (1976), in an older and wonderful article entitled, "A Bill of Rights for Children in Psychotherapy," cited Ross (1974) who specified the following four basic tenets, which are applicable to anyone working with children and hypnosis:

1. Children have the right to be told the truth.
2. Children have the right to be treated with personal respect.
3. The child-client has the right to be taken seriously.
4. The child has the right to meaningful participation in decision making that applies to his or her life.

These recommendations imply that the child is to be taken seriously, listened to, and heard in all professional activities and decision making that involves their well-being. Informed consent and the right to be told the truth need to be communicated in a language readily understandable by the child with sensitivity to his or her developmental level. If this is done appropriately the child will feel respected.

From the early literature in hypnosis, Gill and Brenman (1959) in their classic text *Hypnosis and Related States* have offered that hypnosis is both a transference phenomena and an altered state of consciousness. They noted that hypnotic responsiveness involves several variables or ego-functions. They emphasize the need to appreciate the relationship with the therapist as providing a "holding" function for the patient within the transference. In addition, they note that hypnotic responsiveness involves the capacity of the patient to engage in a light dissociative state, or altered state of consciousness. What is noteworthy for the hypnotic experience is the importance of the therapeutic alliance and transference as a "holding" function allowing the patient to feel secure in promoting the altered state.

Hilgard (1970) studied imaginative involvements, or light dissociative states in college students and found that reading fiction, especially science fiction, involvement in the dramatic arts, and affective arousal to name a few were important antecedent conditions to predict later hypnotizability. She used the capacity to engage in imaginative involvements as her term for these light dissociative states, which is defined as the person's capacity to engage in parallel processing. Olness and Kohen (1996) noted the importance of this variable and its wide application with children. Using imaginative involvements with children, the clinician is engaging the child's capacity to "pretend" in a special way as involvement in the hypnotic experience is generated.

Writing from an interest in the neurobiology of interpersonal experience, Siegel (1999) noted that emotional communication and affective attunement become the medium in which the child's cognitive capacities develop. This would suggest that initial rapport and the development of a therapeutic alliance is co-constructed through affective attunement with the child, thus promoting the child as an ally in the therapeutic process. Siegel (1999) has further stated that emotional communication is also the fundamental manner in which one mind connects with another. This is especially important with children in all phases of treatment and in any hypnotic communication.

Baker (2000), writing from the perspective of the hypnotic relationship, noted that the *interaction* between the clinician using hypnosis and the patient may well be the primary mechanism for the therapeutic action of hypnosis. It is not what the therapist does that is critical; rather it is how "the dyad construes and experiences how they are together which seems most evocative and evolutionary." Again, this is most likely to be accomplished by taking the child and his or her concerns seriously and by being respectful. By communicating the child's right to meaningful participation in the treatment planning and decision-making process, the child's involvement in the therapeutic experience will be vastly increased. With all this communicated in an affectively attuned way, the clinician is more likely to reduce the risks of resistance to treatment and/or early termination by the patient.

A primary issue with children in the healthcare system is the management of their anxiety in an adult world in which the power differential is large. To create an alliance by including them in the development of the treatment planning process reduces the difference in power while strengthening the therapeutic alliance.

The success of any therapeutic relationship is dependent on the management of the three variables: caring, trust, and power. I have addressed the importance of each of these within the framework of and sensitivity for the ethical considerations in working with children and adolescents. As clinicians, we make a difference in many ways. The crucial difference is the meaning the child and his or her parents attach to their relational experience with us. Given the power of this relationship, it is mandatory that we maintain our allegiance to our ethical codes of conduct so that they not only guide our professional behavior but also for appropriate and effective treatment planning. This simultaneous awareness of ethical considerations and the development of clinical decisions creates a "double helix" that co-determines the development of our treatment planning. Nowhere is this more important than with children as we assist them to pursue what Gibran (1976) has so eloquently defined as "the sons and daughters of life's longing for itself." To guide this longing our best hope is to become considerate ethically, compassionate emotionally, and relevant clinically.

References

Adrian, C. (1996). Therapist sexual feelings in hypnotherapy: Managing therapeutic boundaries in hypnotic work. *International Journal of Clinical and Experimental Hypnosis*. Vol. XLIV, 1, 20–30.

Baker, E. L. (2000). Reflections on the hypnotic relationship: Projective identification, containment, and attunement. *International Journal of Clinical and Experimental Hypnosis*. Vol. 48, 1, 56–69.

Bersoff, D. (1995). *Ethical conflicts in psychology*. Washington D.C.: American Psychological Association.

Coons, P. M. (1988). Misuse of forensic hypnosis: A hypnotically elicited false confession with apparent creation of a multiple personality. *International Journal of Clinical and Experimental Hypnosis*. 36, 1, 1–11.

Fisher, C. B. (2003). *Decoding the ethics code*. Thousand Oaks, CA: Sage Publications.

Gibran, K. (1976). *The prophet*. New York: Alfred A. Knopf.

Gill, M. M., & Brenman, M. (1959). *Hypnosis and related states: Psychoanalytic studies in regression.* New York: John Wiley and Sons.

Grisso, T., & Vierling, L. (1978). Minors' consent to treatment: A developmental perspective. *Professional Psychology, 9,* 412–426.

Gutheil, T. G., & Gabbard, G. O. (1993). The concept of boundaries in clinical practice: Theoretical and risk-management dimensions. *American Journal of Psychiatry,* 150:2, 188–196.

Gutheil, T. G., & Gabbard, G. O. (1998). Misuses and misunderstandings of boundary theory in clinical and regulatory settings. *American Journal of Psychiatry,* 155:3, 409–414.

Hambleton, R. (2002). *Practicing safe hypnosis: A risk management guide.* Carmarthen, Wales, U.K.: Crown House.

Hilgard, J. (1970). *Personality and hypnosis–A study of imaginative involvements.* Chicago: University of Chicago Press.

Kalichman, S. (1991). Laws on reporting sexual abuse of children. *American Journal of Psychiatry,* 148, 1618–1619.

Kalichman, S. (1999). *Mandated reporting of suspected child abuse: Ethics, law, and policy.* (2nd ed.) Washington D.C.: American Psychological Association.

Kalichman, S., & Craig, M.E. (1991). Professional psychologists' decisions to report suspected abuse: Clinical and situational influences. *Professional Psychology: Research and Practice,* 22, 84–89.

Knapp, S., & VanderCreek, L. (2003). *A guide to the 2002 revision of the American Psychological Association's ethics code.* Sarasota, FL: Professional Resource Press.

Koocher, G. P. (1976). A bill of rights for children in psychotherapy. *Children's rights in the mental health profession.* New York: John Wiley and Sons.

Koocher, G., Norcross, J., & Hill, S. (Eds.). (1998). *Psychologists' desk reference.* New York: Oxford University Press.

Lakin, M. (1991). *Coping with ethical dilemmas in psychotherapy.* New York: Pergamon Press.

McConkey, K. M. (1995). Hypnosis, memory, and the ethics of uncertainty. *Australian Psychologist*, 30, 1, 1–10.

Nagy, T. (2006). *Ethics in hypnosis*. A workshop presented at the American Society of Clinical Hypnosis meeting in Orlando, Florida, March 2006.

Olness, K., & Gardner, G. (1981). *Hypnosis and hypnotherapy with children* New York: Grune and Stratton.

Olness, K. & Gardner, G. (1988). *Hypnosis and hypnotherapy with children, 2nd ed*. New York: Grune and Stratton.

Olness, K. & Kohen, D. (1996). *Hypnosis and hypnotherapy with children, 3rd ed*. New York: Guilford Press.

Orne, M. (1979). The use and misuse of hypnosis in court. *International Journal of Clinical and Experimental Hypnosis*, 27, 4, 311–341.

Pope, K., & Vasquez, M. (1991). *Ethics in psychotherapy and counseling*. San Francisco: Jossey-Bass.

Relinger, H. & Stern, T. (1983). Guidelines for forensic hypnosis. *Journal of Psychiatry and Law*, 11, 1 69–74.

Ross, A. O. (1974). *The rights of children*. Paper presented at the American Psychological Association Meeting in New Orleans, September 1, 1974.

Scheflin, A. (1997). Ethics and hypnosis: Unorthodox or innovative therapies and the legal standard of care. In W. Mathews & J. Edgette (Eds.). *Current thinking and research in brief therapy: Solutions, strategies, and narratives*, 1, Philadelphia: Brunner/Mazel.

Sheehan, P. and McConkey, K. M. (1993). Forensic hypnosis: The application of ethical guidelines. In J. Rhue, S. Lynn, & I. Kirsch, *Handbook of clinical hypnosis*. Washington D.C.: American Psychological Association.

Siegel, D. (1999). *The developing mind*. New York: Guilford Press.

Stottenberg, C.D., & Delworth, U. (1987). *Supervising counselors and therapists*. San Francisco: Jossey–Bass.

Stromberg, C., Haggarty, D., Leibenluft, R., McMillian, M., Mishkin, B., Rubin, B., & Trilling, H. (1988). *The psychologist's legal handbook.* Washington D.C.: Council for the National Register of Health Service Providers in Psychology.

Wall, T. W. (1991). Ethics—The royal road to legitimacy. *American Journal of Clinical Hypnosis*, 34, 2, 73–78.

Wall, V. J. (1991). Developmental considerations in the use of hypnosis with children. In W. Wester & D. O'Grady (Eds.). *Clinical hypnosis with children* (pp. 3–18). New York: Brunner/Mazel.

Wester, W. C. & O'Grady, D. J. (1991). *Clinical hypnosis with children.* New York: Brunner/Mazel.

Part II

Psychological Applications

Chapter Seven

Hypnosis in Childhood Trauma

Julie H. Linden, PhD

"The best thing for being sad," replied Merlyn, beginning to puff and blow, "is to learn something. That is the only thing that never fails. You may grow old and trembling in your anatomies, you may lie awake at night listening to the disorder of your veins, you may miss your only love, you may see the world about you devastated by evil lunatics, or know your honour trampled in the sewers of baser minds. There is only one thing for it then—to learn." *

Merlyn, advising the young Arthur,
The Once and Future King

The Children

The Trauma of Separation and Divorce

Adam

Adam was 5½ years old when I first met him. His parents were very concerned about his frequent temper tantrums and managing his behavior in new or stressful situations. In addition he was enuretic and since he climbed into bed with them almost every night, they were highly motivated for him to have dry beds. Adam responded very well to learning about the brain-body connection and was quickly using his hypnotic imagination to have dry beds. His extreme

---

*T. H. White. (1958). *The Once and Future King*. New York; G. P. Putnam's Sons.

anxiety about any separations from his parents, along with other symptoms, led to a diagnosis of childhood bipolar disorder. His parents explored medication options to stabilize his moods and to which he was responsive. Then his parents decided to separate. When Adam was told this news he regressed to his old styles of coping. Frequent meltdowns and temper tantrums, oppositionality with adults, and isolated angry play all returned. In play Adam's action figures (children) repeatedly played a game of running away from the parents and surviving on their own. What was the meaning of this repetitive traumatic play? What suggestion did Adam's dolls need to find better ways to cope? After one session in which Adam's monster toy animal killed all of the adult characters with guns and bows and arrows, repeatedly having the child dolls "save the day," I asked him if he wanted to talk about how he was feeling having two homes now. "No," he said, "I am getting used to it, it's okay now."

The Trauma of Chronic Illness

Sandy

Sandy was 12 years old when her kidney failure required her to begin kidney dialysis. She was a bright, affable young lady and well liked by the nursing staff and she took interest in the medical procedures she underwent. When she learned about hypnosis she immediately requested some help with managing painful procedures. She learned to "turn down the dials" and was pleased with how much easier it became to get through the long day of hemodialysis treatment.

The Trauma of Accidents

Jeff

Jeff was badly burned on Thanksgiving Day when he 11 years old. His mother was taking the turkey from the oven and it slipped off the rack and sent burning grease over Jeff's body. Sixty percent of his body was covered in third-degree burns and Jeff spent months in the hospital undergoing painful debridement (removal of dead skin) procedures. In hypnosis, he learned to go to the baseball field and swing his bat during debridement. This helped him diminish his pain and increase the range of motion in his arms so necessary to the rehabilitation of such an extensive burn.

The Need for a Hypnotic Therapeutic Relationship

Childhood is a time we all like to think of as idyllic, safe, and peaceful. Peruse the pictures you have of childhood, or the ones that our society uses to capture this time of life, and you will find they are filled with symbols of love, kindness, and warmth. Icons of childhood include the toddler on Santa's lap, kids building sand castles at the shore, or the smiling small faces on TV ads with milk rings around their mouths. None of us like to think about kids in harms way. That is the stuff of fairytales and scary movies. During the early '70s when child abuse was promoted to a national crisis, building awareness among healthcare professionals was largely a process of addressing denial. We have succeeded in building that awareness and surpassed it with an even more refined understanding of how vulnerable the growing child is, thanks to research on traumatic symptoms in children (Perry 2000; Pynoos, 1994a). This book would be incomplete without attention to the nature, scope, and effects of trauma in childhood and the unique contribution that clinical hypnosis offers for its treatment. Specific techniques are presented in an integrated approach that utilizes the concept of the hypnotic therapeutic relationship.

For every dragon that haunts a child's imagination there is a need for the dragon slayer. For every scary monster there is a guardian angel. With knowledge of trauma and hypnosis, health professionals can help children develop the dragon slayer and guardian angels whose potential resides in each of us.

What is Trauma?

Traumas come in many forms. To the developing child, trauma is often seemingly small or unnoticed by adults, unlike the examples at the beginning of this chapter. The fears that children experience early in life, such as fear of separating from a parent, fear of the dark, fear of heights, snakes, or monsters, can all be traumatic to the developing child (Garber, Garber, & Spizman, 1993).

The definition of traumas often becomes a discussion of whether we mean Trauma with a big "T" or trauma with a little "t." The concept of the little "t" type of trauma (e.g., losing mom in the store) derives from our understanding of developmental responses to the variety of frightening experiences to which a child is exposed. These may form the basis for phobias, habit disorders, and other mental illnesses. Convention refers to big "T" Trauma as events that everyone "gasps" about. These are the events in people's lives about which there is virtually complete agreement on the traumatic nature of the experience. We can think of traumatic events falling into basic categories (Pynoos, 1994a). I have delineated seven major categories that I have found useful for assessment when contemplating clinical treatment:

1. Physical, sexual, or verbal abuse (including homicide, rape, and suicide)
2. Accidents
3. Chronic Illness; Medical Procedures
4. Death-loss of parent, sibling, friend
5. Divorce or separation
6. Natural Disasters (from fears of lightening, fire, etc., to traumas from famine, floods, cyclones, tornadoes, tsunamis, etc.). Terrorism is considered a special kind of disaster.
7. War

While this list is not meant to be exhaustive in terms of all the traumas that can befall an individual, it provides a way to think about the nature of the trauma from the child's perspective. Each category has some elements in common for the "sufferer." For example, traumas from natural disasters usually create a communal response that provides support for the traumatized; however, most humans have greater difficulty healing from traumas at the hand of other humans (i.e., abuse and war) (De Zulueta, 1993). The trauma from chronic illness, medical procedures, and related events presumes an interface with medical personnel and institutions and a specific subset of behaviors for managing those interactions.

Definitions

Defining trauma has proven to be as challenging as determining the types of trauma. Lindemann (1944) defined it as "the sudden cessation of human interaction." This definition, as seen from the perspective of a young child, makes even the "lost in the supermarket child" a traumatized child.

McCann and Pearlman (1990) define an experience as traumatic if it: (1) is sudden, unexpected, or non-normative, (2) exceeds the individual's perceived ability to meet its demand, and (3) it disrupts the individual's frame of reference and other central psychological needs and related schemas. Eliana Gil (1998), a child psychotherapist, defined something as traumatic if it overwhelms the person's perceived ability to cope, debilitates through a central loss of control, and creates the necessity for psychological defenses. It is important that she highlighted the issue of control, since mastery is so intrinsic to child development. A major contribution of Gil's work is that it takes the focus off the trauma and looks at the larger world of the child. Gil concludes that we must have a systemic and contextual lens (1998, p. 8) and understand developmental issues (physical, personality, sexual, emotional, moral, and spiritual) as well as attachment theory in order to know the child's response to the trauma. She concludes that it is the person's response to the event that creates the traumatization.

This inclusion of the *meaning* that someone gives to an event is also captured in the wholist framework for understanding trauma proposed by Valent (1999). He suggests that we need to consider the nature of the trauma (process), the parameters of the trauma (context), and the depth of the trauma (effect of the trauma on human fulfillment). Defining trauma is critical to the assessment of trauma in a child, and our challenge is to understand the various factors that lead to a child experiencing an event as traumatic.

The diagnostic nomenclature (*Diagnostic and Statistical Manual of Mental Disorders–IV-TR*, 2000) for a posttraumatic stress disorder (PTSD) first requires a *recognizable stressor*. The criterion of a recognizable stressor has changed (over the decade since the last update of nomenclature was written) from an event outside the range of normal human experience to one wherein the primary feature is the individual's perception of the event (Daly, 2004).

The Diagnostic and Statistical Manual (2000) then looks at the mindbody response of re-experiencing, avoidance, and arousal. These defensive reactions of the mindbody are expressions of different coping mechanisms of the nervous system. *Re-experiencing* the trauma refers to the intrusive daytime recollections or traumatic nightmares that reflect the persistence of thoughts, feelings, and behaviors specifically related to the traumatic event. *Avoidance* includes denial, suppression, repression, splitting, and the ability to dissociate. Acute stress disorder (ASD) (*DSM–IV-TR*, 2000) is an anxiety disorder characterized by a cluster of dissociative and anxiety symptoms occurring within one month of a traumatic event. Exposure to a *trauma*, which is defined as a stressor that causes intense fear and, usually, involves threats to life or serious injury to oneself or others, is required for a diagnosis of ASD. *Anxiety symptoms* refer to the *arousal* of the psychophysiological state. These symptoms include irritability, physical restlessness, sleep problems, inability to concentrate, and being easily startled. *Dissociative symptoms* include emotional detachment, temporary loss of memory, depersonalization, and derealization.

A third kind of trauma is called *trauma by proxy* (Brooks & Siegel, 1996). This diagnosis is utilized when one feels traumatized as the result of an event that happened to someone else (seeing it or hearing about it) or feels traumatized because of identification with the victim. Children are particularly vulnerable to this kind of trauma.

Acute stress disorder is a newer diagnostic category that was introduced in 1994 to differentiate time-limited reactions to trauma from PTSD. Please note the importance of dissociation in these definitions. The dissociative quality of traumatic response is one of the factors that makes hypnosis a treatment of choice.

Simple vs. Complicated Trauma

Before elaborating on the relationship between dissociative symptoms and the use of hypnosis, it is important to note that traumas can be further defined as *simple* or *complicated* (Brown and Fromm, 1986) or *single* or *double blows* as they are called in the British literature (De Zulueta, 1993). A simple trauma is a single event, it is of brief duration, it occurs later in life after the ego development is solidified, it does not include man-made violence, the person has an active role to play, has advance warning, the symptoms are time limited and can resolve with a facilitative environment and if treatment is needed it is usually of brief duration. Complicated trauma, in contrast, is usually a series of repetitive events, of longer duration, occurs earlier in life, includes man-made violence, the person has a more passive role, the event is sudden and without warning, the symptoms are long lasting and can produce characterological change, requiring treatment, of long duration, and ego-reparative. The very fact that children do not have fully developed egos means they are particularly vulnerable to complicated trauma. In fact, perception is more basic and primitive than is cognition so that in cases of a preverbal experience, the traumatic perception may remain an indigestible part of growing young personality (Eth & Pynoos, 1985).

Assessment

To assess whether a child is experiencing a trauma is not always easy. Adam, in the first vignette, *tells* us everything is fine, while his violent play *looks* otherwise. Sometimes a recognizable stressor is not obvious but awareness of the way behavior manifests itself in children after a trauma is helpful. Children may appear as if they are uninvolved, a kind of emotional numbing. They may be subdued or even mute. Early in my career I was asked to treat a child from the inner city who presented as mute. The youngster had language skills and then suddenly became mute. The family was chaotic and uneducated and there was suspicion of substance abuse. I wondered if the child was traumatized by either neglect or abuse because of the presenting symptom, but the family left treatment before any definitive diagnosis could be made.

When a child is verbal he or she may report a traumatic event in the third person, and it will lack emotion and sound "journalistic." Other signs of avoidance are a sense of foreshortened future or avoidance of activities that arouse recollection of a traumatic event (Terr, 1990). Adam, the child in the vignette enduring his parent's divorce, told his mother that he couldn't sleep because he thought that tomorrow might not come if he was not awake to watch for it. An adult client reported how she was planning for her funeral from the age of 12, sure she would not live through her adolescence. This was a clue that some early trauma had occurred, which was later reported in her treatment.

Children may report a recurring dream or re-enact a specific trauma in their play, both examples of re-experiencing a trauma.

Sally

Sally, age 13, had a repetitive dream about snakes attacking her. She was utterly phobic of snakes and was sure that explained her recurring dream. During treatment she remembered having been sexually assaulted at age 5, after which the recurring dream ceased as did her phobia of snakes.

Symptoms of hyper alertness or arousal that children exhibit include sleep disturbances—an inability to fall asleep, night terrors, or nightmares. There can be irritability or outbursts of anger, memory impairment, or trouble concentrating. Sometimes hyper vigilance is noted and children may be full of guilt. An exaggerated startle response can also be present. When I worked with a group of young teenagers who were brought to the United States during the war in the Balkan countries, one of them described how she jumped out of her dinner chair when a member of the family dropped a fork on the floor. Regressed behavior is also symptomatic of a traumatized child. He or she may go into the parents' bed anew, sleep in strange places, return to an old habit such as thumb sucking, or develop enuresis. All three of the symptom categories of trauma, (re-experiencing, hyper arousal, and numbing/avoidance) are responsive to hypnotic procedures that will be discussed in more detail below.

According to the research of John Briere (2003), only 15–25% of all of those exposed to a traumatic event go on to satisfy *DSM* diagnostic criteria for PTSD; extreme traumas may produce higher rates for those directly affected, but rarely over 50–70%. Bruce Perry (2000) reports, "A growing body of evidence suggests that exposure to violence or trauma alters the developing brain by altering normal neuro-developmental processes." He further notes that hypnosis, because it accesses the brainstem in the same place where traumas seem to be stored or encoded, is particularly suitable for treatment of traumas (Perry, 2006).

Hypnosis and Dissociations

Hypnotherapists who deal with the dissociative phenomenon of hypnosis are familiar with the *DSM* (1994) definition of *dissociation*. It is defined as a disruption in the usually integrated functions of consciousness, memory, identity, or perception of the environment. It may be sudden, gradual, transient, or chronic. Dissociation can be seen as a distancing through the repression of *affect* (numbing), the repression of *thought*, the repression of *behavior*, depersonalization (out of body experiences), amnesias and automatisms (e.g., sleepwalking). Early in the development of our understanding of Dissociative Identity Disorder (DID), Braun (1988) presented the BASK model to remind us that dissociation occurs in behavior, affect, sensory experiences and knowledge (cognitions).

There are similarities in altered states of consciousness in victims of trauma and those reported by individuals in a hypnotic context. These include a narrowed focus of attention, dissociation, altered sense of time, and altered sensory perceptions (Cardeña, 2000). It is my experience that the similarity between the hypnotic state and the traumatized state permits the use of hypnosis to access both cognitive and somatic memory. Hypnosis is particularly flexible for working with these accessed memories because of the easy use of imagination to relax, to contain, and to distance from traumatic material.

Cardeña (2000) states that "patients with posttraumatic conditions, as a group, seem to be more hypnotizable than normal controls," and because high hypnotizability is positively correlated with hypnotic effectiveness, PTSD patients are good candidates for hypnotic treatment (p. 226).

Beverly James (1989) has written extensively on childhood trauma. She is emphatic that unless a child's affective state is the same way he or she felt during the initial trauma, during the time new understandings or cognitions are taught, no change in symptoms can occur. This has also been my clinical experience. Hypnosis often reactivates the dissociative state of the child that is necessary to get to the state of the trauma.

There are many advantages of dissociation. We need distance in order to achieve mastery. Dissociating allows us to compartmentalize, separating ourselves from a trauma so that we can continue to function. Dissociation creates a discontinuity in experience that may help us to later identify that something is missing, and then discover what it is. Dissociation helps to maintain, gain, and regain control. In addition, dissociation may allow the body to handle some of the worst responses to trauma (van der Kolk, 1987b). Perry's (2006) work on infant response to trauma introduces the notion of the continuum of adaptive responses to trauma. His research has shown that trauma can affect us from birth (and perhaps even prenatally) and that there are degrees of responses, which supports earlier findings indicating that not everyone develops PTSD symptoms in the face of trauma.

The advantage of hypnosis for the treatment of trauma is that it can get to the original affective state. As stated earlier, James (1989) said this is a requirement of successful treatment. Hypnosis can train the relaxation response, which allows someone to be relieved of the anxiety that often accompanies a response to trauma.

Hypnosis can create endless containment techniques through imagery and can utilize trance logic phenomenon to restore distortions or remove stored negative suggestions (Kluft, 1985). In addition, hypnosis can bridge between the conscious and unconscious, accessing pictorial and sensorial memory ubiquitous to trauma. Clearly hypnosis is an important treatment modality for the clinician treating traumatized children.

The research of Frank Putnam (1997) on hypnosis and pathological dissociation, in contrast to Cardeña's (2000) work, did not find a strong correlation between hypnotizability and dissociation, but did find a strong relationship between dissociation and trauma. Putnam suggests that the research can be grouped into four lines of evidence for concluding that "trauma *causes* pathological dissociation" (1997, p. 62). One of Putnam's significant contributions is his review of the literature that details the antecedents to the development of dissociation in children. These antecedents include: (1) High rates of early trauma; (2) Higher dissociation scores in traumatized compared to non-traumatized subjects for all kinds of trauma; (3) Severity of trauma correlated with dissociation scores and similarly with trauma severity and PTSD scores; and (4) Peritraumatic dissociation predicts PTSD (pp. 62–63).

Play and Hypnosis

Play serves many functions for the developing child (Schaefer & O'Connor, 1983). At a *biological* level it allows the child to learn basic skills, to relax and release energy, to experience kinesthetic stimulation, and to exercise. At an *intrapersonal* level it helps to develop mastery of situations; permits explorations and curiosity, the development of mind, body, and world understanding; it can resolve conflicts through mastery; it uses symbolism and allows for wish fulfillment. At the *interpersonal* level the child can develop social skills through play as well as separation–individuation skills. For example, play can provide distraction as a coping mechanism and help a child to master anxiety. Another function of play is at the *socio-cultural* level where a child can imitate desired roles and learn a variety of rules for engaging in community.

The kinds of play that children engage in can be either alone/with others or structured/unstructured. Play has many therapeutic factors so it is a natural choice for the treatment of children. Play therapy (Schaefer & Cangelosi, 1993) and sand tray work (Boik & Goodwin, 2000) capitalize on the ability of play to help visualize or use fantasy, to communicate, to form attachments, to enhance relationships and build rapport, to learn through metaphoric teaching, to develop competence through mastery, to think creatively and access novelty, to achieve catharsis or abreaction, to develop positive emotion, to help children overcome resistance (which is often an expression of fear), to master developmental fears, to role-play and to develop game play, which helps with socialization. In short, play allows mastery of experiences through fantasizing, symbolizing, and desensitizing.

In my experience, play is an example of spontaneous hypnosis (Spiegel & Spiegel, 1978). Most forms of play for children produce a trance state in which there is narrowed focus of attention, dissociation, absorption, and imaginative involvement. Any one who has tried to get a child's attention while they are deep in play knows how focused and absorbed a youngster may be. Children prefer action to talking, and play is a way for them to actively release tension. As already noted, play allows for mastery of conflicts through symbolism and wish fulfillment, tapping into unconscious mechanisms and bypassing conscious thoughts. The therapist can utilize this spontaneous hypnosis through various play therapy techniques or art mediums, toys, drama, storytelling and make believe in order to introduce corrective suggestions and relieve the anxiety of trauma. There are many similarities between what I refer to as *hypnoidal* play, informal or spontaneous hypnosis, and formal hypnosis. The ability to resolve problems at an unconscious level is done both with hypnosis and play. One can reach into the sub- and unconscious and retrieve those aspects of the self, which are hidden from the child. Both play and hypnosis are meditative, focused, and absorbed states. Frequently one feels time distortion in each. As already discussed, both share the phenomenon of a dissociative state of mind. Hypnosis and play both permit the relatively easy access to the original affect, and each simultaneously uses both lobes of the brain. Identifying or producing hypnoidal play (Linden, 1996; Linden, 2003) and then pairing this with suggestions is the art of treatment for many traumatized children.

Gil (1998) has identified some characteristics of posttraumatic play in children that are useful for assessing a traumatized child as well as determining the nature of the trauma. She notes that there is a compulsive repetition of play. This is akin to the symptom of re-experiencing the traumatic event mentioned in the assessment of trauma. The child plays the same game or repeats the same series of movements over and over again. For example, in one 8-year-old who I was treating, I noticed that every time the child played with the doll house, she had the doll sit on the toilet and wash its hands in the sink. Any intervention I made to change this sequence met with resistance. I made some comments on this play, however, for her unconscious. I said that it was important to wash the hands (validating the behavior) and that the doll would feel better. In posttraumatic play there is an unconscious link between the play and the real event. The goal of hypnotic play therapy is to speak to the unconscious. Material does not have to be made conscious in order to be resolved. In this child's case it was. Some weeks after her repetitive doll house play I got a call from her mother to tell me that her daughter had revealed having been sexually abused by a friend of the family. Her hands had gotten sticky with something gooey, she reported, and hence the hand washing. (She had been made to masturbate the family friend to orgasm.) This case illustrates how literal the play is when it is posttraumatic play.

There is usually a failure to relieve anxiety in posttraumatic play. Instead, the child may actually appear more anxious. Adam, in the first vignette, after having his monster toy animal kill everyone, suddenly said, "...and the monster died" and put the stuffed toy away. He was visibly upset. My intervention was to praise his coping skill, "it is so good to get rid of bad guys," and redirect him on to something less anxiety provoking. Most traumatic play is a depiction of danger. Another youngster, age 2 ½, who at the age of 18 months experienced the death of his 10-year-old brother, played a game of taking an action figure deep into a large hole, "burying" him with blocks, and making noises that conveyed this was very dangerous. He would then suddenly retrieve the figure with a sigh of relief, only to repeat the game over again. Distracting him from this game was difficult. This creates an interesting dilemma for the therapist, because it is hard to know just how much of the post-traumatic play is necessary and useful to understand and treat the traumatic effects and exactly when it begins to overwhelm the child and cause even more traumatic effects. Using hypnotic containment techniques like the Raggedy Ann or Andy relaxation induction (learning to make each limb floppy like the Raggedy Ann doll) (Olness & Kohen, 1996, p. 68) or other kinesthetic, grounding and anxiety-releasing techniques sprinkled liberally throughout play therapy, usually mitigates further traumatization during the uncovery phase of treatment. Finally, in posttraumatic play there is a lack of spontaneity and enjoyment in the play. Depressed or anxious looks, words, posture, or behaviors are present.

Gil (1998) describes interventions for unhealthy play. I have adapted these to be hypnotic interventions for unhealthy play. Almost any kind of physical movement that captures the child's attention, especially if it is novel or surprising, can enhance the dissociative state in a relaxed and safe way. One might ask a child to stand up, take a deep breath, move their arms and legs, and role-play being an animal or hero figure. "Let's be supermen and fly over the sky far away from this place" can take the abreactive child to a place of calm and safety. This can also serve as a pattern interruption to rigid emotional and behavioral constriction.

One can also use a verbal statement about the play that may encourage the child to disengage, to observe (non-interpretive), rather than to be in it. This technique is the child's version of the hypnotic TV screen projective technique (Brown & Fromm, 1986). For example, "Let's pretend that this is on the TV or DVD and we can watch the bad monster from the sofa over here, where it is nice and safe"

Another hypnotic technique is to interrupt the sequence of play by asking the child to take specific roles and describe perceptions, thoughts, or feelings. In sand tray work the child is often asked to be different figures or items in the sand tray. This pretend play is usually normative play for children and may move the child out of constricted behavior. It implies there are solutions—more than one. The therapist can also take on different roles and model other coping skills for the child.

Manipulating the toys and asking, "What would happen if..." to elicit the child's creative imagination and help him or her to consider new options is another way to promote problem solving and mastery in hypnoidal play. Josephine Hilgard (LeBaron & Hilgard, 1984) described imaginative involvement as the absorbed state of trance in children. When there is imaginative involvement I believe it is the child's version of what Rossi calls "novelty." Rossi (1986/1993) has written extensively on the role of novelty in the hypnotic or dissociated state to create mind and body change. The method described here of intervening in a child's play is quite different from the psychoanalytic stance of neutral watching of play or interpretation of a child's play. Trauma treatment is an active process for the clinician.

The hypnotic containment technique of keeping a child grounded in the present while looking at past traumatic material can encourage the child to differentiate between traumatic material and current reality in terms of environmental changes and new coping strategies. A child, particularly a young one or a severely traumatized one, may not be able to use toys as symbolic and may instead view them as realistic objects. The planned evening activity was a "Hawaiian Night" one evening while I working with some Bosnian children at a camp following the Balkan war. The male children all dressed as warriors. Someone organized taking pictures of the costumed children. One very disturbed (traumatized) child took his flimsy stick, torn from a vine, and held it as a harpoon, ready to be launched at the photographer. The toy weapon was very real to him. This is also a good example of how the very behavior expressed is at once corrective (he could now defend himself) and traumatic (i.e., loaded affectively with his fears for survival.)

Perception in all areas of the mind can be affected. Children's perception of time is not the same as adults, and in the dissociated state, the sense of time is further distorted or absent. Hypnoidal techniques can be used to create a safe space that is timeless and thus enduring.

Discussing the variety of trauma models is beyond the scope of this chapter. However it is useful to understand that all of the hypnotic models agree on a phase-oriented treatment. Pierre Janet, who was the first to point out that dissociated states follow trauma (van der Kolk, 1987a, p. 6), recommended three stages in treatment (van der Hart, Brown & Turco, 1990; van der Hart, Steele, Boon and Brown, 1993): First, the *stabilization* of the individual, establishing rapport, creating safety and building trust. Second, *uncovery* work, or learning about, remembering or feeling the trauma, and modifying its terrible effects; and, finally, *processing* the trauma by working through the negative suggestions or conflicts it may have produced, reintegrating the trauma into one's life, and moving forward. The three phases are not linear, but rather more spiral, since after one does some uncovery or abreactive work, there is a need to return to stabilizing and rebuilding trust repeatedly throughout treatment while being mindful that one is in the present, not the past, and moving towards a healthier, safer future.

There are specific hypnotic techniques that can be used with each of the phases of treatment. Tables 7.1, 7.2, and 7.3 list these specific techniques.

None of the techniques in the three phases is limited to that phase of treatment, but I have found them to be particularly useful at that phase. Any type of relaxation or breathing technique that relaxes is a good place to start treatment for stabilization of a child who is in need of treatment for a traumatic experience. In this same vein, establishing a safe place image or place of peace and sanctuary helps to both stabilize and provide a practiced sensation

Table 7.1: Hypnotic Techniques for Stabilization, Building Rapport, and Ego-Strengthening

Phase One: Stabilization

- Relaxation Exercise/Induction Procedures (breathing)
- Safe Place/Sanctuary
- Restructuring Cognition's (dream alteration, storytelling)
- Problem-Solving Procedures (self-efficacy)
- Ego Enhancing (boundaries, modulation of affect)

Table 7.2: Hypnotic Techniques to Uncover and Explore the Trauma

Phase Two: Uncovery/Exploration

- Affect/sensation bridge[1]
- Silent abreaction[2]/Sensorimotor play (mirroring)
- Metaphors–"Garbage Bag"[3]
- Observing from a distance–TV set, puppet show, theatre
- Learning to endure emotions–affect modulation, knobs and controls, Structured Regression: "It's just not fair"[4]
- Ideomotor signals
- Reframing–storytelling
- Ego states
- Substitution procedures—inserting benign adult, soothing imagery[5]
- Sandwich procedure

[1] J. G. Watkins. (1971). The Affect Bridge: A Hypnoanalytic Technique. *International Journal of Clinical & Experimental Hypnosis, 19,* 21–27.
[2] H. Watkins. (1980). The Silent Abreaction. *International Journal of Clinical & Experimental Hypnosis, 19,* 101–112.
[3] B. James. (1989). *Treating Traumatized Children.* Lexington, MA: Heath.
[4] B. James, 1989.
[5] van der Hart, O., et.al. (1990). Hypnotherapy for Traumatic Grief: Janetian and Modern Approaches Integrated. *American Journal of Clinical Hypnosis, 32, 4,* 263–269.

Table 7.3: Hypnotic Techniques for Securing and Maintaining Gains

Phase Three: Reintegration

- Ego Enhancing—Construct purpose and meaning from trauma through hypnotic storytelling. "Making a Friend of a Scar"[1]
- Assertiveness Procedures—Establish healthier world assumptions through hypnotically mediated cognitive therapy. Develop Affirmations (can be PHS)
- Social Skills Building through metaphors or rehearsal
- Future Fantasies—Hypnotic rehearsal of new behaviors using "future" imagery

[1] B. James. (1989). *Treating Traumatized Children.* Lexington, MA: Heath.

that can be used as a containment technique whenever the child is overwhelmed with affect or other sensory arousal. Children often do well with an imaginary place from stories, movies, or their inner archetypal world or one that includes a safe adult (imaginary or real). Whenever a child is reporting a bad dream, helping the child to alter the dream in a way that reduces affect is very ego-strengthening. A useful suggestion is: "This is your dream, made up by your mind. Can you use your mind to make a better, less scary dream?" This intervention is related to any suggestions that increase problem-solving behaviors; for example, using a metaphor that illustrates a child getting out of a difficult situation through action or quick thinking. During play (spontaneous trance) or in a formally induced trance, one can present a dilemma and ask, "What shall we do now?" and follow the child's lead to discover solutions. In this phase, simple non-scary dilemmas are offered. Any of the hypnotic techniques that use modulation, such as dials, knobs, faucets, or instrument panels can be utilized to make a picture fuzzy, tone it down, add too much light so it washes out, etc., as the child learns that imagination can ease dis-comfort and transform *dis*-comfort into ease and comfort.

Beverly James' (1989) play therapy techniques are very useful during Phase Two of treatment, when it is so important to access the strong affect related to the trauma. The "garbage bag" technique begins with the child decorating a large paper bag with "yucky" things to indicate that it is clearly for garbage. The therapist then records on paper the things the child wants to throw out and put in the garbage. The items are then placed individually into the garbage bag, like folded notes, to be retrieved one at a time, later, during the course of treatment. The very act of placing the "garbage" (the notes) into the bag creates containment for the child's memories and affect. When all have been processed, and the bag is ready for disposal, the child has generally worked through the affect of the trauma.

James' (1989) technique, "It's just not fair," involves a child being able to voice these words out loud. Hypnotically this can be done by helping the child to find a place to yell these words in his or her imagination. In spontaneous trance the child often yells these words during play by using action figures to do the yelling. This is often a first step in expressing upset, as it is projected onto the action figure. Ideally, the child must own the affect as his or her own for full resolution of symptoms. Yelling with the child and modeling the voice tone, verbal expressiveness, and non-verbal expressiveness, enhances this technique.

Janet utilized substitution of inert or new memories to replace fixed images and sensations that were maintaining PTSD symptoms during this phase. The "sandwich" procedure refers to pacing the hypnotic intervention so that one begins with safety, does some uncovery work, and ends with safety.

During Phase Three, children rehearse techniques for using their new behaviors in the future. Creating stories about school, home or friend-related places where the child can provide new solutions to old scenarios helps to integrate new learning and growth from the understanding of the trauma experience. I am reminded of a very bright 6-year-old who told the story, "Candy Land: the bad side of town." In his story he mastered his fears by turning each figure from the child's board game into a bad guy and then destroying it. Each technique, of course, must be adapted to the developmental age of the child and personalized for the best results. Jeff, the child burned by the turkey grease described earlier in this chapter, loved playing baseball. The hypnotic suggestion to swing the bat at the pitcher's throws during his debridement and physical rehabilitation stages worked best for him because it was a personal, familiar, and an action memory.

Using hypnosis for the treatment of trauma in children is a natural integration of the active play that children prefer, spontaneous trance, and the dissociative experiences of trauma. Clinicians can utilize their knowledge of hypnotic phenomenon to assess trauma and to treat trauma using a phase-oriented paradigm. In the hands of an experienced clinician, hypnosis is a valuable and, I believe necessary, tool for the successful treatment of trauma in children. In order to remove the monsters that lurk under the bed, to conquer demons and slay dragons we must first walk with the child into the metaphorical closet and enter "Narnia" where all things are possible.

Caveats

Go slowly—The traumatized developing child is frightened of the dependence required to feel safe. Children need to be soothed. They have few self-soothing behaviors.

Unless you get to the affect—the emotion—no change in behavior is likely to occur.

Abreactions that lead to change do not always occur in the office. In fact, with children they often happen at home or school. Prepare yourself, the child, and his or her parents for this possible occurrence.

Resources

www.childtrauma.org—This is the website for Bruce Perry's work. In particular, *see* free course downloads available on the website.

www.sanctuaryweb.com

Sandra L. Bloom (2000). "Treating Traumatized Patients and Victims of Violence," with R. P. Kluft and D. Kinzie. In C. E. Bell, (Ed.) *Psychiatric Perspectives of Violence: Issues in Prevention and Treatment: New Directions for Mental Health Services #86*. San Francisco, CA: Jossey-Bass.

References

Abu-Saba, M. (1999). War-related trauma and stress characteristics of American University of Beirut students. *Journal of Traumatic Stress*, 12, 1, 201–208.

American Psychiatric Association. (2000). *Diagnostic and statistical manual of mental disorders–Text revision* (4th ed.). Washington, D.C.: Author.

Apfel, R., & Simon, B. (Eds.). (1996). *Minefields in their hearts*. New Haven, CT: Yale University Press.

Bar-On, D. (1996). Attempting to overcome the intergenerational transmission of trauma. In Apfel, R. & Simon, B. (Eds.), *Minefields in their hearts* (pp. 165–188). New Haven, CT: Yale University Press.

Bloom, S., & Reichert, M. (1998). *Bearing witness: Violence and collective responsibility*. Binghamton, NY: Haworth Press.

Boik, B. L., & Goodwin, E. A. (2000). *Sandplay therapy: A step-by-step manual for psychotherapists of diverse orientations.* New York: W.W. Norton.

Braun, B. G. (1988). The BASK model of dissociation: Clinical applications. *Dissociation* Vol. 1, No. 2, 16–23.

Briere, J. (2003). *Fact sheet for mental health professionals working with Acute Traumatic Stress.* Retrieved April, 28, 2003 from http://www.johnbriere.com/fact_sheet.htm.

Brooks, B., & Siegel, P. (1996). *The scared child.* New York: Wiley & Sons.

Brown, D. P., & Fromm, E. (1986). *Hypnotherapy and hypnoanalysis.* Hillsdale, NJ: Lawrence Erlbaum.

Cardeña, E. (2000). Hypnosis in the treatment of trauma. *The International Journal of Clinical and Experimental Hypnosis.* 48, 2, 225–238.

Daly, O. (2004). *Stresspoints.* Spring, 18(2), 4.

Dahl, S,, Mutapcic, A., & Schei, B. (1998). Traumatic events and predictive factors for posttraumatic symptoms in displaced Bosnian women in a war zone. *Journal of Traumatic Stress,* 11, 1, 137–145.

De Zulueta, F. (1993). *From pain to violence.* Northvale, NJ: Jason Aronson.

Eth, S., & Pynoos, R. (1985). *Post traumatic stress disorder in children.* Washington, D.C.: American Psychiatric Press.

Ferren, P. (1999). Comparing perceived self-efficacy among adolescent Bosnian and Croatian refugees with and without posttraumatic stress disorder. *Journal of Traumatic Stress,* 12, 3, 405–420.

Friedman, M. (2003). *Post traumatic stress disorder: The latest assessment and treatment strategies.* Kansas City, MO: Compact Clinicals.

Garbarino, J., Kostelny, K., & Dubrow, N. (1991). *No place to be a child.* San Francisco: Jossey-Bass.

Garber, S., Garber, M., & Spizman, R. (1993). *Monsters under the bed and other childhood fears.* New York: Villard Press.

Gil, E. (1998). *Play therapy for severe psychological trauma* [Videotape and Manual]. New York: Guilford Press.

Hadi, F. & Llabre, M. (1998). The Gulf crisis experience of Kuwaiti children: Psychological and cognitive factors. *Journal of Traumatic Stress*, 11, 1, 45–56.

Herman, J. (1992). *Trauma and recovery*. New York: Basic Books.

James, B. (1989). *Treating traumatized children*. Lexington, MA: Heath.

Janet, P. (1889). *L'automatisme psychologique*. (*The psychological automatism*) Paris: Balliere.

Kapor-Stanulovic, N. (1999). Encounter with suffering: Socioeconomic transition, wars, and children–A reminder. *American Psychologist*, 54, 11, 1020–1027.

Kirsch, I. and Lynn, S. (1999). Automaticity in clinical psychology. *American Psychologist*, 54, 7, 504–515.

Kluft, R.P. (Ed.) (1985). *Childhood antecedents of multiple personality*. Washington, D.C.: American Psychiatric Press.

Kluft, R. P. (1993). Basic principles in conducting the psychotherapy of multiple personality disorder. In R. P. Kluft & C. G. Fine (Eds.). *Clinical perspectives on multiple personality disorder*. Washington, D.C.: American Psychiatric Press.

Layne, C. (1998). *School based mental health intervention program in Bosnia-Herzegovina: Preliminary findings*. Paper presented at the ISTSS XIV Annual Meeting, Washington, D.C.

LeBaron, S., & Hilgard, J. R. (1984). *Hypnotherapy of pain in children with cancer*. Los Altos, CA: William Kaufmann.

Lewis, C. S. (1950). *The chronicles of Narnia: The lion, the witch and the wardrobe*. London: Geoffrey Bles.

Linden, J. (1996). Trauma prevention: Hypnoidal techniques with the chronically ill child. In *Munich lectures on hypnosis and psychotherapy*. Peter, B., Trenkle, B., Kinzel, F. C., Duffner, C., & Iost-Peter, A. (Eds.) (pp. 15–26). Hypnosis International Monographs No.2. Munich: MEG-Stiftung. Also in: *Hypnos*. Wikstrom, P.O. (Ed.) 1996, xxiii, 2, 65–75.

Linden, J. (1997). *Transitions: Adolescents, war and hypnosis.* Paper presented at the ISH, San Diego, CA.

Linden, J. (2003). Playful metaphors. *American Journal of Clinical Hypnosis*, 45 (3), 245–250.

Lindemann, E. (1944). Symptomatology and management of acute grief, *American Journal of Psychiatry* 101:141–148.

Linley, A. (2003). Positive adaptation to trauma: Wisdom as both process and outcome. *Journal of Traumatic Stress*, Vol. 16, No. 6, 601–610.

Marmar, C, Foy, D., Kagan, B., & Pynoos, R. (1994). An integrated approach for treating posttraumatic stress. In Pynoos, R. (Ed). *Posttraumatic stress disorder, a clinical review* (pp. 99–132). Towson, MD: Sidran Press.

Marsella, A., Friedman, M., Spain, E. (1994). Ethnocultural aspects of posttraumatic stress disorder. In Pynoos, R. (Ed.) *Posttraumatic stress disorder, a clinical review* (pp. 17–41). Towson, MD: Sidran Press.

McCann, I. L. & Pearlman, L. A. (1990). *Psychological trauma and the adult survivor: Theory, therapy, and transformation.* New York: Brunner/Mazel.

Northwood, A. (1998). *Trauma exposure, Post-traumatic symptoms, and identity in adolescent survivors of massive childhood trauma.* Center for Victims of Torture, Minneapolis, MN. Paper Session of ISTSS Conference, Washington, D.C.

Olness, K., & Kohen, D. P. (1996). *Hypnosis and hypnotherapy with children* (3rd. ed.) New York: Guilford Press.

Perry, B. (2000). *Violence and childhood: How persisting fear can alter the developing child's brain.* Retrieved July 5, 2001 from http://www.childtrauma@bcm.tmc.edu

Perry, B. (2006, March 27). *Understanding dissociative adaptations during trauma: A neuro-developmental perspective.* Paper presented at the annual meeting of the American Society of Clinical Hypnosis, Orlando, FL.

Perry, B. D., & Szalavitz, M. (January, 2007). *The boy who was raised as a dog and other stories from a child psychiatrist's notebook: What traumatized children can teach us about loss, love and healing.* New York: Basic Books.

Putnam, F. (1997). *Dissociation in children and adolescents.* New York: Guilford Press.

Pynoos, R. (Ed.) (1994a). *Posttraumatic stress disorder, a clinical review.* Towson, MD: Sidran Press.

Pynoos, R. (1994b). Traumatic stress and developmental psychopathology in children and adolescents. In *Posttraumatic stress disorder, a clinical review* (pp. 65–98). Towson, MD: Sidran Press.

Riedlmayer, A. (Producer). (1994). *Killing memory: Bosnia's cultural heritage & its destruction.* [42-minute videotape] (Distributed by the Community of Bosnia Foundation, c/o Dept. of Religion, Haverford College, Haverford, PA 19041-1392.)

Rossi, E. (1986/1993). *The psychobiology of mind-body healing* (Rev. ed.) New York: W.W. Norton.

Sells, M. (1996). *The bridge betrayed, religion and genocide in Bosnia.* Berkeley: University of California Press.

Schaefer, C. E. & O'Connor, K. J. (Eds.) (1983). *Handbook of play therapy.* New York: Wiley & Sons.

Schaefer, C. E. & Cangelosi, D. M. (Eds.) (1993). *Play therapy techniques.* Northvale, NJ: Jason Aronson.

Spiegel, H., & Spiegel, D. (1978). *Trance and treatment: Clinical uses of hypnosis.* New York: Basic Books.

Terr, L. (1990). *Too scared to cry.* New York: Harper & Row.

van der Hart, O., Brown, P., & Turco, R. (1990). Hypnotherapy for traumatic grief: Janetian and modern approaches integrated. *American Journal of Clinical Hypnosis, 32,* 4, 263–269.

van der Hart, O., Steele, K., Boon, S., & Brown, P. (1993). The treatment of traumatic memories, synthesis, realization, and integration. *Dissociation, 6,* 2/3, 162–180.

van der Kolk, B. (1987a). *Psychological trauma.* Washington D.C.: American Psychiatric Press.

van der Kolk B. (1987b). The body keeps the score: Approaches to the psychobiology of posttraumatic stress disorder. In Van der Kolk, B., McFarlane, A., Weisaeth, L. (Eds.). *Traumatic Stress* (pp. 214–241) New York: Guilford Press.

Valent, P. (1999) *Trauma and fulfillment therapy: A wholist framework.* Philadelphia, PA: Brunner/Mazel.

Watkins, J. G. (1971). The affect bridge: A hypnoanalytic technique. *International Journal of Clinical & Experimental Hypnosis*, 19, 21–27.

Watkins, H. (1980). The silent abreaction. *International Journal of Clinical & Experimental Hypnosis*, 19, 101–112.

Watkins, J. (2000). The psychodynamic treatment of combat neuroses (PTSD) with hypnosis during World War II. *International Journal of Clinical and Experimental Hypnosis*, 48, 3, 324–335.

Weine, S. & Pavkovic, I. (1995) *The project on genocide, psychiatry and witnessing. Survey of Bosnian students in the Bosnian student program.* University of Illinois at Chicago: Psychiatric Institute.

Weine, S., Becker, D., Vojvoda, D., Hodzic, E., Sawyer, M., Hyman, L., Laub, D., & McGlashan, T. (1998). Individual change after genocide in Bosnian survivors of "ethnic cleansing": Assessing personality dysfunction. *Journal of Traumatic Stress*, 11, 1, 147–154.

White, T. H. (1958). *The once and future king*. New York: G. P. Putnam's Sons.

Yehuda, R. (Ed.) (1998). *Psychological trauma*. Washington, D.C.: American Psychiatric Press.

Chapter Eight

Hypnotic Treatment of Habit Disorders

William C. Wester, II, EdD, ABPP, ABPH

What is a habit? A habit is "a recurrent, often unconscious pattern of behavior that is acquired through frequent repetition" (*American Heritage Dictionary*, 4th ed., 2000, p. 590). The word "unconscious" has continued to be a significant word in the definition when "habit" has been described by various sources over the years. The next most important word in the definition is "behavior." A habit is a behavior that is repetitious and which becomes so much a part of a person that it is done automatically without conscious thought. The therapeutic goal is to disrupt the habituated pattern of behavior by making the child more aware of the behavior contributing to the habit and affording the child a conscious choice to extinguish the behavior. Because this behavior is being driven in part at an unconscious level, hypnosis provides an excellent avenue to help the child regain control.

Children are wonderful to work with because of their ability to utilize their marvelous creative minds. They are excellent hypnotic subjects and do not come to treatment with the same baggage of myths and misconceptions as adults. They want to have fun, and as a result, hypnosis, behavioral techniques, and simple rewards all lead to high success rates. Most children are well aware that their habit behavior/disorder is part of them, and they feel unable to control that behavior.

One way to start working with the child is to ask him or her, "So why do you want to get rid of this habit?" The specific habit should be named (e.g., "So why do you want to stop pulling your hair?") It is important to elicit from the child four or five motivational statements that can be used later as part of the therapeutic hypnotic treatment strategies. Once the motivations/goals are obtained, it is easy to ask them if they would like to learn some ways to let go of this habit and gain control over their behavior. An example of a metaphor for "letting go" is the "Rice Monkey" metaphor (Bassman & Wester, 1997). The following is an abbreviated and shortened version:

> In one part of the country there is a type of monkey called a rice monkey. People in that part of the country cut holes in coconuts about the size of the hand of the average rice monkey and fill the coconuts full of rice. The rice monkeys smell the rice and come running from miles around. They stick their hand down into the coconut and get a big handful of rice but then they can't get their hand out of the coconut. The people come out from behind trees and tease and chase the monkeys. The smart monkeys quickly learn that if they just let go of the rice their hand easily comes out of the coconut and they run off to safety. The very smart monkeys not only let go of the rice and remove their hand but run away with the whole coconut to get at the rice in another way. Your subconscious mind has just learned something very important."
> (pp. 29–30)

As the therapist establishes the "yes set" he or she can begin to explain the process of hypnosis that can be augmented with behavioral charts and simple rewards. One approach to developing rapport and providing an inexpensive reward is to teach the child a simple magic trick at the end of the session. The child can be given his or her hypnotic homework of listening to their audio tape as well as asked to practice the magic trick so that on the next visit he or she can show you how he or she has started to master hypnosis and the magic trick.

Obviously the therapist must look for emotional issues and other factors during the clinical intake that might be contributing to the habit disorder. Many habits are "empty habits" and are not driven by some underlying emotional/psychodynamic factor. The habit may simply be a habituated habit. One must also rule out issues of secondary gain, habits that still serve a purpose, and habits, such as enuresis, that can be related to developmental level issues.

Working on the assumption that "all hypnosis is self-hypnosis," it makes sense to clearly convey to the child that he or she is going to learn a skill to help himself or herself. There seem to be therapeutic advantages of audio taping the session for the child to practice at home. The eventual goal is for the child to use self-hypnosis without a tape but initially using a tape can be reinforcing and consistent with a learning model. This is not a new idea. Gardner and Olness (1981) describe machine-aided induction techniques but also stress that they prefer that children achieve full independence in using hypnosis. Because of the informed consent issues it is important to inform the parent(s) of your treatment objective in using an audio tape. This is also the appropriate time to request that the parent(s) let you work with their child and that their role is just supportive. The parent who has been bribing his or her child to no avail is usually eager to back off during your treatment. It is a good idea to include an introduction at the beginning of the tape to make it clear who has control. For example, "Since I am making this tape for you I want you to remember that you are in total and complete control at all times. If for any reason at any time you need to stop your hypnosis before the end of the tape, just open your eyes and you will be totally and completely alert. For example, if the phone or doorbell rings, or you need to open your eyes for any other reason—just do so and allow yourself to be fully alert. You can then use your tape at some other time."

Hypnosis can be used with children to treat habit disorders, such as body hair pulling, tics, thumb/finger sucking, nail and cuticle biting/picking, tongue thrusting, speech problems, enuresis/encopresis, overeating, bruxism, self-stimulatory behaviors such as head banging/body rocking, nose picking, and other clinically diagnosed habit disorders. The reader is referred to an interesting article by Harte, Vick, and Boyse (2005) entitled "Bad Habits/Annoying Behaviors." This article provides a good summary of various bad habits and annoying behaviors including less frequently seen habit problems, such as nose picking, teeth grinding, tics, breath holding, and unusual form of masturbation. The authors also suggest a variety of non-hypnotic treatment suggestions, such as ignoring the habit behavior, praising good behavior, making changes slowly and one at a time, redirecting behaviors, and following through with natural consequences.

When it is time to begin your hypnotic intervention remember the child's own motivations stated during your clinical intake interview and begin to develop your therapeutic strategies. You have many choices as to strategies depending on the personality of the child and the ways in which the motivations to change the habit behaviors were expressed. The therapist may choose a paradoxical approach, whereby the child briefly increases the habit and then decreases the habit to emphasize that the child has now regained control. If the child can increase the symptom (not for use with a tape recorded session) he or she can decrease the symptom. The therapist can use a variety of direct suggestions aimed at stopping the behavior. Iglesias (2003) describes three cases of trichotillomania that were treated with direct hypnotic suggestion with emphasis on sensitizing and alerting the patients to impending scalp hair pulling behaviors. Like the vignette presented in this chapter, the patients become free to choose to pull or resist the impulse to pull. This approach, augmented by forming contracts with the parents to relinquish their authority as related to the patients' hair (as noted above), provided effective treatment that extinguished the hair pulling. The only downside to the direct approach is that it can sometimes backfire, and if the behavior does not stop, the therapist has lost credibility and the child becomes discouraged. As Iglesias (2003) noted, allowing the patient to be free to choose, solves this problem. Deemphasizing the symptom, shifting the symptom, re-labeling the symptom, or using ideomotor signaling to see if the child wants to give up the symptom have all been described in the early literature (Minuchin, 1974; Gardner & Olness, 1981; Reaney, 1991).

I have had excellent results using the child's stated motivations, reframing techniques, and working with issues of awareness and control. The following vignette, under Trichotillomania (hair pulling), illustrates my approach.

Trichotillomania (Hair Pulling)

Recurrent hair pulling of the scalp, pubic hair, eyelashes or eyebrows are examples of what would be diagnosed in this category. Reaney (1991) indicates that the pulling may be a symptom of anxiety or of some other more serious emotional problem. Zalsman, Hermesh, & Sever (2001) report on three adolescents who responded to Ericksonian suggestions. The adolescents described their hair as weak and vulnerable and in need of protection. "In therapy, the patient was assigned the role of 'patron of the hair' thereby giving him/her control of the situation" (p. 64). Some children ingest the hair but most discard the hair and then try to cover up the bald spot left behind. My own experience suggests that boys tend to pull more on the sides of their head and girls pull mid-line top scalp. They both try to disguise the pulling. There is no question that tension, anger, stress, frustration, boredom, and anxiety can contribute to this problem. Remember that hypnosis is only a tool, and we must rely on our clinical experience and judgment.

Clinical Vignette

T.S.

T.S., an 11-year-old boy, presented as having trichotillomania. He was an A student, "I have never gotten a B," and was in a gifted program. He says his hair pulling is due to tension, frustration, and feeling bored in school. His pulling was top center, and he combs his hair over the bald spot to hide his problem. When asked why he wanted to stop pulling he replied, "It's annoying, humiliating, and it sometimes hurts." He had tried to stop by holding something in his left hand [*his pulling hand*] and his parents tried to bribe him with money to stop. He pulls less in the summer. T.S. loved using the computer, watching *Star Wars*, reading, and playing soccer. We discussed misconceptions, and then he asked, "How are you going to use my subconscious mind to help me stop this habit?" This question was a clear indicator of how bright this child was. I responded, "We are going to work together as a team. It is my job to help you learn a new skill that you can then use to help yourself."

W. Wester [WW]: Just close your eyes, keeping your eyes closed as I talk with you. Since I am making this tape for you let me put a reminder right at the beginning of the tape that you're in complete control at all times. If for any reason at any time while listening to this tape you would need to stop this state of hypnotic relaxation before the end of the tape you can simply open your eyes and do so. Knowing that and knowing that you are in total and complete control use this time as your special time that you have set aside for yourself to help yourself accomplish a very important goal.

I would like to start now by having you take a couple of moments to get in touch with the best thing we all have going for us to help us relax and that is your whole breathing process. Obviously we all breathe, we do that automatically, we don't think about it very much. If you think about your breathing for just a moment you can feel some air coming into the body each time you take a breath. And you can feel just a little bit of air just leaving the body each time you exhale. Just be aware of your very own breathing pattern. It's pleasant and it's regular and comfortable. That breathing process can just begin to help you to relax so comfortably and so easily now.

And then I would like you to think for a moment about the top part of your head and all the muscles in the scalp and allow those muscles to become smooth and comfortable—all across the top part of the head. And then imagine in your mind, because your mind is so creative, that you are taking like a liquid relaxation shower and instead of water coming out of the shower head it is like a wonderful liquid relaxation. The liquid relaxation comes across all of those muscles in the scalp making those muscles smooth and relaxed. And then that feeling just flows down through the body. [*At this point, a standard progressive relaxation technique is used starting from the head downward—see Chapter Five.*]

All of the muscles in the body now from the top of the head to the tip of the toes are relaxed and so comfortable. Always remember that you're in control. If you just count backwards in your mind from 5 down to zero you can let yourself relax even a little deeper. See just how relaxed you can become. And in your mind now see yourself at home. You are at home and wherever your computer is located, or the one you want to work with, allow yourself to be right there. See yourself sitting in front of your computer feeling so relaxed and comfortable now, and instead of having you talk just let me know you are there by raising one of your finger [*finger goes up*]—That's great!

Now, obviously from talking with you it is clear that you are really very good at using the computer. You are an excellent student and you like to use the computer. See yourself turning on that computer and remember that this is your very special computer in your mind. And when you have that computer turned on I would like you to feed in some information on to that computer. And what I want you to program into that computer are your reasons for wanting to stop pulling your hair. So the first thing you might want to program in is just how annoying—type that right in there—just how annoying that is and when it shows through that's just as annoying. The second reason you stated why you want to stop pulling your hair is that people ask you why or they notice it and that's kind of upsetting when that happens. The third reason is that sometimes the pulling even hurts or it presents a problem when you try to comb your hair. So just put into that computer in your mind all of those reasons of why you want to stop, because those are good reasons to stop pulling your hair.

Now that this information is in the computer we are going to give the computer some other commands. You can program this right in, type it right on the screen. The first thing that you can program on your screen is that your motivation, coming out of your own subconscious mind, to stop pulling your hair is at the highest possible level and will remain at the highest possible level. You might want to abbreviate that and just put motivation high for all of those good reasons because this is something you want to do. Secondly, put right on that special computer in your subconscious mind the fact that you are in total and complete control and you are going to feel very comfortable and confident knowing that what you are doing is good and healthy and it is appropriate for you to stop pulling your hair. So allow your subconscious mind to recognize that you are now going to be in total and complete control. You will be feeling relaxed and comfortable, feeling less tension, less stress, or other things that in the past might have contributed to you pulling your hair. There is just going to be less of that because you have learned how to relax now and you have that high motivation and that high control.

And the third thing I want you to put right on that subconscious computer in your mind is that anytime other than washing your hair or brushing your hair, combing your hair—anytime other than that—when your hand moves up towards your head and your hair, your

167

subconscious mind will let your conscious mind know immediately that you are doing that. So your subconscious mind will tell you immediately that your arm and hand is moving up toward your hair and instead of pulling, as in the past without being aware of it, now every time your hand moves up towards your hair your subconscious mind will immediately tell your conscious mind what is happening and that will let you become aware and stop that movement. That will be your special skill and you will get better and better at doing that [*learning model with emphasis on practice*].

Now even though this may sound a little strange on the tape, you will know what I am doing. Remain in this very comfortable state now and I am just going to come around and move your left arm and hand. I want you to notice now as I move the left arm and hand, the arm and hand start to come up towards the hair, notice what the subconscious mind is doing. It's making you very aware of that hand coming up, and so when the hand moves in that direction, like it has in the past, and certainly by the time it actually touches the hair your subconscious mind will tell your conscious mind that you need to stop and that will really feel good [*child experiences this feeling*]. You will feel proud being so much in control. [*I lower the child's arm.*] And when you listen to your tape you will be able to remember what I just did and while using the tape if you want to "test it out" that's OK. You can actually lift your hand when you hear that part but you don't have to because you know what I did to help you understand.

Allow that computer now to do one more thing. Just program into the computer, before we shut it off, that your behavior from this point forward is going to be even better than it has been during the summer because in the summer you have pulled very little. So put that right into the computer. However you want to shorten that is fine. What I want you to do right now—get ready to turn that computer off. Now, before you turn your computer off, run a printout for your subconscious and conscious mind. So it's right there permanently in your subconscious mind, and as soon as it is in your subconscious mind let me know by moving a finger. [*Finger moves.*] That's great! And that's part of you now, and your subconscious mind is just going to begin helping you quickly, almost immediately, and by listening to this tape a few times you will develop this skill so well that you won't even need the tape. All of your hair pulling will stop in a short period of time—perhaps immediately. [*The trance is terminated at this point with a 1-5 counting approach with reinforcement.*]

During the post-hypnotic period I asked T.S. how he felt: "It was kind of weird but I am totally relaxed and my arm got heavy. And when my arm came up it kept flashing in my mind don't, don't, don't, don't." T.S. was instructed to use the tape every other day and complete a behavioral chart. He put an "X" in each day that there was no pulling of any kind. He returned in two weeks with all "X's" on his chart and said that he was now in control. I followed his progress for six months, and there was no relapse.

Elimination Disorders: Enuresis/Encopresis

The elimination disorders are discussed in detail by Linda Thomson in Chapter Seventeen. For an example of another clinical vignette *see* Wester & O'Grady, 1991, pp. 92–94. This example was of a 7-year-old girl, who presented as having an uninhibited neurogenic bladder with an incompetent urethra. Her enuresis was both during the day and at night. A rag doll induction technique was used along with the imagery of a favorite toy. Muscles in the bladder were associated with the muscles used when making a fist. This basic approach together with suggestions of motivation, control, and success were sufficient to stop the enuresis. In addition to hypnotic suggestions, an inexpensive watch with an alarm was used for one week during the day while the child was at school. The teacher understood the problem and permitted the child to use the bathroom each time the alarm went off. The alarm was first set for 15-minute intervals but was soon extended to 30-minute intervals. After two days the child was able to complete a class before going to the bathroom. Within a week the daytime enuresis was extinguished.

Thumb/Finger Sucking

Thumb or finger sucking generally starts within the first few months of life and is very common. In fact, with prenatal ultrasounds we know that some babies frequently begin sucking their thumbs in *utero*. As children develop, many of them replace the thumb or finger with a pacifier or a favorite blanket that is called a variety of names. This habit rarely poses a problem prior to pre-school. The basis for the thumb or finger sucking that continues generally has roots centered in anxiety or oral needs. This habit behavior is frequently tolerated by the parents, as well as peers, until the child starts elementary school. As with all habit disorders, hypnosis can be helpful if the child wants to stop. Motivation and control once again become the significant issues.

Suggestions of how to control this habit vary greatly. Ellis & Roberts (2005) state that approximately 25–50% of 2-year-old children suck their thumbs. This statistic drops to 15–20% of 5- to 6-year-old children. Just like the trichotillomania narrative in this chapter the child can be made more aware of the movement of his or her hand toward the face. The movement of the hand can be a cue to go off to a favorite place. Reaney (1991) describes a technique that appeals to the child's desire to grow up by raising the question of how soon the child will be grown up enough to stop sucking. Many techniques of a paradoxical nature are described in the literature, such as specific times to suck, giving equal time to each finger, and actually scolding the "bad thumb." A negative approach is described by Crasilneck & Hall (1985) where a child is told under hypnosis "that the thumb will begin to taste bitter, and that this will act as a reminder that he or she no longer wishes to suck the thumb" (p. 185). Sugarman prescribes the symptom and tells the child to go ahead and suck his or her thumb and to notice how the mouth and thumb feel so comfortable. He then states that the rest of the body doesn't get to feel this comfortable feeling: "So as you slowly disengage your thumb from your mouth, as your thumb moves away, your whole body feels better." (Laurence I. Sugarman, personal communication, May 2006).

Returning to the premise that if the child wants to stop he or she can express his or her motivation as to why stopping is important, and then this information can be utilized within hypnotic age-appropriate techniques.

Nail/Cuticle Biting

The onset of nail/cuticle biting in children is usually from pre-school age to adolescence and is rare in children younger than pre-school age. The child's biting is often increased by anxiety. According to Ellis & Roberts (2005), from pre-school age to adolescence the rate of nail/cuticle biting can be as high as 45–60%. This habit can quickly become a medical concern in cases of bleeding and/or infection.

Some of the same hypnotic techniques used for thumb sucking can be used with forms of nail biting. By the time a child reaches a professional, a variety of non-hypnotic techniques have probably been used including the use of bitter chemicals, false nails, band aids, gloves, or bribes.

Children who are motivated to stop can give many of their own good reasons to stop. One child stated that she was embarrassed and wanted to grow up having pretty nails. The area around her nails was literally raw, and she experienced frequent bleeding. The key for her was to see some progress. Hypnotic techniques for relaxation, anxiety reduction, self-awareness, and self-control were given within the framework of positive imagery. During each session, instant pictures were taken of her hands and nails and sequentially placed in her scrapbook that she named "My Healthy Nails." She was seen at 2-week intervals allowing for nail growth and time for her to practice her hypnotic imagery tape. There was no relapse, and she actually bragged to people (and showed them her scrapbook) about how she had used self-hypnosis to stop biting her nails.

Overeating/Obesity

Let us be clear from the beginning that, like obsessive compulsive disorders, overeating is a difficult problem for children, adolescents, and adults alike. There are so many variables that can affect the child's progress including the fact that weight loss does not occur in a smooth curve. If you prepare the child/adolescent for that fact that there may be setbacks in the progress you will be ahead of the game. By reinforcing your gains with ego-strengthening techniques and using a variety of behavior modification approaches, you should see continued progress (Russ, 1987).

There have been reports of unsuccessful and successful results in the literature. I have treated many children and adolescents who are obese with no negative effects other than that only 50% reach their goal weight. Parental pressure, social and peer pressure, and self-image and self-concept issues are among the reasons listed as to why they want to loose weight. We are in a cultural time where "thin" is "in" and many adolescents end up with the opposite problem of anorexia or bulimia. The therapist must be extremely careful when wording hypnotic suggestion to lose weight so that one problem is not traded for another.

I believe that it is essential to combine various cognitive and behavioral techniques, such as progress charts and graphs, which can be used to monitor the progress and provide for visual and emotional reinforcement. On the second visit, I record the session and ask the child/adolescent to use the tape at least every other day (Wester & O'Grady, 1991). The first session is usually taken up with clinical intake data, discovering the stated motivation to change, and an initial hypnotic induction to introduce the child/adolescent to the hypnotic process and provide initial support and reinforcement. During the second session, we review the behavioral charts and then I make a client-specific tape using the "Historical Landmark Technique for Treating Obesity" metaphor as outlined in Hammond (1990). With younger children I use a version of this metaphor called "The Magic Castle." This has proven to be a very effective metaphor that also allows for vast individual differences.

Self-Stimulatory Behaviors

Self-stimulatory behaviors in children and adolescents, such as body-rocking and head banging, are usually benign but are generally worrisome to parents. Ellis & Roberts (2005) report a frequency of 3–19% of developmentally normal children who engage in some form of self-stimulatory behavior. Some authors include masturbation in this category. When masturbation is not developmentally or age appropriate professional advice may be warranted. Age, maturity level, developmental issues, and frequency are variables that might qualify masturbation as a self-stimulatory behavior.

Hypnosis can be used when these habits keep children and adolescents from other childhood activities or become public or obsessive. Children can learn to feel stimulation and body movements hypnotically. This is accomplished hypnotically with imagery of rocking movement, such as being on a boat or in a chair. The child or adolescent can be taught to substitute imagery of a favorite place or some self-directed cue, like squeezing the thumb and index finger together, for the actual self-stimulatory behavior. Trading off gross body movements for less obvious movements like finger tapping might be another approach that can be reinforced with hypnosis (Reaney, 1991).

Stammering/Stuttering

Crasilneck & Hall (1985) place emphasis on decreasing fear and tension followed by reassuring statements, such as "Your speech will be soft, secure, and you will be much more relaxed and at ease, pleased that you can speak without stammering or stuttering" (p. 249). Stammering and stuttering is a problem that affects a significant number of children with the typical onset between the ages of 3 and 5. Many patients with this problem respond very well to speech therapy and psychotherapy. The degree of the problem varies and a percentage of children simply outgrow the problem.

Just like certain anxieties, patients who begin to fear the fear itself, the child who stammers or stutters fearfully anticipates his or her problem, thus making the problem more likely to occur (Reaney, 1991). Neurological problems must be ruled out before moving forward with hypnosis because the common view is that stammering/stuttering has a physiological basis. Hypnotic relaxation techniques can be used in combination with speech therapy to break the stammering/stuttering–anxiety–more stammering/

stuttering cycle. There are new mechanical devices available, similar to hearing aids, which are supposed to modify physical factors that affect speech, thereby giving the brain the ability to more effectively control the movement of speech muscles. Frequently, the harder the child tries to stop stammering or stuttering, the worse it becomes. Paradoxical techniques can be used to emphasize the issue of control and self-hypnosis. If a child can make the symptom worse he or she can learn to make it better. He or she can learn to trigger the relaxation response by a post-hypnotic cue. I utilize a 10-point speech scale (similar to the 10-point pain scale) to help the child realize that he or she is slowly gaining control over his or her problem.

Tics

Children and adolescents presenting with tic behavior usually have some underlying issues. Tics are noticed in a multitude of ways, almost as many varieties as there are muscles in the body. Tics of the upper extremities are seen most frequently; however, major body tics can also occur. Treatment approaches are like those for all habit disorders, but it is usually more difficult for the child to verbalize why the tic is happening. He or she usually wants to rid himself or herself of the tic. A good beginning approach is to use ideomotor signaling to see how much of the tic the child is willing to give up. I have seen children who have demonstrated with ideomotor signaling their willingness to immediately give up 50% or more of the tic behavior.

After ruling out possible medical explanations for the tic, hypnosis provides a marvelous way to interact with the child's creative mind. In one case, after ruling out a psychomotor seizure disorder for lip smacking, I used self-enhancing imagery along with suggestions for control and mastery. This 9-year-old girl was motivated to wear lip gloss. This imagery was supported under hypnosis and what had once been a strong habituated behavior extinguished quickly. I used behavioral charts and positive reinforcement—after a month of "stars" on her chart I gave her an inexpensive make-up kit (Gardner & Olness, 1981; Reaney, 1991).

In addition to the habit disorders discussed, other habit disorders include voice problems, intractable cough, sleep walking, tremors, habituated drug abuse, neurodermatitis, smoking, and bruxism. Most of these disorders are treatable with hypnosis. I offer the following treatment outline as a model for dealing with habit disorders:

1. Do a thorough intake interview and rule out any physiological bases for the presenting habit (e.g., seizure disorder).
2. Assess obvious and underlying psychological dynamics contributing to the habit (e.g., secondary gain issues).
3. Elicit the child or adolescent's own motivations for wanting to decrease or stop the habit (e.g., "I don't want the other kids to laugh at me anymore.")
4. Establish a "team" work approach and dispel hypnotic myths by using the "learning" model (e.g., "It's going to be fun learning how to stop your habit.")
5. Choose a hypnotic induction consistent with the child's age and other variable, such as intelligence and personality (e.g., you can use direct suggestions, indirect suggestions, imagery, etc.)
6. Develop your hypnotic strategies and incorporate those strategies and suggestions into the methods you have selected (e.g., "This child may need ego-strengthening, relaxation, etc.)
7. Reinforce, using the method you have selected, the child or adolescent's motivations as described to you pre-hypnotically (e.g., "I want to be normal again.")
8. You can't go wrong stressing motivation and control (e.g., "Each day and in every way you will become more and more in control.")
9. Use adjunctive approaches as appropriate (e.g., behavioral charts, graphs, and audio tapes.)
10. Have the child or adolescent practice, practice, practice his or her new self-hypnosis until the skill is mastered and the habit behavior has been extinguished. The professional should then follow-up as needed.

References

The American Heritage Dictionary of the English Language (4th ed.). 2000.
Boston: Houghton Mifflin.

American Psychiatric Association (1994). *Diagnostic and statistical manual*
(4th ed.). Washington, D.C.: American Psychiatric Press.

Bassman, S. W., & Wester, W. C. (1997). *Hypnosis, headache and pain
control*. Chicago: American Society of Clinical Hypnosis Press.

Crasilneck, H. B., & Hall, J. H. (1985). *Clinical hypnosis: Principle and
applications* (2nd ed.). New York: Grune & Stratton.

Ellis, C. R., & Roberts, H. J. *Childhood habit behaviors and stereotypic
movement disorders*. eMedicine Journal [serial online] 2005. Available at
http://www.emedicine.com/ped/topic909.htm. (Retrieved March 30,
2006).

Gardner, G. G., & Olness, K. (1981). *Hypnosis and hypnotherapy with
children*. New York: Grune & Stratton.

Hammond, D. C., et al. (Ed.) (1990). *Handbook of hypnotic suggestions and
metaphors*. New York: W.W. Norton.

Harte, K., Vick, S., & Boyse, K. (2005). *Bad annoying behaviors*. University
of Michigan Health Systems. Available at: www.med.umich.edu/
1libr/yourchild/badhabit.htm. (Retrieved March 29, 2006).

Iglesias, A. (2003). Hypnosis as a vehicle for choice and self-agency in
the treatment of children with trichotillomania. *American Journal of
Clinical Hypnosis*, 46(2), 129–137.

Minuchin, S. (1974). *Families and family therapy*. Cambridge, MA:
Harvard University Press.

Reaney, J. B. (1991). Hypnosis in the treatment of habit disorders. In W.
Wester & A. Smith (Eds.), *Clinical hypnosis: A multidisciplinary approach*.
Philadelphia: Lippincott.

Russ, W. (1987). Hypnosis in the treatment of obesity. In W. Wester
(Ed.), *Clinical hypnosis: A case management approach*. Cincinnati, OH: BSCI
Publications.

Wester, W., & O'Grady, D. (Eds.). (1991). *Clinical hypnosis with children.* New York: Brunner/Mazel.

Wester W. C., & Smith, A. (Eds.). (1991). *Clinical hypnosis: A multidisciplinary approach.* Cincinnati, OH: BSCI Publications.

Zalsman, G., Hermesh, H, & Sever, J. (2001). Hypnotherapy in adolescents with trichotillomania. *American Journal of Clinical Hypnosis,* 44(1), 63-68.

Chapter Nine

Depression

Daniel P. Kohen, MD, ABMH

The Beginning of the Story...

B

B was 5¾ years old when he was referred by his pediatrician for help with behavioral concerns. Both long-standing and recently escalating, his problems were characterized by his mother as "cyclical since 18 months of age, including "out of control, unpredictable behaviors during which he acts detached, anxious, sad, suicidal, engages in repetitive thinking and religious/theological talk, and has trouble sleeping." A strongly positive history of anxiety, depression, and bipolar disorder on both sides of the family, and a history of depression and suicide attempts in her own adolescence lead *B*'s mother to, as she said, "fear the worst." She called her pediatrician stating that she "desperately" wanted to protect *B* and to prevent serious problems in his future.

Within a few minutes of our initial visit, *B* reflected a rather normative escalation of excitement as well as the ability to calm himself with help. During the first 15 minutes, *B* began to behave in a very silly fashion. When I asked him to come over to stand close to me, he did so readily, and calmed promptly when I asked him directly to "Please put the 'sillies' away...." The effectiveness of this approach was not lost on his mom, with whom I later reviewed this brief but important interlude. In it he/we had demonstrated both *his* ability for self-control and the important ability he had to take cues from adults around him [*thus modeling for his mom what she could, should, and would ultimately learn to, in turn, model for B*].

When he was in preschool, B's teacher thought he wasn't ready to move ahead and developed a "special behavioral modification program only for him," and told B's parents that "...he [B] doesn't do boundaries very well," and could be "slightly autistic." This was, predictably, terribly frightening for the family. Another previous observer had told B's parents that he "might have pervasive developmental disorder (PDD)." In response to this historical information I told B's mother that after my two observations over 1.5 hours I did not believe that B showed *any* evidence of an autism spectrum disorder or PDD. Indeed, B was quite appropriate, bright, verbal, and highly interactive, reflecting normal social reciprocity for his age. He responded appropriately to social cues around him. He took and responded to directions appropriately and was very likeable. His mom expressed concern about what she called "cycling" abnormal behavior. She explained that "B is a rule-bound boy...extraordinarily so...BUT, when he is in those periods it doesn't appear that there's those internal controls in those periods...there is no self-control then... It's continuous, he's hyper, he'll be spinning around...you can't get through."

As she spoke about this, B's mom became increasingly tense, catastrophizing with "What about when he's 12 years old, how will this be manifest then....even if it's not worst-case-scenario you know, manic depression or schizophrenia...I'm a worrier, I want to get it under control and try to control it and fix it...But no one so far has any understanding of the trigger to these episodes...," which start somehow and then "spiral downwards (for hours, days) before they finally stop." B's mom became increasingly agitated, tearful, sat forward, and was defensive and challenging, saying that it was "very hard to come and tell this whole story again to yet another doctor...."

So, how might hypnotic thinking, talking, and processes be of help in approaching and helping B and his mother?

Terms and Types of Diagnoses

This chapter presents an approach to thinking hypnotically about children, and hypnotically helping children and youth to help themselves when they are sad. The approach and conceptualization will apply in form and substance whether that sadness is from the various episodes of grief and bereavement which young people often experience, from periodic and/or prolonged sad mood as in the very common condition of adjustment disorder (e.g., to chronic illness) with depression/depressed mood, from dysthymia, from major depressive disorder (MDD), or from bipolar disorder, or some other form of sadness.

The *DSM-PC Diagnostic and Statistical Manual for Primary Care* (*DSM-PC*) (1996) defines and discusses *depression* in a "user friendly" manner:

> Sadness, irritability, or a loss of interest in normally pleasurable activities is a common and normal response to disappointment, failure, or loss. Such mood changes only represent a problem if they persist more than a few days and if they represent intense distress or significantly impair the child's ability to function or relate to others at home, school or play....Children and adolescents *may not present with sadness, but may report aches and pains, low energy, or moods such as apathy, irritability or even anxiety.* [Italics added] (Wolraich, 1996, p. 153)

In an effort to draw a distinction between bereavement and depression, *DSM-PC* defines *bereavement*:

> Bereavement is an intense grief response after a major loss, e.g. death of parent, and is usually a normal reaction involving mood and sleep or appetite changes. When bereavement symptoms persist for longer than 2 months or are characterized by marked functional impairment, a more serious diagnosis, such as major depressive disorder, may be diagnosed. (Wolraich, 1996, p. 153)

In clinical practice the symptoms of depression and bereavement may be identical or overlap, both may be present, and in either case there may well be a need for intervention (Wolraich, 1996).

Clinicians' antennae should be tuned toward a myriad of important risk factors that may signal or influence the appearance and/or course of childhood depression. These include parental depression (including postpartum depression), strong family history of depression, early onset of a diagnosable anxiety disorder, family and marital discord, alcoholism, substance abuse, poor coping skills, lack of social support, early childhood losses, uncertainty about sexual orientation and a history of previous depressive episodes (Wolraich, 1996).

Depression is 1.5 to 3 times more common among first-degree biological relatives of persons with MDD than in the general population. Depression occurs in approximately 2% of children and 4%–8% of adolescents (American Academy of Child and Adolescent Psychiatry, 1998) with MDD being twice as prevalent in adolescent girls as in adolescent boys. (Emslie, Weinberg, Rush, Adams, & Rintelmann, 1990.) The prevalence of MDD in children and adolescents is said to be 2%–8% (Birmaher, Ryan, Williamson, Brent, Kaufman, Dahl, et al, 1996a). With an estimated 38,000,000 Americans between the ages of 6 and 15 years, 2%–8% represents between 750,000 and 3,040,000 million young people who may meet *DSM-IV* criteria for the diagnosis of MDD.

Review of Literature

In a recent literature review, Kohen and Murray (2006) noted the absence of prevalence data for other forms of depressed mood/ sadness in children and youth. Considering the many different diagnostic categories into which children with sadness and depressed mood problems fall, they estimated it is likely that there are at least 7 to 10 million children with significant symptoms of depression and depressed mood (p. 191). There is little to no epidemiologic information about the prevalence of varying other, and likely more common, forms of depression/depressed mood (e.g., adjustment disorder with depressed mood, dysthymia, grief, and bereavement.) One study (Garland, Hough, McCabe, Yeh, Wood, & Aarons, 2001) identified children from five public sectors of care in San Diego including alcohol and drug services, child welfare, juvenile justice, mental health, and public school services for youths with serious emotional disturbances. Major depression was identified in 8.9%, 4.7%, 4.7%, 5.7%, and 7.9% respectively or overall in 5.1%. The less severe—although more ongoing—

diagnosis of dysthymia was identified in only 0.5% (Garland et al. 2001).

It seems reasonable to predict that the more indolent, "less severe" diagnosis of dysthymia might well "fly beneath the radar" and not be identified as involved in services in these sectors, Also not included in these data are, of course, those large numbers of youth with other expressions or kinds of depression and depressed mood who may be served in private or community mental health-care, or who have otherwise been simply and sadly unrecognized. As Kohen and Murray (2006) observed, "Particularly when we understand the accelerating prevalence of problems which chil-dren encounter that may be best characterized as adjustment dis-order with depressed mood, it is not unreasonable to consider that, as with the adult population, sadness and depression in chil-dren and youth are of large and still growing proportions" (p. 191).

Research supporting the use of self-hypnosis/hypnosis in treating depression is lacking and pertinent research involving children and adolescents is practically non-existent. A search of Medline and PsychInfo databases for "depression" and "hypnosis" identi-fied studies directed at the treatment of another illness with changes in mood reported as a secondary outcome, if at all (Kohen & Murray, 2006, p. 193). The specific value of hypnotherapeutic approaches for depressive symptoms associated with other ill-nesses was described for youth with irritable bowel syndrome (Gonsalkorale, Miller, Afazl, & Whorwell, 2003) and children with chronic pain (Zeltzer, Tsao, Stelling, Powers, Levy, & Waterhouse, 2002).

As Yapko (2006) observed, "Depression in children was histori-cally considered so unlikely that no such category was included in diagnostic classification systems until *DSM–IV*. As a result, the sci-entific literature on children's depression is underdeveloped" (p. 213–214). In addition to the obvious need for increased research in depression in children and adolescents, there is clearly a need for prospective trials of self-hypnosis in the treatment of depres-sion, especially in children and adolescents. Yapko (1992; 2001) has extensively addressed how hypnosis may be appropriately inte-grated with cognitive behavioral therapies for depression.

Clinical Diagnosis and Strategies

The clinical diagnosis of sadness/sad mood/depression begins with an understanding of parental (and/or school) observations and concerns. Signs and symptoms should trigger the clinician to wonder about the possibility of depression as either a primary or contributing cause or concern related to the presenting complaint. In children and adolescents the so-called classical or typical "vegetative" signs of depression (low energy, hypersomnolence, sad mood, and apathy) are much less common than they are in adults. More commonly—and one of the reasons that forms of depression diagnoses have for so long been under- or undiagnosed—is that children reflect signs and symptoms that are vague, or more subtle. It becomes our challenge, therefore, to increase our proverbial "index of suspicion." In addition to recognizing what is "typically" or "obviously" diagnostic of depression, we need to attend to more subtle cues and suggestions that have not traditionally alerted us. These should capture our attention and lead us to additional diagnostic inquiries and/or evaluations that identify those children in need of intervention.

In *DSM–PC* (p. 156) a "sadness problem" is defined and offers guidance regarding the kinds of symptoms that should indeed get our attention in clinical practice. Symptoms of a sadness problem may include irritable or sad mood, diminished interest or pleasure in usual activities (in this regard clinicians and parents should be alert to the reality that *any* new and especially sustained behavior may indeed be a sign or symptom of as yet unrecognized or undiagnosed depression or depressed mood; weight loss or gain or failure to make developmentally appropriate expected weight gains, insomnia or hypersomnia, psychomotor agitation or retardation, fatigue or energy loss, feelings of worthlessness or excessive or inappropriate guilt, diminished ability to think or concentrate.

Perhaps even more importantly, in school-aged children (6–12 years old) commonly occurring, recurrent, and/or persistent somatic complaints, such as chronic or recurrent headaches, or recurrent abdominal pain may well represent the first indication that the clinician should begin to consider and inquire about depressed mood and related feelings. Additionally, it is essential to keep in mind that while bereavement is normal, symptoms from bereavement that are intense and/or prolonged (e.g., beyond 2 months) may well benefit from further evaluation and intervention whether or not they officially qualify for a diagnosis of a "depressed" state.

With this grounding in mind, it behooves clinicians to refine their thinking accordingly in order to trust their clinical judgment and intuition when first noticing, and then thinking about, kids being sad. Ultimately this means developing personal confidence and comfort while acknowledging the importance of making time to ask kids to talk about sad feelings, and to consider implementation and utilization of various screening tools to support and verify one's clinical and diagnostic perspectives.

Beyond the valued use of the *DSM–PC* (Wolraich, 1996) as a resource, useful diagnostic tools include the *Child Depression Inventory (CDI)* (Kovacs, 1992), the *Beck Depression Inventory (BDI)* (Beck, Steer, & Brown, 1996), the *Achenbach Child Behavioral Checklist* (parent–CBCL), and the *Achenbach Youth Self Report (YSR)* (Achenbach, 1991), and the *Pediatric Symptom Checklist* (Jellinek et al., 1988). Kohen and Murray (2006) have recently described the use of these as adjuncts to clinical evaluation (pp. 192–193). Their particular value seems to be in situations where the child's clinical presentation doesn't seem at first to be depression. When, upon further consideration, the clinician's index of suspicion rises, such tools may be very helpful. As Kohen and Murray (2006) note, "…one should never rely only on such inventories to arrive at a diagnosis of depression or depressed mood" (p. 192).

If depression is suspected clinically, appropriate and timely therapeutic intervention should proceed, even if one of these inventories yields a "normal" result (Birmaher, Brent & Benson, 1998). When one clinically suspects significant depression/depressed mood, and an inventory does not support the "official" diagnosis, one should nonetheless proceed, of course, to provide appropriate supportive and therapeutic intervention. Thus, as we consider how best to craft hypnotic approaches to help young people manage sad feelings, it is, of course, essential to honor and ensure their awareness of their own sadness, and not nearly as important (or even necessary) to discern or label the precise diagnostic category.

It should be a natural part of the educational and therapeutic process to also ensure the young person's awareness of manifestations of his or her sadness/depression (e.g., anxiety, somatic complaints, acting out). Thus, for example, as our rapport develops I expect to find a way to explain to a child (or, better, to have *him or her* discover for himself or herself) that his or her headaches or acting up, or not sleeping are, indeed, his or her sadness "coming out sideways." It is, of course, important that both the young person's awareness and acknowledgment of this logically flows from his or her history and our conversations, and not from my interpretation of his or her symptoms. The young person should ultimately reflect *his or her* understanding and formulation of the reasons he or she is feeling and behaving that way, and his or her expectations and motivations for getting well again. Most importantly, it's critical to assess if the young person has the energy/wherewithal to do the emotional/hypnotic work necessary to improve. This is important particularly in helping the clinician to decide whether, if, and when the patient might also or necessarily have medication added to the treatment program in order, for example, to facilitate sufficient functionality to be able to work clinically. I believe the same kind of thinking is applicable whether the medication that is being considered is anti-depressant, anxiolytic, and/or analgesic (Kohen & Murray, 2006).

As also described in Chapter Fourteen, the evolution of successful hypnotic strategies rests upon an implicit understanding of the critical role of the clinician's rapport with the young person, their understanding of their personal history in the context of an understanding of their developmental trajectory, and the clinician's commitment to noticing, remembering, and utilizing the unique aspects of each child and their problem. A commitment to noticing carefully within the context of rapport and a developmentally sensitive history will allow physicians to "find the hypnosis in the encounter" (Sugarman, 1997/2006; *see also* Chapter Fourteen).

As Kohen and Murray (2006) recently noted, "'Finding the hypnosis in the encounter' means considering that children, particularly those who are suffering, hurting, and sad—may *already* be in a hypnotic state, one with many if not the same characteristics of an 'induced' hypnotic state, i.e., focused narrowly and intently (albeit negatively so), on their sadness, their loss, their pain, their self-image/self-esteem, their perception of the existential futility of their life" (p. 194). In their negative hypnotic state of depression they are internally absorbed, less attentive or inattentive to surrounding stimuli, but nonetheless ready to listen; and likely hoping that the clinician will say the right thing that allows them to proceed toward some relief and hope for improvement.

Much as in conditions of emergencies (Kohen, 1986), recognition of these spontaneous hypnotic states, as discussed in Chapter Fourteen, allows the clinician to just be hypnotic, to shift according to the communicated needs of the child, to honor their perspectives, and to help them move from a negative to a positive focus. Attention to what the child gives us, and particularly to their precise uses of language, will allow the clinician to refine not only finding the spontaneous hypnosis in the encounter, but also to know when a more direct approach and teaching of formal hypnotic strategies may be preferable to "just" being hypnotic with reframing of language and indirect techniques.

Following the Ericksonian dictum to "go with the child" allowed me to ask B to "Please put the sillies away," and saying so with kindness, sensitivity, competence, and authority allowed him to receive and understand (unconsciously) the positive expectancy that it indeed *would happen*, and so it did. Further examples of this and the integration of other hypnotic strategies are illustrated in the rest of the story of B below.

The Rest of the Story...

B

Early in this therapeutic relationship B's mom not only said that she wanted a preventive approach to help B, but also tearfully added, "But I don't want helping him to be therapy for *me*...and I get the feeling you're saying he's normal and it's something *we* are doing, and I don't want us to be in therapy...." Therapeutically responding to this potential barrier, we reviewed concepts of normal child development, noting that he is dynamic not static, and that we don't usually get an advance warning when a child shifts stages in development (i.e., they just do it) and then we—as parents—have to "catch up." Thus, what was true 6 months ago may not be true today. I emphasized this, noting that he *will* be different 6 months from now, and that while there are not everyday changes as there were (for example, at 12 to 36 months of age), there are a lot. These developmental changes and challenges—which may feel like burdens to us as parents [*purposeful use of universalizing "us" in an effort to join with B's mother*]—would be true whether or not there is an underlying disorder, mild or severe.

Responding to the fact that B's mother didn't want to be the one who was getting therapy for "his" problem(s), I emphasized that "...helping B is about helping him in the context of his family and his community, and that means talking with and helping parents and not only the child. B's mom was consciously unaware of her tendency to catastrophize and to be burdened by memory of how things were before and, therefore, expectations that they will again. We discussed "just because a behavior was there before doesn't mean that it will be again."

At the end of the first two visits the official diagnoses included:

1. Anxiety—Normal behavior during first visit;
2. Concerns about Possible Depression by history;
3. Concerns about "Obsessive/Compulsive Behavior" by history, but none observed;
4. History of Nightmares and Night Terrors—incompletely explored
5. History of Sleep Onset Insomnia—not yet discussed;
6. Strong Family (Maternal) History of Anxiety and Depression.

Early in our second visit B said, "I want to ask you something...how come when you rest your brain your hand gets warm?" and then closed his eyes, went into a spontaneous hypnotic trance with eyelid flutter, stillness, eye movements, and palms upward on his lap. I asked him how he knew that his hands got warmer and he said he could feel it, and when I asked him why he thought that was so, he began to talk about "chemicals in the brain send a message down there I think." I complimented him and used this as a natural and appropriate segue to introduce him to computerized biofeedback.

Using electropmyography (EMG) on his forearm as a measure/reflection of voluntary muscle control and electrodermal activity (EDA)[1] he was able to achieve dramatic physical relaxation. EDA was monitored from the right palm and explained as "mind relaxing" and "imagination." He began at a fairly aroused state at 27.5 micromhos, dropped to 17.5 micromhos, briefly went up to 20 micromhos and then down to 17.5 micromhos during suggestions for eye closure. When he accepted the hypnotic suggestion that he could change his EDA with his imagination, his skin conductance dropped dramatically from 27.5 to 5 micromhos. I gave him printouts of graphs of this wonderful decreased activation and offered the waking suggestion that "it would be good to put these up on the wall in your bedroom to remind yourself that whenever you need to you can calm down so well so fast, just like in my office today..." His response was that maybe he could put them up in the living room! I asked him to discuss that with his mom.

It was apparent that a major factor in this child's behavior challenges was his mother's fear about the possibility that B might have manic-depressive illness (bipolar disorder) or schizophrenia and that somehow she had "given it" to him (i.e., "I don't want him to go through what I have gone through, being in and out of therapy, etc...."). Both B's mother and father believed that they were helpless to prevent and/or respond to this. It seemed reasonable and apparent that one way that she could learn that she was not helpless was by seeing that B was not helpless, and that as he improved and was able to learn to calm himself, that she, too, could not only become calm but also could become able to be more receptive to hearing about how to calm herself, and, in turn, help him.

---

[1] Electrodermal activity, galvanic skin response, or skin conductance, measures conductance of electrical current through sweat glands. Sweat gland activity is tightly linked to sympathetic nervous system arousal (the "fight or flight response") so that EDA provides direct and immediate feedback about the subject's level of autonomic nervous system activity.

Two months later

B's mom reported that when his dad comes home from work B "breaks into such excitement that he seems to 'go somewhere else'...he's excited and can't seem to contain it. He'll run around, bump into things and laugh hysterically and often won't stop until threatened (with deprivation of something special)" at which time he may often "melt into tears and protest (that thing can't be taken away, etc.)" During these times, he is reportedly not attentive to what's going on. Sometimes he'll also stop when he falls down (and then cries). Mother characterized this as an over-reaction to simple stimuli. though of course most parents can describe having had similar experiences. Dad used the word "dissociated"...and Mom said, "He gets manic...." Ignoring the temptation to latch onto these diagnostic-labeling invitations, I suggested alternative approaches, such as holding him gently, with her face close to his, and saying, "Please STOP NOW" firmly, once. I was able to demonstrate this shortly thereafter when, during the 30 minute visit, B was quite "on the go" throughout the 30 minutes. He was flitting about, jabbering, and was quite distractible. I asked him to come close to me:

> **D. Kohen [DK]:** Want to see something cool? [*interrupting the "set"*] ...come over here please...Great. Now [*directive*], pretend [*meaning "go into trance"*] it's winter [*easy to do in Minnesota!*] Now... be a snowman....right! [*to do this he had to stop what he was doing and shift...and he did, readily, demonstrating to his mom and to himself that he is able*] Great...Now Mr. Happy Snowman all frozen and stiff and icy, the sun is going to come out and it could get warm and you might start to melt slowly [*with no further instruction, his muscles began to relax*]...all the way down your body [*and he began to "droop" to the floor*] 'til you are a puddle of fresh water...and that water can then be springtime and it will help seeds to grow into a big, strong tree [*metaphor for growth, ego-strength, control*] with strong branches....So, you can be a snowman just the same way, to relax whenever you need to.

Understanding his orientation to play, and the fluid boundaries between fantasy and reality at his age allowed for offering suggestions that operate at multiple levels of meaning, from the challenge (but really the ease) of becoming abruptly quite still (frozen snowman) instead of restless/active, relaxing (instead of tense), calming, then growing to a sturdy tree (= a strong, confident boy) as future projection suggestions, and all without formal hypnotic induction or formally shifting from "Now I'm doing my history and *now* I'm guiding and teaching [self-] hypnosis."

Six months later

Now 6½ years old, B's behavior was reported to have been and, indeed seemed, much more normal. He had navigated the preceding 6 to 8 months very well. The previously observed/reported inattention, distractibility, and impulsivity no longer seemed to be prominent and, therefore, I thought, diagnostically, that he was a pretty normal boy with some anxiety. I no longer believed that his behavior could or might represent bipolar disorder or ADHD. There seemed to be no evidence of depression, or OCD. While there was some reported increase in nightmares, he was going to sleep much more easily. Not surprisingly, his parents, too, were improved.

Six months later

Now 7 years old, B continued to do very well. In a very intellectualized fashion for a 7-year-old he asked, "What should you do when you're doing something you know is not right but it's hard to stop?" In therapeutic response, finding the opportunity for the hypnosis in the encounter, I directly suggested:

> **DK:** Just close your eyes... [*He went quickly into trance, as reflected in slowing of respirations, spontaneous muscle relaxation and stillness, and, most importantly, his subsequent engagement with and report of believed-in imagination.*] Now, picture a STOP sign. [*He did so with guidance, and in trance described a red background, the S-T-O-P letters as white and, in response to suggestion, he let it "get bigger and bigger" until it filled the screen in his mind's eye. This was offered as a way to STOP unacceptable behavior, or stimulus responses when feeling "wild."*]

Finally, I asked him to picture a traffic light and to see what color it was while he was messing around screaming and jumping on Daddy when he comes home. B knew…and said that it was green, and without any prompting, he said, "Oh, I get it, I should make it be yellow and then red, right?" Right.

Seven months later

In last meeting and my observation 7 months earlier, B's behavior did not meet the criteria for the diagnosis of either ADHD or bipolar disorder. Today, by contrast, his Mom reported recent escalation, and B demonstrated dramatic impulsivity, distractibility, fidgetiness and motoric hyperactivity, and inattention. In addition, he told me privately that he was sad and mad about how he was acting, that he "couldn't help it" and sometimes thought he shouldn't be alive. In view of this and his mother's interim history, I began to think again that perhaps he did have ADHD or that perhaps this was hypomania and reflective of bipolar disorder. We agreed upon watchful waiting, during which he effectively and often used his STOP sign and traffic light "strategies."

Six months later

Now 7½ years old, we were talking about B's "out of control" behavior and I asked him to close his eyes and think about it, and he explained—opening and closing his eyes—that when he practices his imagination "sometimes it's baseball, sometimes it's something else, you know?!" I encouraged him to use the "Ruler Imagery" (i.e., measuring on a 0–12 ruler with 12 = most wild behavior and 0 = none) saying while he was in spontaneous hypnosis that "You know, I'm not sure where that ruler will be, perhaps in the clouds, or floating in air, or in the bushes, or on the side of the tube while you're tubing or wherever…" and he said, "Hey, you just gave me an idea, the ruler is on the baseball bat and whenever I hit it (in my mind) it goes down!" and I, of course, congratulated that.

I invited him to practice this regularly because "the more you practice the better you get…" and suggested to him directly that (1) You use the STOP sign to stop the worry about the smell of fire that you used to worry about, (2) and also to STOP any not-so-great-feeling and (3) when that part of you starts thinking stuff like you don't want to live or that you feel hateful, then another part of you can have a conversation back and say 'STOP that!' " He really liked this idea. And so it was that he was offered these post-hypnotic suggestions, ego-strengthening praise for success, and opportunity to mobilize internal resources in the form of "another part of you" that has the controls he needs.

Additionally, *B* was taught what he would come to call his "3's and 6's," a simple relaxation/imagery/self-hypnotic technique of focused attention on breathing:

> **DK**: Close your eyes. Focus on your breathing only. Breathe in through your nose...slow...and easy...and slowly count to 3 to yourself as you breathe in and your tummy pushes out...that's right...and then let your breath out very slowly...and your tummy goes in, slowly count to 6 as you breathe out...that's right. Now...do it again yourself, and notice as you do it that you get very, very relaxed and comfortable because you're doing it right and because you want to...Good!

One year later

When *B* was 8½, his Mom called out of the blue and said that *B* was "Cycling out of control and we want him to see a psychiatrist to see if he really does or doesn't have bipolar disorder." Over the ensuing weeks and months psychiatric consultation was arranged. A diagnosis of ADHD was made initially and after substantial consideration *B*'s parents agreed to a trial of atomoxetine (Straterra) for ADHD. It was completely unsuccessful, with no discernible improvement. Thereafter a neuroleptic (Trileptal) was prescribed, also with no discernible benefit. Risperidone (Risperdal) was offered and, to his parents' great relief, *B* had *remarkable improvement*. His parents (and I) were reassured by the psychiatrist that this did not represent a "missed" diagnosis, but rather a condition whose diagnosis was unclear and was evolving, ultimately reaching some clarity with this successful trial of medication.

Three months later

Now 8¾, *B* and I talked about how he sometimes has scary dreams; and we talked about the mind's ability to "program your own dreams." He described his various self-hypnosis techniques:

> ***B***: I use the 3's and 6's, I use the STOP sign, and I use that balloons thing [*a levitation technique*] to get rid of bad feelings.

Conclusion

And so it is that *B* goes to school, has friends, fights with his brother, challenges his teachers intellectually, and his parents emotionally, but has far fewer mood and behavior swings than in the past. While it is clear that he benefits from low dose risperidone, it is also clear that from his and his parents' perspectives, his medication is adjunctive to the benefit he derives from a variety of self-hypnotic/self-regulation techniques that initially he learned both independently and from/with his parents as models/guides when he was younger, and that he now cues himself to do in order to become calm when he is agitated, or worried, or can't fall asleep as easily as before. Hypnotic techniques were tailored to his developmental age and abilities and in the context of diagnostic considerations. They helped him to identify and characterize his feelings, to modulate unpleasant and unacceptable behavioral responses, to orient (himself) toward problem solving, and in the process to promote the requisite ego-strength for continued healthy maturation.

His clinical improvement can be attributed, of appropriate necessity, to a blend of effective parent counseling and guidance, skill development training in self-hypnosis, and intermittent and adjunctive use of medication, all in the context of his and his family's history, and where he was/is maturationally. While various official diagnoses were appropriately considered, successful therapy for his (and his parents') sadness came ultimately from asking and providing answers to the questions "So what?" and "Now what?" These days when *B* asks himself "Now what?" both he and his parents invariably answer with spontaneous application or modification of his various self-modulation skills or with requests for help in so doing.

Caveats

As recent epidemiologic surveys suggest that children and adolescents represent the fastest growing group of individuals suffering from depression, clinicians must keep depression and sadness-related diagnoses on their radar at all times (i.e., if we don't think of it, we can't/won't make the diagnosis). Both because of the strong biologic heritability of depression and because of the risk of negative attribution styles and avoidant coping being modeled through parents' behavior, having a depressed parent is a strong risk factor for a child developing depression (Yapko, 2006, p. 214).

Providing high-quality care for children who are sad requires an understanding and awareness of the research literature and rec-ommendations regarding the care of children with depression, including recommended practice parameters and approaches (Birmaher et al., 1998; Jellinek & McDermott, 2004), evidenced-based treatments (Hamrin & Pachler, 2005; Pavuluri, Graczyk, Henry, Carbray, Heidenreich, & Miklowit, 2004) and medication approaches (Keller, Ryan, Strober, Klein, Kutcher, et al., 2001; Emslie, G., Heiligenstein, Wagner, Hoog, Ernest, Brown, et al, 2002; Wagner, Robb, Findling, Jin, Gutierrez, & Heydorn, 2004).

It is my impression, as noted earlier, that it is more important to notice the sadness and respond to it therapeutically than it is to necessarily provide a specific "label" or "diagnosis" per se. Ongoing follow up will allow for monitoring the evolution of symptoms, their response to intervention (hypnotic or otherwise), and for the possibility of evolving diagnosis, as exemplified by *B* in the foregoing case.

References

American Academy of Child and Adolescent Psychiatry. (1998). Practice parameters for the assessment and treatment of children and adolescents with depressive disorders. *Journal of the American Academy of Child and Adolescent Psychiatry*, 37(Suppl):63S–83S.

Achenbach, T. (1991). Integrative guide for the 1991 CBCL/4-18, YSR, and TRF. Burlington, VT: University of Vermont, Department of Psychiatry.

Beck, A., Steer, R., & Brown, G. (1996). *Beck depression inventory* (2nd ed.), San Antonio, TX: Psychological Corporation.

Birmaher, B., Brent, D. A., & Benson, R. S. (1998). Summary of the practice parameters for the assessment and treatment of children and adolescents with depressive disorders. *Journal of the American Academy of Child and Adolescent Psychiatry, 37*, 1234–1238.

Birmaher, B., Ryan, N. D., Williamson, D. E., Brent, D. A., Kaufman, J., & Dahl, R., et al. (1996a) Childhood and adolescent depression: A review of the past 10 years. Part I. *Journal of the American Academy of Child and Adolescent Psychiatry, 35*, 1427–1439.

Birmaher, B., Ryan, N. D., Williamson, D. E., Brent, D. A., Kaufman, J., & Dahl, R., et al. (1996b) Childhood and adolescent depression: A review of the past 10 years. Part II. *Journal of the American Academy of Child and Adolescent Psychiatry, 35*, 1439–1447.

Emslie, G. J., Heiligenstein, J. H., Wagner, K. D., Hoog, S. L., Ernest, D. E., Brown, E., Nilsson, M., & Jacobson, J. G. Fluoxetine for acute treatment of depression in children and adolescents: A placebo-controlled, randomized clinical trial. (2002). *Journal of the American Academy of Child and Adolescent Psychiatry, 41*(10): 1205–1215 .

Emslie, G. J., Weinberg, W. A., Rush, A. J., Adams, R. M., & Rintelmann, J. W. (1990) Depressive symptoms by self-report in adolescence: Phase I of the development of a questionnaire for depression by self-report. *Journal of Child Neurology, 5*: 114–121.

Garland, A. F., Hough, R. L., McCabe, K. M., Yeh, M., Wood, P. A., & Aarons, G. A. (2001). Prevalence of psychiatric disorders in youths across five sectors of care. *Journal of the American Academy of Child and Adolescent Psychiatry, 40*(4): 409–418.

Gonsalkorale, W. M., Miller, V., Afzal, A., & Whorwell, P. (2003). Long term benefit of hypnotherapy for irritable bowel syndrome. *Gut, 52*(11): 1623–1629.

Hamrin, V., & Pachler, M. C. (2005) Child and adolescent depression: review of the latest evidence-based treatments. *Journal of Psychosocial Nursing and Mental Health Services, 43*(1): 54–63.

Jellinek, M. S., & McDermott, J. F. Formulation: Putting the diagnosis into a therapeutic context and treatment plan. (2004). *Journal of the American Academy of Child and Adolescent Psychiatry, 43*(7): 913–916.

Jellinek, M., Murphy, J., Robinson, J., Feins, A., Lamb, S., & Fenron, T. (1988) Pediatric symptom checklist: Screening school age children for psychosocial dysfunction. *Journal of Pediatrics, 112*, 201–209.

Kaffman, M. (1981*).* Monoideism in psychiatry: Theoretical and clinical implications. *American Journal of Psychotherapy* 35(2): 235–243.

Keller, M. B., Ryan, N. D., Strober, M., Klein, R. G., Kutcher, S. P., Birmaher, B., Hagino, O. R., Koplewicz, H., Carlson, G. A., Clarke, G. N., Emslie, G. J., Feinberg, D., Geller, B., Kusumakar, V., Papathodorou, G., Sack, W. H., Sweeney, M., Wagner, K. D., Weller, E. B., Winters, N. C., Oakes, R., & McCafferty, J. P. (2001). Efficacy of paroxetine in the treatment of adolescent major depression: A randomized controlled trial. *Journal of the American Academy of Child and Adolescent Psychiatry,* 40(7): 762–772.

Kohen, D. P. (1986) Applications of relaxation/mental imagery (self-hypnosis) to pediatric emergencies. *International Journal of Clinical and Experimental Hypnosis,* 34:4, 283–294.

Kohen, D. P., & Murray. K. M. (2006). Depression in Children and Youth: Applications of Hypnosis to Help Young People Help Themselves (pp. 189–216). In Yapko, M. D. (Ed.), *Hypnosis and Treating Depression—Applications in Clinical Practice.* New York: Routledge.

Kovacs, M. (1992). *Children's Depression Inventory Manual.* North Tonawanda, NY: Multi-Health Systems.

Myers, K., & Winters, N. C. Ten-year review of rating scales, II: Scales for internalizing disorders. (2002). *Journal of the American Academy of Child and Adolescent Psychiatry,* 41(6):634–659.

Pavuluri, M. N., Graczyk, P. A., Henry, D. B., Carbray, J. A., Heidenreich, J., & Miklowitz, D. J. (2004). Child- and family-focused cognitive-behavioral therapy for pediatric bipolar disorder: development and preliminary results. *Journal of the American Academy of Child and Adolescent Psychiatry,* 43(5): 528–537.

Rossello, J., & Bernal, G. (1999). The efficacy of cognitive-behavioral and interpersonal treatments for depression in Puerto Rican adolescents. *Journal of Consulting and Clinical Psychology,* 67, 734–745.

Sugarman, L. I. (Producer) (1997/2006). *Hypnosis in pediatric practice: Imaginative medicine in action.* [DVD and Learning Guide]. Carmarthen, Wales, U.K.: Crown House.

Wagner, K. D., Robb, A. S., Findling, R. L., Jin, J., Gutierrez, M. M., & Heydorn, W. E. (2004). A randomized, placebo-controlled trial of

Citalopram for the treatment of major depression in children and adolescents. *American Journal of Psychiatry*, 161,1079–1083. Available at: http://ajp.psychiatryonline.org/cgi/content/abstract/161/6/1079

Wolraich, M. (Ed.) (1996). *Diagnostic and Statistical Manual–Primary Care, Pediatrics (DSM-PC)*. Elk Grove Village, IL: American Academy of Pediatrics.

Yapko, M. (1992). *Hypnosis and the Treatment of Depressions*. New York: Brunner/Mazel.

Yapko, M. (2001).*Treating Depression with Hypnosis: Integrating Cognitive-Behavioral and Strategic Approaches*. New York: Brunner/Routledge.

Yapko, M. D. (Ed.) (2006). *Hypnosis and Treating Depression—Applications in Clinical Practice*. New York: Routledge.

Youngstrom, E. A., Findling, R. L., Calabrese, J. R., Gracious, B. L, Demeter, C., Bedoya, D., & Price, M. (2004) Comparing the diagnostic accuracy of six potential screening instruments for bipolar disorder in youths aged 5 to 17 years. *Journal of the American Academy of Child and Adolescent Psychiatry*, 43(7): 847–858.

Zeltzer, L. K., Tsao, J. C., Stelling, C., Powers, M., Levy, S., & Waterhouse, M. (2002). A phase I study on the feasibility and acceptability of an acupuncture/hypnosis intervention for chronic pediatric pain. *Journal of Pain and Symptom Management*, 24(4): 437–446.

Chapter Ten

Hypnotic Treatment of Anxiety in Children

William C. Wester, II, EdD, ABPP, ABPH

What is anxiety? Anxiety is "a state of apprehension, uncertainty, and fear resulting from the anticipation of a realistic or fantasized threatening event or situation, often impairing physical and psychological functioning" (*American Heritage Dictionary*, 4th ed., 2000, p. 590). The words "uncertainty," "fear," "anticipation," and "threatening event" are key words for the child or adolescent (hereafter referred to as the child) experiencing symptoms of anxiety. It is generally agreed that anxiety involves a psychological and physical response to a perceived danger, with the differences being the type of danger and whether the response is appropriate.

The medical community should "rule out" neurological factors, respiratory factors, metabolic factors, endocrinology factors, or other medical causes of the symptoms. Psychological symptoms are rarely entirely ruled out. There is no question about the body-brain connection when dealing with anxiety. The nervous system is brought into action and triggers the "flight or fight" response we all learned about in general psychology.

Anxiety disorders are not necessarily connected with a specific external danger and, therefore, give the symptom(s) a unique quality. In many situations, the child knows that there is no specific reason for his or her response, and, as a result, feels not only anxious but less in control (Eppley & Tepe, 1990). Hypnosis has been used to treat anxiety disorders in children, with one of the earliest published accounts being Mason's 1897 report of treatment of a child who was too frightened to cooperate with medical treatment (Schultz, 1991).

I believe that anxiety needs to be quickly reframed and dissociated from the otherwise normal child. Children become identified with their symptoms by family and peers. An example would be parents who refer to their child as "my anxious child" or peers who give their best friend a variety of names such as "freak," "buzz," or "hyper." Everyone seems to forget that the child has a name and is a person who happens to be experiencing symptoms of anxiety.

During or at the end of my clinical intake interview, I ask the child if it is okay to refer to his or her symptoms in a different way. He or she is happy to do this, and as I pull an ugly looking monster toy from my desk I say, "I would like you to meet the "It Monster." From that point forward I refer to his or her anxiety symptom(s) as the "It Monster." This dissociative technique automatically reframes the anxiety and increases his or her sense of control and provides the child with an opportunity to change the symptom.

I usually do not use the "It Monster" term with very young children without first checking out their perception of a monster. As one young child said to me, "We can call it the 'It Monster' because monsters only live in books." This obviously gave me another opening as well in terms of his treatment. Most children look at the ugly model and think it is cool to rename their symptom. This is all part of the fun and game playing when working with children. I explain the rationale for doing this and how looking at things in a different way will be helpful to them. Once this new pattern is established the next step is an easy one: namely asking, "Would you like to learn how to control the 'It Monster' instead of the 'It Monster' controlling you?" I then introduce the concept of hypnosis and discuss any myths and misconceptions.

I review the child's motivations, which I obtained during the initial interview, and consider incorporating them later into the hypnotic procedure. Even though children do not have the same misconceptions as adults, they still watch television where they see a variety of misconceptions related to hypnosis.

It is important to present the learning model, skill building, and team approach. "I am going to be helping you learn a very special skill so that when the 'It Monster' tries to raise its ugly head, you will be in control and use your skills to help destroy the 'It Monster.'" I give the child a handout entitled, "Destroy the 'It Monster'" to take home. I discuss the handout with the child and share it with his or her parent(s). Then I ask the child to find the hidden message in the handout and share it with his or her parent(s) and then with me at the next visit. (The first letter of each statement spells out "Self-Hypnosis Now." A copy of the handout is at the end of this chapter.)

Both children and adults feel out of control and unprepared when their symptoms strike. I want the child to know that he or she now has a plan to deal with the anxiety. Having a plan is far better than not having a plan. In addition, it is important to talk about his or her need to try out his or her plan, which includes self-hypnosis and confronting the "It Monster."

My typical comment is, "Every time you confront the 'It Monster' it gets weaker and you get stronger." For the child who needs to see something happening, I use an imagined 10-point scale or switch technique (dissociative technique). Ten represents the highest level of anxiety he or she has ever experienced and zero is little or no anxiety. The child is in charge and in complete control of the scale or switch.

At the beginning of the session, he or she is asked to identify the level of his or her anxiety at that time. At the end of the session, following the hypnotic intervention, the child is asked once again to identify his or her level of anxiety. The post-hypnotic level is always lower and helps the child learn that what he or she has been doing has been helpful, and that he or she is really gaining control. This is an important experiential step versus taking the therapist's word that there will be a change.

Finally, I ask them to give themselves a pat on the back and to verbalize at least three cognitive reframing statements. Examples of such statements include, "I did it," "It worked," "Wait till I tell my therapist about this," "I made more out of my anxiety than it was worth," "It's getting better each time I do this," "I'm pleased with me," "I changed the 8 to a 4," or "Come and try to get me 'It Monster,' I now have a plan to deal with you." Both the "It

Monster" and the scale or switch techniques are dissociative with emphasis on the child's ability to notice change. Dissociative approaches work and increase the child's sense of control.

Clinical Vignette

The Balloon Technique

A.P.

To emphasize the points I am making, I refer to the case of A.P., a 12-year-old boy whom I saw for a total of four sessions. He presented as having a panic disorder with agoraphobia (American Psychiatric Association, 2000). This young man described how scared he was of going into rooms with no windows, being afraid that he would be locked in the room. He also expressed worries about robbers and "things" coming into his room. The symptoms increased to the point where he was so afraid that he was unable to leave his home. His treatment was very successful.

He and his parents arranged to come back for a free reinforcement session and to be videotaped for teaching purposes. Before the actual hypnotic induction, he described what he had learned from coming for help:

> **AP**: I learned how to relax and how to relax very quickly. I also learned how to control my fears and how I can control them and they cannot control me. I use my review tape and control meter and turned down any anxiety to one. I can now go on elevators and go into the small band practice room at school. I learned how to think logically. I now know self-hypnosis and can just sit down and go back to my special place at any time.

Keep in mind that the following transcript is a reinforcement session about four months after therapy was terminated. The induction method was selected to support the child's control and ability to use self-hypnosis.

W. Wester [WW]: Prop your feet up again [*a recliner chair with a foot rest*]. It might be interesting before I say very much at all for you to show me how you have been doing this yourself. It might be a good place to start and when you feel you are in that relaxed state let me know by just moving one of your fingers. So right at this moment you will not have to talk. You can just move a finger to tell me you are in that special place. So just go ahead and do that and I will watch for that finger to move" [*It took over a minute for the finger to move, which was a great indicator to me that he was taking his time and processing what he had learned—finger moves*]. That's fine—Very good. Just begin to relax a little more comfortably and a little more deeply and as you relax a little more deeply your mind can begin to remember everything that you have learned about hypnosis and how you have been able to use this very special skill that you now have [*reinforces learning model*].

And it is very nice to hear and observe how well you have learned this skill and that you have been able to use this with and without your tape [*reinforces self-hypnosis*]. For those times and situations in the past where you were scared or frightened or where you were feeling that anxiety that we called the "It Monster," you have learned ways in which you can relax and control that "It Monster." And now, several months later, you find yourself highly skilled and being able to do what you need to do at any time to help yourself. And what's really nice to know is that this is a skill that you will have with you your whole life. If for any reason at any time in the future you feel any undo anxiety, whatever the reason might be, you now have a skill that you can utilize and it will always be part of you. Sometime, maybe in school or if you go to college—whatever the case might be—you might have to give a talk—whatever the situation might be—you are in charge and you are in control. All of that learning that has taken place will be with you and will stay with you from this point forward.

As you experience this real pleasant comfortable feeling now I would like you to just learn a couple of other things about hypnosis and how powerful that very special part of your subconscious mind is. You really have already learned that, but I would like you to experience that in a little bit different way. For example, you can use that creative part of your mind right now. You can think about, for a moment, your right arm and your right hand and simply by using your mind you can think about a piece of string being tied around your wrist and attached to that string is a very colorful balloon. There may even be more than one and those balloons are filled with a special kind of helium gas that will make that right arm and hand a little bit lighter and lighter. It is going to be interesting to you when that arm begins to just slightly move upward—that balloon just kind of tugging away at the wrist and just starting that arm and hand to slowly begin to move upward feeling a little lighter and lighter now. That's right.

And any time you need or want to add a balloon to make it even lighter—that's okay. That's right—just allow it to come up now to a level that you are comfortable with. Notice as the arm and hand comes up now you continue to relax even more deeply because you are in control the whole time. It's fun to use that special part of your mind in that way because your subconscious mind, that very special part of you, has already been able to show you how you can control feelings and emotions and how it has been helpful to you to change your thinking by allowing yourself to think rationally and calmly [*reinforcement of his new skill and what he has accomplished*].

As situations present themselves you will continue to think rationally, calmly, making good choices and good decisions for yourself. Just enjoy that feeling of lightness now and if you have more than one balloon attached to your arm and hand just let go of one at a time. If there is just one balloon allow the air to come out of that balloon very slowly and the arm and hand will now get heavier and heavier and just come back down to rest comfortably on the arm of the chair. That's very good. [*At this point I did one other trace ratification procedure, namely a circle silver dollar anesthesia, which involves drawing a circle with your finger, about the size of a silver dollar, on the back of the hand and giving suggestions of that area becoming numb and insensitive as you rub that specific area. This was tested with ideomotor signals and then the hypnotically produced anesthesia was removed.*]

Allow yourself to enjoy this very comfortable and pleasant state and remember everything that I have said and all that you have learned. What you have learned is now part of you, a skill that you have learned. You have done very well and you are no longer afraid, no longer anxious and able to do the kind of things that you have really wanted to do but now you can do those without fear or concern. You will continue to make good judgments using that very logical and rational part of your mind that we talked about earlier. You will always know that you are in control. Take just a couple of moments and then in your own mind count from one to three and when you reach three you will open your eyes—you will be totally alert. You can begin counting now.

Following this session A.P. stated:

AP: I had three balloons on my arm and it felt like the balloons were really pulling on the arm. They were multicolored. I felt no discomfort when you drew the circle on my hand, made it numb and squeezed it. I feel great now!

WW: [*I then asked what he would recommend to other boys and girls his age in terms of hypnosis.*]

AP: Well, I would tell them it's not like what you see on television and stuff where some people make other people act in weird and strange ways. It helps you to relax and teaches you things other people don't know. It makes you feel good. I would recommend it!

Panic Disorder

The vignette you have just reviewed was that of a 12-year-old boy who met the criteria for panic disorder with agoraphobia. A panic disorder is the broader codable disorder such as panic disorder with or without agoraphobia. There is a fine line between a panic disorder and a panic attack. *Panic attacks* are sudden episodes of, usually intense, fear meeting at least 4 of the 13 symptom criteria as described in the *Diagnostic and Statistical Manual of Mental Disorders–Fourth Edition–Text Revision (DSM-IV–TR, 2000).* These symptoms include rapid heart rate and palpitations, unusual sweating, shaking or trembling, shortness of breath or a smothering feelings, choking sensations, significant chest pain or discomfort, nausea or stomach distress, feeling lightheaded or dizzy, feelings of unreality or being detached from oneself, fear of losing control or actually going crazy, fear of dying or imminent death, numbness or tingling sensations, and hot flashes or chills.

This 12-year-old experienced a significant number of the above symptoms but also experienced a fear of being in places or situations from which escape would be difficult or in which help might not be available in the event of a panic attack. Remember from the vignette presented, that his symptoms had progressed to the point where he could not leave home. An attack usually peaks over a 10 to 15 minute period and this fact becomes part of the cognitive restructuring with and without hypnosis. It is interesting to note in the case of the 12-year-old how he took control of the "It Monster," controlled his fears, used his "control meter," and learned to think logically and rationally. The child can be taught what irrational beliefs are and that they are the result of faulty thinking. All-or-nothing thinking, catastrophizing, overgeneralization, minimizing self-accomplishments, and "should messages" are reviewed with the older child.

Specific Phobia

This disorder used to be referred to as a simple phobia. The specific phobia is a persistent and excessive fear of a specific object and is probably the most common diagnoses in the general population. The most common phobias tend to be related to more common objects such as animals, storms, bridges, elevators, and planes. Adolescents frequently have a phobia of blood.

The most common hypnotic treatment of phobias is patterned on basic desensitization where hypnotic relaxation and suggestions of safety are paired with the feared situation/object. When the therapist gives suggestions of increased control, and the fact that the child now has a plan, this reduces the physical experience and psychological negative imagery of the feared stimulus.

Hypnotherapy can also provide for *in vivo* desensitization. In an older study, Ambrose (1968) has the child make a fist and the child is told that he or she has all of the fears and problems clasped in his or her fist. On the count of three, the fist will open and all of the anxieties will disappear. This suggestion is followed by positive ego-strengthening statements of feeling happy and confident.

Good self-talk learned under hypnosis is as follows. "Here comes the anxiety. This is my cue to focus my concentration. I can handle this. This is just anxiety. It will pass soon. I must not worry. Worry will not help. I will focus on my breathing and relaxation and ride it out. I will wait for it to pass. I am fine" (Eppley & Tepe, 1990, p. 71).

Social Phobia

Social phobias usually do not affect young children and tend to emerge in early adolescents. The incidence of social phobias is about equal between males and females. There is a persistent and unreasonable fear of a situation that could prove embarrassing or humiliating. This might be classroom speaking, eating in public, or a more generalized fear of saying something really stupid.

In the case of school phobia, the problem is usually connected to anxiety about leaving parents rather than a fear of school. Other precipitating factors such as underlying dynamics must also be explored (Schowalter, 1994). Many of the hypnotic experiences previously described in this chapter can be used. *In vivo* desensitization is an excellent technique to use within the hypnotic model. The critical importance of hypnotic imagery (visualization) is working toward the adolescent's goal. In imagery, he or she can see himself or herself mastering the goal, happy, confident, smiling, taking one step at a time, and imaging every positive detail. The key element of treatment is, once again, motivation and control.

Separation Anxiety

Separation anxiety is usually seen before adolescence, and to meet diagnostic criteria, the symptoms must be present for at least 4 weeks. Many related phobias such as school phobia or sleep problems may fall within this category. The major criteria is the recurrent significant distress as a child is separated from home or a major attachment figure (American Psychiatric Association, 2000).

Hypnosis can be used to decrease the anxiety via relaxation, positive imagery, and mastery of a skill to help the child help himself or herself. Look for specific symptoms and work with hypnosis to reduce the specific symptom, thereby reducing the overall feeling of separation. In Chapter Five, I used a separation anxiety case as an example of a television technique induction together with sports imagery. Even though the diagnosis is separation anxiety, the specifically felt symptom was "butterflies in the stomach." The therapy centered on this symptom and extinguished the separation anxiety.

Obsessive-Compulsive Disorder

Obsessive-compulsive disorder (OCD) in children and adolescents was at one time thought to be quite rare. Approximately 2% of the general population, children and adults, have OCD. This computes out to several million people in the United States alone. Familial patterns are usually seen during the intake interview that clearly support the biochemical aspect of this disorder. It is estimated that 50% of children with panic/anxiety disorder have at least one relative, frequently a parent or sibling, affected with an anxiety disorder. Children know something is wrong but lack the understanding or insight to alter their behavior.

Diagnostically, there is a clear distinction between obsessions and compulsions. Simply put, thoughts are obsessions, and acts (behaviors) are compulsions. To meet criteria for obsessions, the child's thoughts must be persistent and recurrent, not just excessive worries; the child attempts to suppress them, and usually is aware that such thoughts are a product of his or her own mind. In French OCD is *maladie la doubt*, which is to say the "sickness of doubt." Although the child knows these thoughts are different, there is always the question that he or she might really be wishing them. The child cannot relax by finally dismissing the thought (Eppley & Tepe, 1990).

To meet criteria for compulsions, the therapist must see repetitive behaviors in which the child feels driven to perform and that the behaviors are aimed at preventing or reducing distress. In addition to the obsessions or compulsions or both, the child must have some recognition that his or her thoughts or behaviors are excessive. Finally, the thoughts or behaviors are not only highly stressful but consuming to the point of interfering with the child's normal routine, academic functioning, or social activities, or relationships (American Psychiatric Association, 2000).

Compulsions are behaviors that are often the result of obsessions. The resistance to the compulsion usually triggers increased stress and tension, and giving into the compulsion decreases stress and tension and thus the compulsion is further learned and reinforced. Typically in children we see such compulsions as hand washing, counting, arranging, repeated rituals, checking, touching, hoarding, and cleaning.

When working with hypnosis to treat OCD, I recommend treating the entire "forest fire" as opposed to treating the "brush fires." Brush fires, like specific phobias, are quite easy to treat only to find another brush fire starting up in its place. You might feel great in that you have helped stop a specific behavior such as checking, only to find out in the next session that the child has substituted excessive grooming or ordering in place of the checking. Remember the learned and reinforced aspect of this type of behavior.

Medications can be extremely helpful in treating the biochemical part of this disorder, but medications alone will not change all of the learned patterns. Treating the "forest fire" means to use hypnotic procedures to treat the learned aspect of the OCD. Talk with the child on a learning level, something he or she certainly understands, together the two of you can work as a team to learn new ways to manage and/or destroy his or her OCD.

Once again, the "It Monster" can be part of your strategy. Learning hypnotic relaxation techniques, specific helpful imagery or knowing how to think differently (good cognitions) all begin to give the child a sense of empowerment over his or her OCD. Keep the treatment process fun and one of learning skills to defeat the "It Monster." Listen for changes in the child's thinking and build upon and reinforce these changes. For example, the child who says, "The 'It Monster' tried to come out several times but I just used what you showed me (some cues) and I was able to trigger my relaxation and It went away." Finally, have the child learn how to use self-hypnosis and self-talk (with or without his or her eyes closed). For example,

"Here comes the doubt. It isn't me. It is the disorder that makes me doubt. I can handle it. I am a good person. My thoughts are the problem. When I can control them, I can control my anxiety. I can change my thinking. I can manage this. I will use thought stopping. No negative thoughts. I don't need anyone's reassurance. I can trust myself. It's just the OCD that makes me think I can't trust myself. I can handle this."

Generalized Anxiety Disorder

Includes Overanxious Disorder of Childhood
Excessive worry or anxiety that persists for "more days than not for at least 6 months," worry that the child can't seem to control, and worry that is associated with at least one of the following symptoms meets the criteria for Overanxious Disorder of Childhood. The symptoms include restlessness, fatigue, poor concentration, irritability, muscle tension, or sleep disturbances (American Psychiatric Association, 2000). Some professionals may miss this diagnosis unless these symptoms are more severe.

Adjective checklists are frequently used on the intake form to be completed by the parent or child (depending on the child's age) prior to the first session. Recently, I came across such a form that had a section entitled, "Checking In (check the words that apply to you)." Included were such items as "Trouble going to sleep," "Feel worried," "Feel afraid," and stomachaches (Professional Pastoral Counseling Institute, Inc., 2003). Adding some of the symptoms described above, such as "Feel on edge," "Feel tired," "Have trouble concentrating," and "Irritable," might round out the criteria as described. Remember that for children only *one* symptom must be present in order to meet criteria. I like the idea of including such a checklist on the intake form that might "red flag" something that needs to be checked further.

In terms of hypnosis, I do not usually use the "It Monster" slogan because these symptoms are frequently not as severe or as focused. The learning model together with simple education about anxiety starts the reframing process. Learning new skills including relaxation, developing skills of turning down or off the anxiety (such as an anxiety dimmer switch), or substituting a favorite place at the time of the anxiety feeling can go a long way in helping the child control his or her feelings.

Just as in real estate where things hinge on "Location-Location-Location!" when treating anxiety in this way takes "Practice-Practice-Practice!" Bassman and Wester (1997) list one of the "Ten commandments" for coping with chronic pain as "Relax-Relax-Relax!" Listen to a relaxation tape or just sit down, close your eyes, and imagine a favorite place" (p. 64). Some of the other commandments might be reworded to fit generalized anxiety, such as "Use your cognitive skills and remind yourself that the anxiety will decrease"; "Remember the control you do have in managing your anxiety"; and finally, "Practice your self-hypnosis to decrease the level of anxiety" (p. 64).

Posttraumatic Stress Disorder

Children and adolescents are also prone to posttraumatic stress disorders by being exposed to a traumatic event in which the experienced or witnessed significant event could have or actually resulted in a death or serious injury. The child may then experience intense fear and exhibit his or her symptoms by disorganized or agitated behavior. The trauma is then re-experienced in a variety of ways, such as flashbacks, frightening dreams, and avoiding any associated stimuli.

Children tend to avoid anything associated with the trauma, such as places or people, which stimulate recollections of the traumatic event. The final part of the criteria that must be met is that there are "persistent symptoms of increased arousal" such as hyper vigilance or an increased startle response (American Psychiatric Association, 2000, p. 220).

Trauma comes in all forms. For example, childhood posttraumatic stress disorder in complicated bereavement is a condition that results from the loss of a loved one when the death comes about from some traumatic means, such as a parent killed in an automobile accident and the child survives, or a shooting occurs in the child's school and close friends are killed. Iglesias and Iglesias (2006) present two cases of single session treatment with clinical hypnosis of PTSD resulting from the traumatic loss of the parental figures. They used a "Hypnotic Trauma Narrative" that includes the telescope metaphor that allows the child to view the traumatic loss through a distant vantage point to help narrow, constrict, and blur painful details. This method also provides for a more unstructured indirect age progression aimed at allowing the child to look forward to future possibilities (Phillips & Frederick, 1992). Iglesias and Iglesias's (2006) follow-up a week later and a telephone follow-up two months later demonstrated the resolution of traumatic manifestations and the spontaneous beginning of the normal grief process.

Crasilneck and Hall (1985) present their treatment of an adolescent girl suffering from psychogenic amnesia after a major trauma. (The actual protocol can be found in Crasilneck and Hall, 1985, p. 315.) The case is mentioned here because in Olness and Kohen's hypnotherapeutic work with amnesic patients they give additional permissive suggestions for reinstatement of the amnesia. For example, "When you come out of hypnosis, you can remember as much as you are now ready to cope with, now ready to face" (Olness & Kohen, 1996, pp. 114–115). Working forensic cases with children or adults, this type of statement is extremely important so that the victim or witnesses can have time to work through these issues with their therapist.

As a young psychologist I remember having a wonderful hypnotic session with a hospitalized patient suffering from PTSD. The important information was clearly remembered. While charting, the head nurse asked what I had done to my patient because she was agitated and upset. I had opened the floodgate (flooding) and did not remember to use such procedures as described above by Crasilneck and Hall. I immediately worked with the patient and used a similar permissive technique and the patient was fine. I still refer to this case today to illustrate this point to my graduate students.

Obviously I do not use the "It Monster" metaphor with children who have experienced a traumatic event. PTSD is treated non-hypnotically in a variety of ways, including bereavement work, bereavement group work, behavioral therapy, and/or medications. Hypnotherapeutic techniques have been frequently used when treating posttraumatic stress disorder. The hypnotic induction usually involves components of relaxation which, in and of themselves, reduce anxiety associated with the trauma. Bereavement work and behavioral methods that depend upon relaxation and mental imagery are often greatly enhanced by hypnosis (Elkins, 1987).

The hypnotic treatment of anxiety in children can be exciting and rewarding. In most cases, children want to learn and, if you have fun with the process, they will react with their own excitement. Always assess their own motivation for change, not the motivation of others, and use this information creatively when developing your hypnotic strategies. Build upon and use the non-hypnotic techniques you have learned during your training for the treatment of anxiety but use these techniques within a hypnotic model.

Reframing, dissociation of the anxiety, changing irrational thinking to rational cognitive thinking, general anxiety reduction, skill building, ego strengthening, cues, images of favorite places, and many other creative approaches can be used within the hypnotic model. You have already seen in Chapter Five how reframing can be used to treat a symptom that represented a young man's separation anxiety. Let your creative mind open up and do what you do best within a hypnotic framework when treating children with anxiety.

References

Ambrose, G. (1968). Hypnosis in the treatment of children. *The American Journal of Clinical Hypnosis, 11*, 1–5.

The American Heritage Dictionary of the English Language (4th ed.). 2000. Boston: Houghton Mifflin.

American Psychiatric Association. (2000). *Diagnostic and statistical manual of mental disorders–Fourth edition–text revision*. Washington, D.C.: Author.

Bassman, S. & Wester, W. (1997). *Hypnosis, headache and pain control*. Chicago: American Society of Clinical Hypnosis Press.

Crasilneck, H. B. & Hall, J. A. (1985). *Clinical hypnosis: Principles and applications* (2nd ed.). New York: Grune and Stratton.

Elkins, G. (1987). Hypnotic treatment of anxiety. In W. Wester (Ed.), *Clinical hypnosis: A case management approach*. Cincinnati: BSCI Publications.

Eppley, S. R. & Tepe, K. T. (1990). *Success: 1-2-3! The behavioral and pharmacologic treatment of anxiety disorders*. Cincinnati: BSCI Publications.

Iglesias, A. & Iglesias, A. (2006). Hypnotic treatment of PTSD in children who have complicated bereavement. *American Journal of Clinical Hypnosis, 48*(2–3), 183–189.

Mason, R. D. (1897). Educational uses of hypnotism: A reply to Professor Lightmer Witner's editorials. *Pediatrics, 3*, 97–105.

Olness, K., & Kohen, D. (1996). *Hypnosis and hypnotherapy with children* (3rd ed.). New York: Guilford Press.

Phillips, M., & Frederick C. (1992). The use of hypnotic age-progression as prognostic, ego-strengthening, an integrating technique. *American Journal of Clinical Hypnosis, 35*(2), 99–108.

Professional Pastoral Counseling Institute, Inc. (2003). Cincinnati, OH. Available at: www.pastoral-counseling.org

Schowalter, J. E. (1994). Fears and phobias. *Pediatrics in Review, 15*, 384–388.

Schultz, J. (1991). Hypnosis and anxiety in children. In W. Wester and D. O'Grady (Eds.), *Clinical hypnosis with children*. New York: Brunner/Mazel.

Destroy the "It Monster"

Stay in the present

Exercise reduces muscle tension, uses energy

Let go, float, and flow

Feelings are normal bodily reactions

Handle "IT"—nothing terrible will happen

You will feel better; plan what to do next

Positive self-talk to calm yourself

Notice how "IT" fades when you stop thoughts

Opportunity for progress, use "IT" to cope

Slow down

I can handle "IT"; I am in control

Slowly breathe through your nose

Nothing happening, only thoughts and feelings

Optimistic thinking; use your skills

Wait for anxiety to pass, accept "IT"

Chapter Eleven

Hypnotherapy for the Treatment of Childhood Somatoform Disorders

Gary Elkins, PhD, ABPP, ABPH
Michelle M. Perfect, PhD

Perhaps more than any other health professionals, those who practice hypnosis and psychosomatic medicine with children are confronted with the emotional and psychological aspects of disease etiology and symptom presentation. In medical practice, children are generally brought by their parents and the focus is usually on a physical symptom or a complex of symptoms. The healthcare provider must have considerable expertise in discerning the physiology of disease. However, expertise in pathophysiology alone is not enough. The child's presentation of symptoms is often affected by psychological factors as well. In clinical practice, the dynamics of the child's family, stressful events in the child's life, and school or environmental concerns may be of primary importance in understanding the cause of symptoms and in planning treatment. The practitioner of hypnotherapy for childhood psychosomatic disorders should be especially cognizant of these influences. A short case history, taken from the early work of Anton Mesmer (often regarded as the father of hypnosis), illustrates this point.

Among patients treated by Mesmer (Tinterow, 1970) was a teenage girl whose complaints included poor sight, depression, rage, and episodes of delirium and seizures. Mesmer began to treat the girl using his technique of "therapeutic passes" and "mesmerism." The therapy was successful; the girl's sight was restored, and she was reported to be symptom free. The father then stopped

217

treatment prematurely as the girl's disability pension was to be terminated. The presenting symptoms returned. Mesmer again was asked to treat the patient, and once again her symptoms were removed. However, after the girl returned home, she relapsed again. Mesmer speculated that parental influences were of primary importance and that the girl had been urged to generate symptoms.

What is Psychosomatic?

Diagnosis of a *somatoform disorder* denotes that there are physical symptoms or impairments in sensory or motor functioning without an organic or physiological cause. In the fourth edition of the *Diagnostic and Statistical Manual of Mental Disorders* (*DSM-IV-TR*) (American Psychiatric Association, 2000), *somatoform disorders* are defined as:

> [T]he occurrence of one or more physical complaints for which appropriate medical evaluation reveals no explanatory physical pathology or pathophysiologic mechanism, or, when pathology is present, the physical complaints or resulting impairment are grossly in excess of what would be expected from the physical findings. (p. 445–446)

Somatoform disorders are further subdivided into: Body Dysmorphic Disorder, Conversion Disorder, Pain Disorder, Hypochondriasis, Somatization Disorder, or Somatoform Disorder, Undifferentiated.

Since somatoform disorders are based on there being psychogenic causes, several theoretical perspectives have been espoused to explain the emergence and maintenance of symptom. For instance, the psychodynamic formulation proposes that repression or suppression of threatening emotions leads to physical symptoms. Accordingly, the patient tends to hold emotions inward so that the emotion is expressed symbolically through the physical symptom (Bhatia, 2004). This view relates specific personality characteristics, interpersonal conflicts, and emotions to specific psychosomatic symptoms. For example, a patient who states that a conflict in the family "makes me sick" may develop abdominal pain and nausea. Hypnotherapy may be directed toward uncovering and resolving the underlying emotional conflict.

An alternative view is that of social learning theory. This formulation emphasizes the effects of modeling and social reinforcement. The child may learn a "sick role" that is then reinforced through attention and social support. Typically an adult or another child with physical complaints models a behavior that the child unconsciously learns to imitate. For example, consider the child who has difficulty in school and whose parent has chronic headaches. The child's complaint of headache (learned from the parent) may bring about an exemption from school (avoidance learning) and increased attention and nurturing from family, peers, teachers, and physicians (social reinforcement). This theory is further supported by the fact that symptom presentation may change following a child's witness of another person who actually experiences the disorder (Stores, 1999).

A third conceptualization may be referred to as a "stress-coping model" of psychosomatic disorders. Although the definitions of *stress* have varied, it has generally been characterized as physiological and psychological consequences that occur when the demands placed on a person exceed his or her individual and social resources (Cicchetti & Walker, 2001). *Coping* is defined as a way to manage the stressful situations. Problems arise when the individual attempts to cope with a stressful situation but feels overwhelmed when existing coping mechanisms are inadequate. Therapeutic approaches such as stress management, self-control relaxation, and self-hypnosis are used to teach the patient specific skills to enhance a greater sense of control and self-efficacy.

The biopsychosocial model (now often thought of interchangeably with the concept of mind-body interactions), posits that underlying somatoform disorders are an integration of the physical, psychological, and sociocultural factors (Borrell-Carrió, Suchman, & Epstein, 2004). Further, as advances in technology and neuroscience have emerged, greater consideration has been given to implications of underlying neurological processes for somatoform disorders. For example, a conversion disorder may stem from disconnection between higher and lower order processes in the brain. Tallabs (2005) reviewed data from two previous neuroimaging studies, one targeted people diagnosed with a conversion disorder (defined later in this chapter) with paralysis and the other focused on people who received suggestions for paralysis as part of a hypnotic induction. Interestingly, in both studies, increased activity was observed in the right anterior cingulate and the right orbitofrontal cortex, whereas decreased activity was identified in the right primary motor cortex. The author explained that the primary difference between these experiences is that in contrast to a conversion disorder, hypnotically suggested paralysis ceases at a participant's will (Tallabs, 2005). Further, the onset of a conversion disorder is typically tied to traumatic circumstances or emotional turmoil. Reports of hypnosis being used to evoke somatic symptoms and case histories describing employment of hypnotic suggestions to remedy non-organically caused physical symptoms, provides support that a hypnotic intervention would facilitate patients with various somatoform disorders gain control over their symptoms and provide them with an avenue to process their distressing emotions (Van Dyck & Hoogduin, 1989).

Literature Review

Review of all possible psychosomatic symptoms in children would probably fall short of its goal. The range is so great that some investigations have suggested that virtually all physical disorders are at least partly psychosomatic. This review, therefore, will be limited to a few of the more investigated and clinically common problems among the pediatric population. Chapter 18 is devoted to a discussion of hypnosis for recurrent pain in children.

Conversion Disorder

A conversion disorder is characterized by "an alteration or loss of physical functioning that suggests a physical disorder, but is actually the expression of some psychological need or conflict" (Moene, Spinhoven, Hoogduin, & Van Dyck, 2003, p. 30). Conversion disorder was initially conceptualized as "hysteria"

(Tallabs, 2005). Symptom presentation may include a variety of sensory and motor dysfunctions, such as blindness (Braaic, 2002), motor paralysis or weakness (Oakley, 1999), intractable sneezing (Bhatia, Khandpal, Srivastava, & Kohli, 2004; Maloney, 1980); mass psychogenic illness (Elkins, Gamino, & Rynearson, 1988), or coughing (Elkins & Carter, 1986). In terms of demographics, there have been reports that conversion disorders are more common in females, though one study found a greater incidence among male children (Malhi & Singhi, 2002). Psychogenic symptoms are less likely in children under age 10, though it is possible that a conversion disorder may be observed in those younger (Malhi & Singhi, 2002).

Maloney (1980) conducted a review of 105 cases of conversion reactions in children seen at a large medical center. The majority of children came from families in which depression and conflict were common. Additionally, over three-fourths of the families demonstrated difficulty with emotional expression and communication. Interestingly, the onset of conversion symptoms was almost uniformly (97 of 105) related to familial stress (Maloney, 1980).

The prognosis for treatment of conversion disorders is generally positive, but becomes less favorable when the condition becomes chronic or treatment is delayed. Thus, the focus should be on early intervention. The diagnosis of conversion reaction depends on recognizing the limits of an organic etiology of the patient's symptoms. For example, a 14-year old girl with arm paralysis and numbness was referred to GE for psychological assessment and hypnotherapy. Neurological evaluation had previously indicated that the symptoms followed no known anatomical or neurological pathways and, as a result, conversion disorder was suspected. The symptoms had begun suddenly while she was at home one evening and had continued despite hospitalization for several days. GE utilized hypnosis to explore possible stresses and to reduce symptoms. An early hypnosis session revealed that the conversion symptoms were brought on by feelings of anxiety following an episode of inappropriate sexual behavior by a family friend. The conversion symptoms appeared to provide an expression of feelings as well as protection from the situation. The symptoms resolved with the reassurance of support by her parents after these dynamics were acknowledged.

There has been at least one randomized controlled clinical trial (Moene et al., 2003) that examined hypnosis for adult patients with conversion disorder, motor type. The hypnosis intervention consisted of a preparatory session, 10 weekly hypnosis sessions, homework, and instructions for self-hypnosis. The researchers found that compared to wait-list control condition, participants in the hypnosis intervention group, experienced a significantly greater reduction in physical and social impairments and that the improvements were maintained at 6-month follow-up (Moene et al., 2003). Hypnosis for treatment of conversion disorders needs to be further evaluated through rigorous research. Moreover, investigations focusing on adults can only provide some insight into possible benefits for children, but in the absence of studies targeting youth, a clinician must rely on a theoretical and case study approach to design an intervention utilizing hypnotic techniques.

In 1978, Olness and Gardner described a case report of an 8-year-old boy who had presented with progressive pain and weakness in his arms and legs in the absence of a medical cause. After two weeks of symptom presentation, he was hospitalized because he was unable to walk or use his hands. An assessment indicated that issues of autonomy were causing conflict between him and his parents. The physical symptoms were targeted first as to reduce the potential for secondary gain. Two hypnosis sessions, consisting of suggestions "to recall previous good health and transfer these feelings to the present" (Olness & Gardner, 1978, p. 231) contributed to restoration of functioning in his arms and legs and no re-emergence was noted. Follow-up therapy targeted family dynamics that had contributed to the conversion symptoms. More recently, Bloom (2001) described the use of hypnosis with a 12-year-old girl and 15-year-old boy to aid in resolution of complete or partial paralysis. The author also underscored the importance of individualizing hypnosis based on the unique experiences of the patient, though certain hypnotic techniques can be applied across patients.

Elkins and Carter (1986) described the use of hypnotherapy in the treatment of childhood psychogenic coughing. The patient, Larry, was 11 years, 10 months old. He had a chronic cough of such severity that it resulted in his missing about one month of school.

The patient's symptoms began with a sore throat and mild cough. He was tested by his pediatrician, which resulted in a positive strep screen, and he was treated with penicillin. However, his cough became even worse. He was seen 14 days later complaining of severe episodes of coughing that lasted up to five hours at a time. The cough continued to worsen despite medication trials with promethazine, codeine, and guaifenesin syrup. On one occasion, his parents brought him to the emergency room, where he received an injection of morphine that stopped the cough, but only for a few hours. The coughing, described by the father as a very distracting "loud barking," was of such severity that Larry was unable to attend school. The symptoms had continued for seven weeks before referral for hypnotherapy. Prior to referral, all medical and laboratory tests were normal.

The patient was an only child and a good student. He stated that he wanted to return to school, but expressed some reluctance to return until he "was well." The use of hypnosis was discussed with both the child and parents, and they were interested and supportive of "anything that would help."

During the initial visit, it was learned that the patient enjoyed movies and especially liked the movie *Star Wars*. This provided the basis for a "science-fiction imagery" (Elkins & Carter, 1986) technique. Larry was asked to take a deep breath and close his eyes. He was led, via mental imagery, on an imaging journey into space with "Luke Skywalker," where he met a friendly "Dr. Zargon" who provided a "wonderful medicine" to "cure his cough." At this point, with Larry's permission, the therapist lightly touched him around his neck with suggestions for relaxation, and "as the medicine is applied, your cough becomes less and less." The imagery resulted in immediate symptomatic relief as the coughing stopped. The patient was instructed in the daily practice of hypnosis using a tape recording. He then returned to school full time. The parents were asked to award him a special prize after he was able to attend school for a full week and to give daily praise for school attendance. The symptoms gradually stopped over the next seven days. At a 7-month follow-up, he had no symptoms or cough, was involved in school and extracurricular activities, and showed no symptom substitution. It was hypothesized that excessive parental attention and school avoidance had been contributing to the patient's intractable cough.

Anbar and Hall (2004) reported on the effectiveness of teaching self-hypnosis for 51 children presenting with "habit coughs." The instructions for self-hypnosis included a self-induction, relaxation imagery, cough-related imagery (e.g., "imagine a switch in the head that turns the cough on or off"), validation (e.g., "Notice how the cough diminishes or resolves during and after hypnosis"), and encouragement for daily practice for a period of at least two weeks (Anbar & Hall, 2004, p. 214). A retrospective chart review revealed that 78% of the children stopped eliciting the habit coughs during or immediately after the initial hypnosis instruction session, 8% ceased within one week, and 4% within one month (Anbar & Hall, 2004).

Pseudoseizures

Conversion disorders can be further classified according to the presenting physical symptoms. For instance, *pseudoseizures* may occur. Some other terms that have been used to describe pseudoseizures include nonepileptic seizures, psychogenic seizures, hysterical seizures, or hysteroepilepsy (Oakley, 1999; Stores, 1999). It is estimated that 7% to 25% of children seen in epilepsy centers are non-epileptic. Although, these patients are more likely to be female, particularly as they move into adolescence and adulthood, males are more likely to present with pseudoseizures after sustaining a mild-to-moderate head trauma (Barry & Sanborn, 2001). The interesting aspect of pseudoseizures is that the types of "seizures" are quite varied in their presentation and behavioral attributes. For instance, one child may exhibit vocalizations, such as grunting and moaning, during the apparent seizure, whereas another child may demonstrate significant gross motor movements (Stores, 1999). One seizure emitted by a child whom I [MP] saw for a neuropsychological evaluation had been described as mimicking an absence seizure, yet the staring off into space lasted almost 20 minutes, far longer than a typical absence event.

The challenge to diagnosing pseudoseizures arises from the fact that it is a difficult undertaking to distinguish among purely neurogenic seizures, seizures of a hysterical or psychogenic etiology, and a combination of these factors. The physical presentations are similar and may be indistinguishable through observation alone. Even the duration of an "episode" cannot be an absolute determinant. In the case with the prolonged staring off into space above, that information was but one piece of information to support a diagnosis. Electroencephalographic (EEG) monitoring is also a critical part of the evaluation as changes in rhythmic patterns in recordings would not be expected when evaluating someone with pseudoseizures, although a normal recording does not rule out an organic cause for the seizures (Stores, 1999). There has also been some evidence to suggest that individuals who experience convulsions are more likely to manifest pseudoseizure, complicating the diagnosis even further (Bhatia, 2004).

Outcomes for children diagnosed with conversion disorders with seizures are favorable, provided there is early identification and appropriate treatment (Bhatia & Sapra, 2005). For example, Bhatia and Sapra (2005) described the characteristics of 110 children who presented with conversion disorder, 50 of whom experienced pseudoseizures. The average age was 8.2 years in boys (44%) and 9.4 years in girls (56%), with a typical duration of pseudoseizures for 1 to 3 months. When the patients were put on appropriate drug treatment and/or psychotherapy for 3 months, 72% remitted, 20% showed a decrease in frequency of pseudoseizures, and 8% did not improve (Bhatia & Sapra, 2005, pp. 617–619).

Several researchers (e.g., Barry & Sanborn, 2001; Martinez-Taboas, 2002) have discussed how hypnosis might be used to distinguish organically based seizures from pseudoseizures. Martinez-Taboas (2002) reported on a small sample of eight adults who had been referred for a psychological evaluation because they exhibited seizures without evidence of an organic cause. The author emphasized the importance of collecting data before, during, and after the seizure episode. The hypnosis was described to patients as a "pleasant relaxation state;" the clinician used suggestions for imagery and experiences of physical sensations associated with the convulsions. Further, since the induction took place as part of an assessment, the clinician permitted seizure episodes to manifest, but did include a prompt (i.e., tap on the shoulder) to stop a seizure if an episode progressed more than a few minutes (Martinez-Taboas, 2002). Each patient experienced a seizure during the 10-minute procedure, and in all cases, the seizure stopped in response to the prompt. The author noted that a simple gesture would have been ineffective had those been epileptic seizures.

We relate the following case example, seen by GE, to further illustrate how hypnosis can facilitate differential diagnosis in children.

Kevin

Kevin, a 10-year-old boy, was admitted to the physical-medicine unit because of uncontrolled seizures. He had missed seven weeks of school owing to almost daily seizures. The patient had been diagnosed as having a seizure disorder five years earlier and was placed on a regimen of phenytoin—initially with good results. However, his seizures began to recur two years prior to the hospital admission after the death of a younger brother who had fallen from the back of a moving truck in which both he and the patient had been riding. The patient was observed by the nursing staff to be very clinging and he would have seizures (up to 14 per day) when his requests for attention were not immediately met. Psychogenic seizures were suspected; his seizures consisted of trembling movements in his arms and legs.

I [GE] was consulted to assist with further diagnosis and treatment. Kevin proved to be an excellent subject and quickly responded to hypnotic suggestions. During the hypnotherapy session, I suggested that he could begin to have a seizure when he was touched on the forehead. The patient responded to this suggestion and then was able to terminate the seizure when requested. In addition, a post-hypnotic suggestion was given that when his pediatrician later touched his forehead, seizure activity would again result. The next day during an EEG recording, the sequence of hypnotic induction and suggestion was repeated. The EEG tracings were normal through the "seizure." During later sessions, the patient was taught self-hypnosis with suggestions for control of his seizures. Kevin was an avid science fiction fan. The imagery used was of his being in a spaceship with the mission of shooting down enemy "rockets." Suggestions were given that

---

each "rocket represents a part of a seizure" and "as you shoot down each rocket, the seizure becomes less and less as you relax more and more.

Abdominal Pain

Recurrent abdominal pain has been reported to be the most common complaint in childhood, with estimates ranging from 10% to 17% of school-aged children (Banez & Gallagher, 2006). Although reports of symptoms presentation have varied, one classification system developed in the past decade gives some guidance on diagnostic criteria. First, clinicians should determine the frequency, duration, and level of interference with daily functioning, posed by the symptoms (e.g., three or more pain episodes in at least 3 months, pain interferes with functioning). If a diagnosis of recurrent abdominal pain appears warranted, the clinician should provide further information regarding the etiology. For instance, a subgroup may be depression related (Banez & Gallagher, 2006).

Although it has been noted that organic causes of abdominal pain are likely underidentified, historically less than 10% of those presenting with abdominal pain were found to have an identifiable organic etiology (Apley, 1975; Banez & Gallagher, 2006). In terms of demographic profiles of youth presenting with abdominal pain, they are more likely to be female and middle school age. Although there may be physical causes that contribute to the gastrointestinal complaint, many cases are also manifestations of psychological processes. More often, emotion is found to be expressed as "my stomach hurts." The complaint may become chronic as secondary gain factors enter the picture. Studies examining the impact of abdominal pain have noted that these children are likely to experience frequent school absences, other somatic complaints, high levels of healthcare utilization, and symptoms of mood disorders (e.g., anxiety and depression) (Blanchard & Scharff, 2002; Walker, Garber, Van Slyke, & Greene, 1995).

Browne (1997) presented anecdotal evidence from 51 children and adolescents who presented with externalizing, internalizing, enuresis, or abdominal pain that supported the use of hypnosis to bolster self-confidence and assertiveness. Thirty-nine of the youth experienced a resolution of symptoms, including all 7 of those who had experienced abdominal pain. Most noteworthy was the convenience factor with this type of intervention as most of the hypnosis sessions (range of 3 to 9 for each patient, plus use of an audiotaped induction) lasted only five minutes each.

One article (Anbar, 2001) described the benefit of self-hypnosis for abdominal pain without a physiological cause among five children. Individual sessions included provision of inquiry to obtain preferences for imagery, instructions for self-hypnosis, identification of cues for relaxation, and reinforcement of successful control of the abdominal pain. Four of the children experienced resolution of symptoms within 3 weeks of the first session. One, who was reported to have only practiced self-hypnosis at home two times compared to daily or alternating days reported by the others, did not experience relief from symptoms. The case presented was about a girl with a pseudonym of Allison. She had excelled at school and participated in various extracurricular activities. Symptoms developed after having gastroenteritis. She had reported experiencing stomach pain sometimes in the morning and frequently after school; symptoms interfered with her attending a family sailing trip. After symptoms had persisted for years, she attended the session to teach her the self-hypnosis. Symptoms subsided following the initial session. She attended a follow-up session one month later, and her symptoms did not reemerge for at least the subsequent 11 months (Anbar, 2001).

The studies reviewed thus far reveal that a variety of hypnotherapeutic methods are employed with positive results. There are some common features among the differing approaches. Following are descriptions of our approach to assessment and the planning of hypnotherapeutic interventions, which will be illustrated in a more detailed case study.

Diagnosis of Childhood Somatoform Disorder

Assessment

When children develop symptoms of a psychosomatic nature, the first avenue of professional contact is within a medical milieu (Kreipe, 2006). Generally, children are first evaluated by their pediatrician and then appropriate neurological and laboratory studies are carried out. As much as possible, organic causes of symptoms should be ruled out before the institution of psychological intervention and treatment. For example, the child with headaches should first receive a thorough and complete medical evaluation. The diagnosis of somatization or conversion disorder cannot be made on the basis of psychological testing or a psychiatric interview alone without ruling out medical conditions (Kreipe, 2006).

The second step is a thorough psychological assessment. This may include intellectual and personality test batteries as indicated by the clinician's judgment. In the initial consultation, the goal should be to understand and make sense of both the origins of the patient's symptoms and the factors that contribute to its maintenance. Several areas should be covered, such as (1) stress factors, (2) modeling effects, (3) family dynamics, (4) reinforcement and secondary gain factors, and (5) the child's own motivation and interests. When determining suitability for a hypnosis intervention, an assessment of hypnotizability, inquiries regarding expectations toward hypnosis, and preferences for imagery should be obtained. At the forefront of the assessment process is the ability of the clinician to gain the family's trust and foster their confidence. Garralda (1999) explained that parents often express anxieties regarding the possibility of a physical condition that remains undiagnosed.

In the consultation with the child and family, the therapist looks at any stress in the child's environment or major changes that have occurred. Green, Walker, Hickson, and Thompson (1985) found that patients with recurrent pain without organic etiology reported significantly higher life stress than comparison patients with organic findings. Negative events most commonly experienced in their study included failing grades, arguments between parents, family illness, peer conflicts, death in the family, sibling rivalry, arguments with parents, and losing a friend.

Family dynamics should also be explored. The clinician may inquire as to whether anyone else in the family has a similar problem. It is useful to determine whether anyone else serves as a model for the child's symptoms and behavior, and also to ask or observe how the parents and siblings respond to the patient. Several key questions or areas of exploration may provide useful information as part of this evaluation. Does the symptom result in reinforcement? For example, when the child complains of headaches, is he or she cuddled and given ice cream? Also, what do the parents believe about the problem? Are they resentful of psychological referral? Are they angry? What have they heard from their pediatrician? And, importantly, what are the parents' and child's beliefs and attitudes toward hypnosis? During this interview, I explore the child's interests, likes and dislikes, and development level in order to formulate an appropriate hypnotic induction.

Neuropsychological screening instruments or tests are particularly appropriate as they also provide reassurance to the family regarding examination of any underlying neurological etiology. There are also a variety of self-report measures that capture components of emotional expression, mood disturbance, coping styles, family relationships, somatic complaints, and personality characteristics. Projective techniques may be particularly useful to reveal underlying dynamics that the child is not openly willing to disclose, or for that matter, may not have adequate self-awareness.

Family Conference

A family conference is usually indicated to gather further assessment information, provide feedback, and to assist with treatment planning. A conference is held with the parents and child (and may include grandparents or other family members), and may include the referring physician as well. It might be helpful to see the family first. Without at least a minimal degree of parental support, the most skillful hypnotic intentions are likely to fail.

The goal of this meeting is to (1) give the diagnosis and (2) formulate and agree upon a treatment plan. Apley (1975) refers to the commonly held "triple fallacy," which states that (1) physical symptoms must have (2) physical causes, which must have (3) physical treatments. The aim is to move from viewing the symptoms from a physical problem to a predominately psychological one (Garralda, 1999). The clinicians should first encourage the family to express understanding and then try to present the diagnosis in a way that fits the child's and parents' models of the world that is acceptable and nonoffensive to them. The family is helped to understand the contribution of psychological factors, and the use of hypnosis is openly discussed and a treatment plan outlined.

Behavioral Management/Family Counseling

As with most psychological disorders, a multimodal approach can be very helpful in treating somatoform disorders (Garralda, 1999). A holistic approach to diagnosis and treatment involves a combination of diverse approaches, such as behavioral therapy, family counseling, hypnosis, and pharmacotherapy. Behavioral strategies may help target secondary gains afforded to the child's somatic complaints. For example, two adolescent girls were reported to have developed intractable sneezing in response to psychological stressors. Due to the onset of their symptom, they each received special attention from teachers and family members, were able to avoid school, and were not expected to perform as well academically (Bhatia et al., 2004). Should it be determined that a child is receiving rewards and attention for symptomatic behavior (e.g., being sent home from school following an attack), then the parents are asked to ignore the behavior and instead to reinforce appropriate coping (McCleen & Dyer, 2003). For instance, once the child has been able to attend a full week of school, the parents may be asked to give a special reward. If it is found, for example, that the child's behavior is really symptomatic of an underlying marital problem, or if the parent is excessively dependent on the child, then marriage and/or family therapy is also recommended.

Hypnotherapy

Hypnosis is presented to the child as *a skill to be learned and mastered*. The emphasis is on enhancing the child's sense of self-control. This "teaching model" of hypnosis gives the child greater control over and responsibility for symptoms. A nonauthoritarian approach is usually taken that avoids forcing and instead gives the child the opportunity to learn hypnosis. The actual induction is individualized to suit the child's level of development, interests, fantasies, and likes. Hypnotherapy can help the child alter symptoms, uncover psychodynamics, and learn self-hypnosis.

The initial hypnotic induction allows the emergence of some general idea of the child's responsiveness to hypnosis as a treatment. Hypnosis is a potent intervention and the possibility of rapid change and self-control is communicated to the child and parents. It is suggested during the preinduction talk that significant change may occur after the first hypnotherapy session.

It is not necessary to use standardized hypnotic susceptibility scales. However, it is often useful to demonstrate some "tests" of hypnotic responsiveness such as arm levitation or glove anesthesia. This helps to increase the child's confidence and conviction in his or her ability to exert control. In order to demonstrate the child's degree of control, the child may be asked to produce symptoms (i.e., "the abdominal pain begins now") and then to reduce the symptoms (i.e., "as you now relax, the pain grows less and less") during the hypnotic induction and hypnotherapy.

In virtually all instances, the child is taught self-hypnosis. Usually, this also means making an audiotape recording of a session and giving it to the child for home practice. It is the child's responsibility to remember to practice hypnosis. The parents are usually asked to avoid reminding the child or otherwise trying to "take over" the child's responsibility (Olness, 1976). Rather, the parental role is to avoid attention to symptoms and to provide a supportive environment for the child's mastery of hypnosis.

The process of hypnotic induction and hypnotherapy is demonstrated in the following case example of a child with chronic tension headaches who had been seen by GE. The accompanying narrative illustrates the type of induction, use of personal imagery, deepening, direct suggestion for symptomatic control, and self-hypnosis emphasizing the child's sense of mastery.

Larry

Larry was a 14-year-old boy admitted to the hospital because of persistent and severe headaches. He had made numerous visits to the emergency department and pediatric clinic because of the headaches. Neurological and medical studies had been carried out, including an EEG, computed tomography scan, and a spinal tap, which were entirely normal. He was on acetaminophen with codeine and cyproheptadine. He had missed 8 weeks of school prior to the consultation and was on a homebound program.

The headaches were bilateral and associated with neck tightness and shoulder stiffness. The parents denied any significant stress or conflict at home or school. He had maintained good grades and verbalized that he enjoyed school. In his discussion of medical problems, he was very conversant. For example, he stated during the initial visit, "I have the classic symptoms of allergy," and "My migraine headaches are in the usual localized areas." It was noted that the mother also had chronic headaches. In fact, the mother did not attend that session because she was at home "in bed with a sick headache." It was supposed that there was a component of identification with the mother with regard to headache symptoms and that school avoidance had become a secondary problem.

The parents did accept a partial psychological explanation of the headaches. In fact, they told me that after receiving the diagnosis of psychogenic headaches and the recommendations at the family conference that he return to school, the following events took place that evening at home.

"Larry became upset at this, angry, and his headache started getting worse," they said. The parents reacted by trying to get him to calm down, having him sit in a whirlpool, and so on. But, in their words, he "worked himself up into a headache." By this they meant he became very nervous and was "trying to hyperventilate." They eventually got him to calm down by giving him a great deal of attention, reassurance, and compassion; administering acetaminophen and diazepam; and calling the family doctor. Larry had not returned to school.

The patient was then seen for hypnotherapy. The goal of the session was to gain symptomatic control of his headache and to instruct him in the use of hypnosis for self-control. Further, it was emphasized to the parents that Larry should return to school and that they should avoid reinforcing his headaches by paying special attention to him or allowing absence from school.

The following is a transcript of one hypnotherapy session with Larry. It illustrates specific hypnotic suggestions and a rapid hypnotic induction that may be useful with some children or adolescents.

G. Elkins [GE]: First take in all the air you can hold in your lungs. Hold, and as you exhale, now let your eyelids come down, closing. That's right. All the way down. Very good. Exhale. Relax. Deeper and deeper. Relax. Each time you feel pressure on your right shoulder, Larry, that will be a cue to go into an even deeper state of hypnosis. Drifting deeper and deeper. Just like you were drifting down, just kind of drifting down like you were in an elevator.

You are on the tenth floor in an elevator and every floor that you pass, going deeper and deeper in a deeper state of hypnosis as you do with each breath you exhale. More relaxed. Ten ... nine ... eight. Head, neck, and shoulders relax. Shoulders slumping. Arms beginning to feel heavy. Eight—breathing each time you exhale, relaxing more. Seven. Elevator going down past the floors. Seven. Six. Five. Halfway there. Twice as relaxed. Four. That wave of relaxation spreading down to your legs. Feet beginning to feel heavy. Three. Two. All the way down now to one. Any tension that remains can be released now.

Now, Larry, a part of your mind can begin to drift. Just letting your mind drift to another place and that might be to go fishing. A part of your mind is able to relax you and let go of tension. While you go on a fishing trip now and see that happen. There you are at the river.

Notice whether or not it's a warm day. And whether or not the water is cool; certainly it is cooler than the air around you so that you cannot only breathe the air, but feel it on your face and skin. Perhaps even a slight breeze, Larry, that blows through and that breeze can be so relaxing so that the muscles of your forehead just begin to relax. That's right. Doing very well. So that as you're there you may want to watch what's happened with the fishing and get ready to enjoy catching some fish. As you cast, the line goes out into the water and you get a bite and catch the first fish. You set the hook and begin to reel it in, bringing the fish in. And if it's all right with you, Larry, each time you cast out, as you reel it in, the headache becomes less and less, less and less. Any discomfort becoming less and less and you are able to relax even more.

And so I'll know where you are, whenever you're aware of any sense of headache, I'd like for you to raise one finger on your right hand or your thumb, whichever is right for you. That's right. Any amount of headache that you can feel now. Just raising that finger, or perhaps you've already gotten rid of the headache, and if that's occurred, I'd like for you to raise your thumb. Very good. Very good. That's right, just let that thumb come back down and just continue each time you cast out and you reel in, the headache becoming less and less. Feeling the tension go out of your shoulders. The muscles of your neck relax. Breathing slowly and more comfortably. Drifting all the way down, deeper and deeper, relaxed.

Just as relaxed as you need to be, just as relaxed as you want to be. Feeling of spreading comfort, and as you are fishing there, finding that it's warm enough, that your throat may feel a little dry, thirsty, and you may find yourself going back to the shore. There is some cool water there, delicious, cold, clear, fresh water, and it's hot today and feeling the warmth of the sunshine on the top of your head so that by the time you get there, you just want to sit down under a shade tree. And as you're there under the tree, drinking that cool water and enjoying it. Noticing how relaxing and comfortable it is to be there. Noticing the taste of the cold water, and noticing how refreshing cold water can be. While you are sitting under that tree and the shade, watch the water of the river flow past. Maybe seeing the fish down at the bank that you've caught. Feeling more and more relaxed so as you're there, just resting under a tree, and watching the river flow by.

Larry, any time in the future that you begin, just begin, to have a headache, you now have a way of controlling it by thinking the word "relax" and creating a feeling of relaxation across your forehead, neck, and shoulders. Learning more and more so then, as you practice self-hypnosis, becoming better and better at it. You can become so deeply relaxed whenever you want by practicing self-hypnosis. Alerting now as I count from three to one. Relaxed, three, becoming consciously alert. Two, more alert. One, alert, relaxed, and feeling good and normal in every way.

Conclusion

This chapter reviews the use of hypnosis for the treatment of psychosomatic disorders in children. Hypnosis is usually well accepted and is a feasible intervention for many psychosomatic problems. However, medical and physical causes should be carefully evaluated and ruled out before proceeding with hypnotherapy. Hypnosis can be useful in altering symptoms as well as in clarifying dynamic issues. The clinician should integrate hypnosis into an overall treatment plan that considers family issues, stresses, psychopathology, and secondary gains that may be associated with psychosomatic symptoms. Hypnosis is presented as a skill that gives the child or adolescent greater insight and control of their symptoms. The existing literature suggests that when appropriately applied, hypnosis may be an effective tool in the treatment of childhood psychosomatic disorders.

References

Alexander, F. (1950). *Psychosomatic medicine*. New York: W.W. Norton.

Anbar, R. D. (2001). Self-hypnosis for the treatment of functional abdominal pain in childhood. *Clinical Pediatrics*, 40, 447–451.

Anbar R. D., & Hall H. R. (2004). Childhood habit cough treated with self-hypnosis. *Journal of Pediatrics*, 144(2), 213–217.

American Psychiatric Association (APA). (1994). *Diagnostic and statistical manual of mental disorders* (4th ed.). Washington, D.C.: Author.

Apley, J. (1975). *The child with abdominal pains* (2nd ed.). Oxford: Blackwell Scientific.

Banez, G. A., & Gallagher, H. M. (2006). Recurrent abdominal pain. *Behavior Modification*, 30(1), 50–71.

Barry, J. J., & Sanborn, K. (2001). Etiology, diagnosis, and treatment of nonepileptic seizures. *Current Neurology and Neuroscience Reports*, 1, 381–389.

Bhatia, M. S. (2004). Pseudoseizures. *Indian Pediatrics*, 41(7), 673–679.

Bhatia, M. S., Khandpal, M., Srivastava, S., & Kohli, G. S. (2004). Intractable psychogenic sneezing: Two case reports. *Indian Pediatrics*, 41(5), 503–505.

Bhatia, M. S., & Sapra, S. (2005). Pseudoseizures in children: a profile of 50 cases. *Clinical Pediatrics*, 44(7), 617–621.

Blanchard, E. B., & Scharff, L. (2002). Psychosocial aspects of assessment and treatment of irritable bowel syndrome in adults and recurrent abdominal pain in children. *Journal of Consulting and Clinical Psychology*, 70, 725–738.

Bloom, P. B. (2001). Treating adolescent conversion disorders: Are hypnotic techniques reusable? *International Journal of Clinical and Experimental Hypnosis*, 49(3), 243–256.

Borrell-Carrió, F., Suchman, A. L., Epstein, R. M. (2004). The biopsychosocial model 25 years later: Principles, practice, and scientific inquiry. *Annals of Family Medicine*, 2, 576–582.

Braaic, J. R. (2002). Conversion disorder in childhood. *The German Journal of Psychiatry*, 5(2), 54–61.

Browne, S. E. (1997). Brief hypnotherapy with passive children. *Contemporary Hypnosis*, 14, 59–62.

Cicchetti, D., & Walker, E. F. (2001). Stress and development: Biological and psychological consequences. *Development and Psychopathology*, 13, 413–418.

Elkins, G. R., & Carter, B. D. (1986). Hypnotherapy in the treatment of childhood psychogenic coughing: A case report. *American Journal of Clinical Hypnosis, 29*, 59–63.

Elkins, G. R., Gamino, L. A., & Rynearson, R. R. (1988) Mass psychogenic illness, trance states and suggestion. *American Journal of Clinical Hypnosis, 30*, 267–275.

Garralda, M. E. (1999). Practitioner review: Assessment and management of somatisation in childhood and adolescence: A practical perspective. *Journal of Child Psychology and Psychiatry, 40*(8), 1159–1167.

Green, J. W., Walker, L. S., Hickson, G., & Thompson, J. *(1985).* Stressful life events and somatic complaints in adolescents. *Pediatrics, 75*, 19–22.

Kreipe, R.E. (2006). The biopsychosocial approach to adolescents with somatoform disorders. *Adolescent Medicine, 17*, 1–24.

Malhi, P., & Singhi, P. (2002). Clinical characteristics and outcome of children and adolescents with conversion disorder. *Indian Pediatrics, 39*, 747–752.

Maloney, M. J. (1980). Diagnosing hysterical conversion reactions in children. *Journal of Pediatrics, 97*, 1016–1020.

Martinez-Taboas, A. (2002). The role of hypnosis in the detection of psychogenic seizures. *American Journal Clinical Hypnosis, 45*, 11–20.

McLean, T., & Dyer, C. (2003). Treatment of psychogenic pseudoseizures in an adolescent with a history of epilepsy. *Clinical Psychologist, 7*(2), 109–120.

Moene, F. C., Spinhoven, P., Hoogduin, R. A. L., & Van Dyck, R. (2003). A randomized controlled clinical trial of a hypnosis-based treatment for patients with conversion disorder, motor type. *International Journal of Clinical & Experimental Hypnosis, 51*(1), 29–50.

Oakley, D.A. (1999). Hypnosis and conversion hysteria: A unifying model. *Cognitive Neuropsychiatry, 4*, 243–265.

Olness, K. (1976). Autohypnosis in functional megacolor in children. *American Journal of Clinical Hypnosis, 19*, 28–32.

Olness, K., & Gardner, G. G. (1978). Some guidelines for use of hypnotherapy in pediatrics. *Pediatrics, 62,* 28–32.

Stores, G. (1999). Practitioner review: recognition of pseudoseizures in children and adolescents. *Journal of Child Psychology and Psychiatry, 40,* 851–857.

Tallabs, F.A. (2005). Functional correlates of conversion and hypnotic paralysis: A neurophysiological hypothesis. *Contemporary Hypnosis, 22*(4), 184–192.

Tinterow, M. M. (1970). *Foundations of hypnosis: From Mesmer to Freud.* Springfield, IL: Charles C. Thomas.

Van Dyck, R., & Hoogduin, K. (1989). Hypnosis and conversion disorders. *American Journal of Psychotherapy, 43*(4), 480–493.

Walker, L. S., Garber, J., Van Slyke, D. A., & Greene, J. W. (1995). Long-term health outcomes in patients with recurrent abdominal pain. *Journal of Pediatric Psychology, 20*(2), 233–245.

Chapter Twelve

Hypnotic Treatment of Behavior Disorders

Charles G. Guyer, II, EdD, ABPP

The following vignettes provide useful clinical settings for a discussion of hypnosis in the treatment of behavior disorders. The course of treatment and outcome will be discussed later in this chapter.

Vignette 1

J.P.

J.P., an 8-year-old male, was having problems following directions at school and home. His mother reported that he was unable to focus on any task, "jumped from one thing to another," and was "never" still long enough to sit down and have dinner with the family. His teachers reported that J.P. was "always" out of his seat and disruptive to other students. During the intake interview J.P. demonstrated some of this behavior by crawling on the furniture and rolling on the floor. After listening to a full history and obtaining the proper consents, his pediatrician was contacted. The doctor reported that there were no underlying medical explanations for J.P.'s behavior and that he had prescribed a variety of psychostimulants for J.P. but none was very helpful. He added that he believed J.P. met the *DSM–IV* criteria for Attention-Deficit/Hyperactivity Disorder (ADHD) and that this had been compounded by poor parenting. At the time of the interview, J.P.'s father was deployed with the United States Marine Corps.

Vignette 2

G.T.

G.T. was a 17-year-old male whose biological parents had physically, sexually, and emotionally abused him. He had sexually molested his two younger siblings. He was taken from his biological parents and placed in a foster home where he repeatedly molested another adolescent boy. He was subsequently transferred to a group home with male and female residents. He molested a younger female there. Finally, he was moved to an all-male group home with tighter security. At school, G.T. gained a reputation for being a "tough kid." He had physically forced another boy into a trash can in the school bathroom. In the group home, he delighted in attempting to "beat the system." He continually tried to sneak by the alarms on bedroom doors and disable the video cameras in the hallways. There our therapy started.

Vignette 3

M.T.

M.T. was an 11-year-old boy whose parents characterized him as "explosive." He would fight with peers, talk back to teachers, lie, and steal. He had been arrested for stealing at school and from a convenience store. M.T. exhibited little motivation for change.

Vignette 4

M.R.

While serving in the United States Navy, I was stationed at Marine Corps Recruit Depot, Parris Island, South Carolina. This Marine

Corps "Boot Camp" is a very stressful environment for the 18- and 19-year-old new recruits. One evening, I was paged to the Emergency Room to see an 18-year-old recruit, M.R., who had lost all feeling in her body from the waist down. She said, "I don't know what happened, I just sat down on my bunk this evening and then I could not stand up." M.R. did not react to a surprise pinprick to the top of her foot. The medical evaluation revealed no organic cause for her paralysis. She told me that she was raised in a small town in rural West Virginia and her parents and friends were very proud of her for becoming a Marine. The Drill Instructor reported that M.R. was "always complaining and whining about something," so that she slowed the progress of the entire platoon. As a result, many of the recruit's peers were angry with her. The Drill Instructor believed that M.R. would be held back, something no recruit wants—a consequence tantamount to failure.

Definitions

Educators and special educators originally used the term "behavior disorder" because it was considered to be less stigmatizing than "mentally ill" or emotionally disturbed (Guyer, 1991). This seems to have changed. In recent years the meaning of "behavior disorder" has broadened greatly to include a myriad of behaviors with psychological complications or etiologies. Persons now referred with behavior disorders have a huge spectrum of problems (violent offenders, sex offenders, ADHD, intermittent explosive disorder, oppositional defiant disorder, childhood bipolar disorder, Asperger's Syndrome, and others). "Behavior disorder" has morphed into its predecessor, "emotional disturbance." Terms may change, but behaviors remain constant. For example, the term sociopath was meant to replace the term psychopath, supposedly because it had less negative connotations. The behavior it described remained the same and thus, sociopath came to have the same negative connotations as psychopath. *Webster's New World Dictionary–College Edition* (1966) offers no definition of a behavior disorder, nor does Stedman's Medical Dictionary (1978) or English and English's *Dictionary of Psychological and Psychoanalytic Terms* (1974).

In her 1986 book on behavior disorders, Coleman listed tools used to identify behaviorally disordered children and adolescents including the Rorschach Ink Blot test, the Children's Apperception test, Sentence Completion tests, Human Figure Drawing tests, the Thematic Apperception test, and other personality tests. Many of these tests are utilized to aid psychologists in determining a differential diagnosis between psychopathologies.

Guyer (1991) defined a behavior disorder as "a behavior that violates societal expectations in a specific setting." This definition includes many diagnostic categories, is situation specific, and places the power to label someone with a behavior disorder in the hands of persons in authority (e.g., teachers, police, physicians, psychologists, etc.). This last characteristic is problematic. For example, a person who engages in an activity that is creative but does not follow the situational expectations is labeled as having a behavior disorder and his or her creativity may be stifled as a result. Another reason for concern is that a person in control may use labeling of an individual to expand their power. Authority figures may control a person by defining their behavior as inappropriate and removing them from a given situation.

Several factors then determine who is defined as being behaviorally disordered. These include, but are not limited to: (1) the person in authority's tolerance for various behaviors; (2) the setting in which the behavior takes place; (3) the persistence of the behavior over time; (4) the training and background of the authority figure observing the behavior (Guyer, 1991).

Tolerance is of interest because this varies from person to person and culture to culture. Helton and Oakland (1977) found that teachers in public schools preferred to teach children who are passive and conforming; Coleman and Gilliam (1983) found that teachers had unfavorable attitudes toward aggressive children. This contrasts with the educational culture of a Montessori school with its emphasis on the training of the senses and self-education through guiding rather than controlling the child. This environment is much different from the more traditional public school classroom.

If a behavior deviates *persistently* from a setting's expected norm (e.g., talking in math class), it is more likely to be viewed as a behavioral disorder. The longer a deviant behavior persists, the more it is likely to be labeled "disordered." An authority figure may overlook a one-time digression, but may not overlook ongoing aberrant behavior.

The person who is in charge of the setting (e.g., teacher, physician, psychologist, etc.) also has an experiential past that affects his or her view of acceptable behavior. Hobbs (1975) noted that the same child "may be viewed as mentally ill by a physician, as emotionally disturbed by a psychologist and as behavior disordered by a special educator" (p. 54).

Review of Relevant Literature

Olness and Kohen (1996) write that "there are fewer reports of child hypnotherapy for primary psychological problems than for medical and surgical problems" (p. 99). This statement is as true now as it was in 1996. There are many non-hypnotic approaches to psychotherapy with children and adolescents who have been diagnosed with behavioral problems. These include, but are not limited to, the following:

- Group psychotherapy—Bates and Johnson, 1972; Glasser, 1975; Guyer and Matthews, 1981; Morris and Cinnamon, 1975; Houck, King, Tomlinson, Vrabel and Weeks, 2002; Salloum, Avery and McClain, 2001; Hanson, 2000; Feindle, 1998
- Multisystemic psychotherapy—Littell, Popa, and Forsyth, 2005; Boris and Zeanah, 2005
- Family systems psychotherapy—Robbins, 2005; Miklowitz, 2004; Miklowitz, George, Axelson, Kim, Birmaher, Schneck, Bersford, Craighead and Brent, 2004; Miklowitz, Simoneau, George, Richards, Kalbag, Sachs-Ericsson and Suddath, 2000; Aman, 2001
- Psychosocial treatments—Murphy, 2005; Smith, Gorman-Smith, Quinn, Rabiner, Tolan and Winn, 2004
- Parenting training—Bor, Sanders, Markie-Dadds, 2002

- Behavior modification programs—Bandura, 1969; Skinner, 1953; Pelham, Wheeler and Chronis, 1998
- Social skills training—Pfiffner and McBurnett, 1997; Frankel, Myadt, Cantwell and Feinberg, 1997
- Art therapy—Henley, 2000
- Medication management—van de Wiel, van Goozen, Matthys, Snock and van Engeland, 2004; Murray, 2001

In addition, several authors discuss combining medication management with family and/or group psychotherapy—Miklowitz, George, Richards, Simoneau and Suddath, 2003; James and Javaloyes, 2001; Steifel, 1998.

All of these modalities may be helpful in treating persons labeled as behavior disordered. One must then ask what advantage is gained by implementing hypnotherapy alone or with other techniques. Araoz (1979; 1982; 1985), Zarren and Eimer (2002), and Yapko (1992; 1997) have noted that when cognitive/behavioral techniques are effective, hypnotic techniques may be more effective. Williams (1979) believed that hypnosis may accelerate the therapeutic process and lead to a quicker elimination of symptoms. It appears that the characteristics of a hypnotic state lend themselves readily to working with children and adolescents diagnosed with a behavior disorder.

Attention-Deficit/Hyperactivity Disorder (ADHD) has received a great deal of attention over the past 10 to 15 years. Given the popularity of this subject, there have been surprisingly few papers published concerning hypnosis as a treatment modality for ADHD. *The Diagnostic and Statistical Manual of Mental Disorders–4th Edition–Text Revision* of the American Psychiatric Association (*DSM-IV-TR*, 2000) describes the symptoms of ADHD. These are offered in two sections: (1) one for inattention that includes nine criteria of which six must be met; (2) another section for hyperactivity-impulsivity listing six criteria for hyperactivity and three criteria for impulsivity of which six must be met. It is also noted that symptoms must be manifested by 7 years of age, and some impairment from symptoms must be present in two or more settings (e.g., school, daycare, home, etc.).

Calhoun and Bolton (1986) studied the effectiveness of hypnotherapy in the treatment of Attention-Deficit/Hyperactivity Disorder by psychologists and physicians. Their study included seven boys and four girls enrolled in a special day classroom for hyperkinesis and behavior problems. The children were being treated with methylphenidate (Ritalin). The researchers first attempted a group induction, but were unsuccessful. Eventually, individual inductions were utilized. These researchers reported a significant improvement from pre- to post-hypnotic meetings with the children. They did not include a control group.

Illovsky and Friedman (1976) conducted a study in which 48 hyperactive adolescents received recorded hypnotic suggestions. These authors reported that their modified hypnotic technique helped 45 of the 48 children to lower frustration level and an increased attention span. This study also reported no control group.

Crasilneck and Hall (1985) describe their intervention with an 8-year-old female, who most likely would be diagnosed with Attention-Deficit/Hyperactivity Disorder. They reported that the etiology of the problem was determined to be "minimal brain injury" (a term for these behaviors that preceded the *DSM-III*–1980 definition of ADHD). They focused on decreasing the child's anxiety and improving her sense of confidence. Suggestions were given that the child would find herself wanting to study more and would feel gratified from doing a good job. She was reportedly given suggestions while in a trance that some of the energy that was self defeating for her would be directed to more useful work. She was also given suggestions of improved concentration and better peer and parent relations. At the end of nine weeks, she was reported to have improved a letter grade on most subjects and she seemed more able to attend and concentrate. Her interpersonal relationships improved. Crasilneck and Hall (1985) state "In an organ as complicated as the human brain, injuries that do not produce gross abnormalities, such as paralysis, may still underlie subtle changes in the functioning of the child. Such injury, often attributed to the difficulties of birth, may be correlated at times with a problem of hyperactivity" (p. 254). This very fact may be why there are so few reported studies utilizing hypnosis with

ADHD. If indeed minimal brain injury underlies many ADHD diagnoses, then as these authors point out, hypnosis is not the treatment of choice. This, of course, is just one case and generalization is limited.

Dunn and Howell (1982) reported that after 10 sessions of relaxation training, 10 boys diagnosed as hyperactive exhibited reduced muscle tension and changes in behavior that were easily observable by parents and researchers. The authors did offer control sessions prior to treatment. There was no formal control group.

In recent years, there has also been a move toward implementing computer assisted biofeedback in the treatment of ADHD. Since Miller (1969) first described the operant conditioning of the autonomic nervous system (e.g., blood flow, heart rate, etc.) biofeedback has moved into a position of prominence as a treatment modality. It has become so popular that Olness and Kohen (1996) devoted an entire chapter of their book to the interaction of biofeedback and hypnosis. These authors state: "It is noteworthy that manuals provided with biofeedback equipment invariably include relaxation imagery or hypnotic inductions to be used in the training process" (p. 319). Loo and Barkley (2005) echo this sentiment and emphasize that more research is needed in the use of electrophysiological methods as a treatment modality. After reviewing the literature on this topic, Monastra, Lynn, Linden, Lubar, Gruzelier, and LaVaque (2005) agree with Loo and Barkley.

Blanton and Johnson (1991) report their use of biofeedback with three children (two 11-year-olds and a 10-year-old) diagnosed with ADHD. Their goal was to improve these children's self-control. These children were selected by their teachers and their principal as showing "the most ADHD-like behaviors." These patients were treated with biofeedback sessions lasting up to 20 minutes. These sessions included 2 minutes of baseline, verbal instructions for 2 minutes, a relaxation tape for 8–12 minutes, and a relaxation period of 2 minutes. Results showed that all three children were able to relax with computer assisted biofeedback, and one student for which on-task behavior was gathered, exhibited an increase in on-task behavior after this intervention. There is no mention of a control group in this paper.

Tansey (1993) reported quite impressive results in which a 10-year-old boy who was diagnosed as hyperactive and had failed the fourth grade in a special education class. Tansey noted that this child also presented with a "developmental reading disorder" along with being diagnosed with Attention-Deficit/Hyperactivity Disorder and being "perceptually impaired." The child was trained in EMG biofeedback and with an EEG 14-Hz biofeedback regime. Training also included what appeared to be hypnosis and/or relaxation training. The child was reported to be symptom free in only three sessions. What is more impressive is the fact that the patient remained symptom free at a 10-year follow up. This is a case report and no control group was utilized.

Other diagnostic headings that fall under the title of a behavior disorder have been treated by similar means. The problem of injecting children with vaccines is well known in the medical community, and is a short-lived, situation specific behavioral problem. Children often react with distress, anxiety, fear, increased motor tension, and some may even run from the doctor's exam room or hide behind furniture. These behaviors not only make it difficult for healthcare providers to deliver the vaccine, but also interfere with parental cooperation and aggravate anti-vaccine sentiment in the general public (Jacobson, Swan, Adegbenro, Ludingten, Wollen, and Poland, 2001). These authors found that combined with an attitude of empathy, informal methods of hypnosis (distraction, calming, etc.) reduced the negative effects of a child receiving vaccine. They found formal hypnotic inductions, which combined a deep state of relaxation with focused imagery and suggestion, were even more helpful in aiding children and adolescents to prepare for, cope with, and tolerate the pain and anxiety associated with the delivery of vaccine through a needle.

J. Sommers-Flanagan and R. Sommers-Flanagan (1996) described an approach that they entitled "Wizard of Oz" hypnotherapy for use with children 8–13 years old who are generally difficult to treat, because of their intermittent, inattentive impulses and oppositional characteristics. The authors reported they have used this approach as an adjunct to cognitive/behavioral psychotherapy both individually and in a small group format. The authors noted that this approach appeared to facilitate personal problem solving, improved self-regulation skills, and enhanced self-esteem. They feel this was accomplished because the metaphor strengthened the therapeutic alliance, increased the child's interest in therapy procedures, and generally improved the child's cooperation with treatment.

Culbertson (1989) asserts that hypnotherapy may sometimes be helpful in ameliorating the behavioral characteristics of Tourette's Disorder. A case study of an adolescent male who was referred by his physician for hypnotherapy is presented. Culbertson outlined a 4-step approach to treatment that involved progressive relaxation, fingertip temperature feedback using a biotech finger band, Spiegel's eye-roll procedure, and imagery. This treatment encompassed nine sessions over a period of six months. At the end of this period, the adolescent's tics and vocalizations were minimal to nonexistent. A follow-up report 6 months later indicated that the adolescent had applied to the Air Force and had been accepted with no mention of Tourette's Disorder as an issue during the Air Force examination. This was an anecdotal paper and no control group was utilized.

Goldbeck and Schmid (2003) investigated the influence of autogenic relaxation training in a "mildly disturbed" population of children and adolescents with mostly "internalizing symptoms" and/or some aggressive, impulsive, or attention deficit symptoms. Their study included 50 children and adolescents from southern Germany with a mean age of 10.2 years old and a range from 6–15 years old. This study included a waiting list control group. They measured behavioral symptoms with the child behavior checklist (CBCL) and psychosomatic complaints were measured by the Giessen Complaint List. The level of stress was assessed before and after the intervention or before and after the waiting period. Individual goal attainment was evaluated at the end of the intervention and in a 3-month follow up. At the end of the intervention, 56% of the children and 55% of the parents reported partial goal attainment, 38% of the children and 30% of the parents reported complete goal attainment; 71% of the parents reported partial goal attainment 3 months post intervention.

Baumann (1970) utilized visual imagery induction techniques to treat drug use in adolescent patients. Reporting the incidence of marijuana use in middle schools as high as 30–40% and in college as high as 80%, he described a technique in which he used revivification of an earlier "good trip" for a happy drug experience. Baumann found this technique was not successful with marijuana users. He considered this might be attributed to their lack of motivation to change as most of them did not believe marijuana was harmful to their health. Baumann did find that his approach worked with users of Lysergic acid diethylamide (LSD) and of amphetamines, as these users did understand that their drug of choice was dangerous.

Lawlor (1976; 1978) suggested that hypnosis can be effective with school phobic children. She described the case of a 5-year-old boy, the eldest in a sibship of three. He became fearful and had tantrums each morning before going to school. Under hypnosis, the child revealed a fear of sibling rivalry and fearfulness that his mother would die while he was away at school. It was revealed that his grandmother, with whom he was very close, had died shortly before he began school. In Lawlor's approach, hypnosis was utilized as an uncovering technique. Once difficulties were identified, she established a behavioral program that included the parents and school personnel. The child responded positively and was able to enter school without difficulty the following year. This is a case study and included no control group.

When reviewing the literature in the area of hypnosis and the treatment of behavior disorders, it becomes clear that there still are few articles published in this area that are empirically based. The majority of published articles are case studies (often single case) or do not have sufficient experimental designs to withstand the scrutiny of the scientific community. Milling and Costantino (2000) called shortcoming the major limitation preventing child hypnosis from qualifying as "efficacious" according to the criteria for empirically supported therapies (EST). There is a current movement within the American Psychological Association to support EST interventions. Should this movement succeed, therapeutic interventions that do not meet the empirically supported therapies' criteria will lose support. EST guidelines require treatment specification via a manual or its equivalent. This sounds an alert for those who utilize hypnotherapy in our treatment of children and adolescents. Not only do most clinicians who utilize hypnotherapy with children or adults prize creativity, openness to new methods, and clinical acumen instead of manuals or cookbooks, the use of creativity and novelty in hypnotherapeutic approaches may be a critical element in their success (Rossi, 2002).

Clinical Strategies

When making a clinical intervention, it is imperative that the child's parent/guardian sign an informed consent for treatment, and an informed consent for hypnotherapy/hypnosis. This informed consent agreement should make clear to the parent/guardian, the adolescent and the child when possible, the limits of confidentiality. This must be explained in such a way the responsible party understands what can remain confidential and what cannot. If for any reason a case is court ordered (e.g., an acting out violent teenager, the law has been broken, etc.), the clinician must explain in detail that all information will go back to the judge. If a case is referred by a Department of Social Services, the clinician should explain that a report containing most of the information will go back to a social worker for that agency. It is also important to explain the policies of the clinic, hospital, practice, etc., where the evaluation or psychotherapy is being conducted. All should understand that when hypnosis is utilized, information gained during a hypnotic state, and possibly after a hypnotic state will most likely not be admissible in court (Hammond et al., 1994).

In my practice, I give the responsible party a brochure so they can review it and fully understand the policies and procedures of the office. When hypnosis is to be utilized, I give the responsible party and the child (if appropriate) a brochure that was prepared by Wester (2006) entitled, "Questions and Answers about Clinical Hypnosis." This brochure is given to aid in dispelling myths that the parent/guardian, adolescent or child may have about hypnosis. The brochure is then sent home with them and they are asked to read it again on their own so that we can discuss any new questions in our next session.

When a minor child between the ages of 10 to 18 is the patient, I generally have them sign an informed consent as well as their parent/guardian. I have found many children feel more invested in the therapeutic intervention simply by going through the informed consent process. Some children have indicated that they feel more secure knowing exactly what will be done with the information they and their parent/guardian provide. In the first meeting, I clarify with the child and the parent/guardian what information the child offers that will be shared with the parent/guardian and what information will not. These practices vary from case to case, but are always agreed upon by all parties before the first session ends. Children often gain a sense that they are respected by being involved in this process. This is vital for future self-concept building and our rapport.

Next, I conduct a structured clinical interview to establish a working diagnosis and gain a thorough history. Many writers feel that a thorough psychosocial history must be completed before any form of psychotherapy, but especially when hypnotherapy is undertaken (Crasilneck and Hall, 1985; Brown and Fromm, 1987; Barber, 1996a; Bonica and Loeser, 1996; Kroger and Fezler, 1976; Guyer, 2000; Zarren and Eimer, 2002). This allows for a therapeutic intervention to be tailored to the patient and avoids blundering into unknown areas with untoward results.

Guyer (2000) has offered the following headings to aid in collecting information:

1. Presenting Problem and Referral Source
2. Primary Care Physician—name, telephone number and office street address
3. Mental Status Examination
4. Medical History
5. Psychological History
6. Social History
7. Legal History
8. Substance Abuse Screen (history and current data). This is very important when dealing with pre-teens and teenagers.
9. A working diagnosis using the *DSM-IV-TR*, AXIS I through V.
10. Medical and Psychiatric Consultation, when requested.

11. Development of a safety plan, verbal rehearsal, and home-work to rehearse the safety plan between this meeting and the next meeting (this is used when the child or adolescent has violent outbursts. This is established for the protection of the patient and other family members).
12. Treatment Plan
    • Goals of Treatment
    • Objective Outcome Measures
    • Planned Interventions
    • Date of Next Appointment
    • How to Contact the Evaluator, Therapist or Backup Person in the case of an emergency, 24 hours a day, 7 days a week

With this background review completed, we return to the vignettes that started this chapter to illustrate the integration of hypnosis in the treatment of behavioral disorders. There are, of course, as many treatment strategies as there are patients and psychotherapists.

J.P.—Treatment

In the first vignette, J.P. presented with classic symptoms of Attention-Deficit/Hyperactivity Disorder. He had been cleared by his physician of medical problems. In consultation with his mother and his physician, a treatment plan was established that employed hypnotherapy, the establishment of a behavior modification program in the home and continued medication management by his physician. The behavior modification program consisted of a contingency management contract (Zimbardo, Weber, & Johnson, 2003) that the therapist helped J.P.'s mother establish for him and his 6-year-old sister. J.P.'s mother also gave her consent for him to engage in hypnotherapy.

One of J.P.'s favorite hobbies was collecting quarters that had been produced with an image representing each state on one side of the quarter. This seemed to make the coin induction technique (Olness and Kohen, 1996) a natural. J.P. was asked to pick his favorite coin and to stare at it until it dropped. He easily learned how to place himself in a trance. While in a trance, he was given suggestions of relaxation, peace, tranquility, and how to recognize these feelings in his daily life and enjoy them. He was also asked to envision himself at school sitting in his seat listening to the teacher and moving only his leg or foot, but not leaving his chair and how good that might feel. He was also given suggestions that reading would be easier, more enjoyable and he would find pleasure and satisfaction in doing the very best job possible. He was told, while in trance, that the drive/energy that had caused him difficulty while in school would be automatically channeled into a new more productive direction. He was also told while still in a hypnotic state that when the situation was appropriate (e.g., outside at home or on the playground) he could move freely and that would help him expend any "left over energy" in a safe way.

J.P. showed improvement throughout the next nine weeks and his grades improved significantly. Most of his grades were C's with two A's. Before, his grades had been mostly F's with an occasional D. The teacher and his mother both reported that his behavior had greatly improved. At school, he was much more cooperative with the teacher and hardly ever left his seat at inappropriate times, rarely talked back to the teacher, and no longer disrupted other students. His mother said the same was true at home. J.P. was taught self-hypnosis and asked to practice it each day.

A telephone call to J.P.'s mother one year later revealed that she felt most gains had continued, although his grades had been up and down over the year.

G.T.—Treatment

In the second vignette, the group home staff and the Department of Social Services worker who had custody of G.T. asked if I would treat him. They were aware that I utilized hypnosis in treating sex offenders. A psychiatrist had been prescribing psychotropic medications for G.T. and continued to do so. G.T. was placed on aripiprazole (Abilify). G.T. was then involved in a 7-stage program for treating sex offenders that I had developed while on active duty in the United States Navy (Guyer & vanPatton, 1995). This therapeutic model has also been applied to spouse abusers (Guyer, 2000).

This program was adapted to meet G.T.'s specific needs and progressed as follows:

Stage 1. First, the legal system was reinvolved. The courts had placed G.T. in Department of Social Services custody and then placed him in a group home and done little else. It was imperative to the treatment of G.T. (as with any other sex offender) that he understand that he had broken the law. G.T. was made aware of the fact that if he had been over the age of 18 when he sexually abused his sisters and the other teenage boy he would now be in jail. He was confronted with the reality that he is fast approaching the age of 18 and that if he perpetrates any sexual crime after that age, he will go to jail (Glasser, 1975). The judge, who he had seen in previous cases, called G.T. into his chambers to explain this clearly and specifically to him.

Stage 2. In this stage, G.T. was confronted with the fact he is totally responsible for his sexually abusive behavior to his sisters and to the boy in the foster home.

Stage 3. The third stage of G.T.'s treatment involved traditional cognitive-behavioral psychotherapy. In this stage, G.T. was taught techniques for effectively coping with the stress in his life and methods for dealing with obsessive thoughts and compulsive behaviors. He was also trained in appropriate conflict management techniques. Using the cognitive behavioral model with sex offenders has been shown to have much lower recidivism rates than other therapeutic interventions. Therapeutic interventions in general with sex offenders have a recidivism rate of 14%–28% (McCary & McCary, 1982). With exposure to cognitive-behavioral approaches, recidivism rates fall to 5%–15% (Traven, Bluestone, Coleman, Culler & Melella, 1986; Traven, Bluestone, Coleman & Melella, 1986).

Stage 4. This stage focused on having G.T. understand that his biological parents were poor examples of how to interact within a family and that role boundaries were not made clear by them (Goldenberg & Goldenberg, 1985, pp. 183-203). Since G.T. had no current family to engage in systems psychotherapy to clarify family roles, he was enrolled in a parenting program. It was hoped that this would help to clarify each person's role in a "normal" family and help him understand how parents are expected to treat their children. There is data from the spouse abuse literature to suggest that persons who are abusive decrease both physically and emotionally abusive behavior after completing a parenting course (Navaco, 1975; Schinke, Schilling, Barth, Gilchrist, & Maxwell, 1986; Stacy & Shupe, 1983). G.T. was taught these skills in individual sessions following the systematic training for effective parenting model of Dinkmeyer and McKay (1976). G.T. reported that he actually enjoyed this training, and he began to compare his parents to what he now viewed as "regular parents."

Stage 5. In stage five, a hypnotherapeutic intervention was carried out. There are many similarities between cognitive-behavioral therapies and hypnotically based interventions (Araoz, 1979; 1982; 1985; Zarren & Eimer, 2002; Yapko, 1992; 1997). These authors feel that in circumstances where cognitive-behavioral techniques are effective, hypnotically based techniques may be even more effective. The hypnotic technique used with G.T. involved seven steps as follows:

Step 1. G.T. began this step by being introduced to the hypnotic procedures that would be utilized. Once he understood completely what this entailed, he was asked if he agreed to engage in the treatment. He did agree. Even though he was underage in the State of North Carolina, he signed an informed consent for the use of hypnotherapy. An example of the consent form can be found in Hammond et al. (1995, p. 50–51).

Step 2. G.T. became proficient in the development and use of imagery techniques (Guyer, 1991). A hypnosis tape was made for him to use at home (Guyer & Guyer, 1984). He reported that he practiced hypnotic imagery at home twice a day. He also practiced heterohypnosis twice a week in my office.

Step 3. G.T. was next involved in working with imagery specifically designed to focus on his anger with his parents, fear of rejection, anxiety with interpersonal interactions and his poor self-concept. These all appeared to be major influences for his aggressive and sexually abusive actions. G.T. frequently teared throughout this process. He appeared to gain great insights during this portion of his treatment program.

Step 4. In this portion of the hypnotherapeutic intervention, an age regression (Kroger & Fezler, 1976) was undertaken. G.T. regressed to when he was a young child (around 1½ to 2 years old). This was his first memory of his father physically abusing him. He also recalled his mother sexually abusing him about the same age. He reported that these types of abuse continued until he was removed from his biological parents' care at the age of 13 years old. The therapy focused on his acknowledgment of his anger and ways to resolve this anger so that it might be expressed in more socially acceptable ways.

Step 5. At this point, an attempt was made to re-educate G.T.'s inner child (Araoz, 1982). This was accomplished by again age regressing G.T. to his early childhood when the physical and sexual abuse started. This regression was very emotional for G.T. and he cried hysterically throughout this process. While G.T. was in a regressed state, G.T. as a child was introduced to the 15-year-old boy he sexually abused at the foster home with the boy appearing as a young child. The images of the two young children were given suggestions for becoming friends, caring for one another, protecting one another, and seeing one another as equals. The images of the two young children were then merged into one young child. G.T. signaled by raising his right forefinger that this merger was fully completed. This new unitary child is now G.T. as a child. The 17-year-old G.T. was then reintroduced into the scene. The 17-year-old G.T. then gave advice and guidance to the young child G.T. and through this experience, re-educated the young child G.T. so that he would not again repeat new sexually abusive behaviors/ offenses. The 17-year-old G.T. was then removed from the scene, and G.T. as a young child slowly age progressed back to the age of 17 years old. Post-hypnotic suggestions for empathy, caring, understanding and equality of people were made during the age progression back to G.T.'s current age of 17 years old.

Step 6. This portion of the intervention entailed an age progression to a time in the future when G.T. accepts responsibility for his behaviors, handles all interactions with others non-violently, has no obsessive thoughts, and no compulsions. Post-hypnotic suggestions were given for confidence, a decreased need to manipulate others, a decreased need for power and control of others, ego strengthening, and normal interactions with persons of both sexes.

Step 7. G.T. was then reoriented to the therapeutic setting. In future sessions, we dealt with his emotions concerning the age regression, merging of the children, and age progression. Much of this was accomplished through cognitive-behavioral psychotherapy.

Stage 6. At this stage of therapy, G.T. had been in psychotherapy for one year. He had continued by his own desire after he turned 18 years old. He verbalized that he felt more empathy for his past victims, specifically for the 15-year-old boy, and he exhibited what appeared to be genuine remorse. Over the period of that year, G.T. was not without some behavioral issues. He had run away from the group home once when he was still 17 years old. He had difficulty transitioning to independent living and was placed in an adult group home. He, however, had not molested another person of either sex and he exhibited no violent behavior. G.T. appeared to still be struggling with many sexually related issues, but felt he would not act on these inappropriately. He still had no girlfriend or love relationship. He had dated several girls on and off, and stated that since he had turned 18, he had consensual sex with a girl he had dated who was 21 years old. That experience had not gone well for him with him ejaculating prematurely. The girl ridiculed him.

Stage 7. This stage was the closure of the therapeutic alliance. G.T. eventually moved from the city where I practiced. I have had no follow-up information on him. I did feel that he was in need of continued psychotherapy. He did resolve many of his issues, but I still viewed him as a high risk for sexually reoffending.

M.T.—Treatment
In vignette 3, 11-year-old M.T.'s parents made it clear to him that if he did not choose to change his fighting, stealing, lying, and disrespectful behavior, he would be sent to a therapeutic camp for children with conduct problems. M.T. was assessed by a psychiatrist.

He was placed on aripiprazole (Abilify). A reality therapy approach was utilized (Glasser, 1975; Lipsett and Lipsett, 2000) in which M.T. was confronted with the fact that he had broken the law and the school was going to press charges if he did not agree to be involved in psychotherapy.

When the idea of hypnotherapy was brought to M.T.'s attention, he appeared excited about it. He had a vivid imagination and easily learned imagery induction techniques. While in a trance, M.T. was given suggestions of calming, relaxation, peace, and empathy for others. Suggestions of change in a positive way were also given. He was asked to imagine himself talking openly and freely with his parents and other authority figures. In these images, his parents and the other authority figures would hear what he was saying, work with his frustrations, and help him resolve his concerns. Suggestions of ego-strengthening and ego enhancement were also given. M.T. was given a recording to help him practice hypnosis at home (Guyer & Guyer, 1984).

On one occasion after a trance session, M.T. spontaneously shared with the therapist that he was angry because he did not think his parents loved each other or him. He said he knew they wanted to be apart because they had separated when he was 4 or 5 years old. This was confirmed from the intake history. During the intake interview, his parents downplayed that event and M.T. denied that it had bothered him. In a separate interview with his parents, it came to light that neither parent had been happy in the relationship since that split. They had stayed together for M.T.'s sake. His parents entered couple's counseling and decided to separate. M.T. remained in psychotherapy (both cognitive and hypnotherapy) to help him adapt to his parents' impending divorce. While he was saddened by his parents' separation, his overall anger decreased, as did his acting out behavior. Therapy ended after his parents' divorce and there were no reported major conduct problems at a one-year follow-up telephone call. His parents agreed to joint custody.

M.R.—Treatment

The fourth vignette was the case of M.R., the 18-year-old paralyzed female Marine treated in the Emergency Room. When I met with her, I explained that we needed her to relax more and I was going to teach her how to do this. We spoke about hypnosis and she agreed to use it. I induced a trance by using passes over her arms and face because when we spoke of using hypnosis, she described this technique. She was not touched, but I moved my hands a few inches above her arms and face. M.R. easily entered trance. While in trance, she was told she could open her eyes, move her head, talk, and hear clearly.

I explained to her that she had a disease called spinoneurogitus (I made it up). She was then told that there was a cure for this disease, and that it required only one shot of medication for a total cure. The emergency room physician administered saline solution with a small bore needle. M.R. was then told that due to her illness, she would have to be separated from the United States Marine Corps and that we were sorry, but this was the law. She said that she understood. She was told that she would gain feeling back in her legs and would be able to walk again in the course of approximately two hours. I explained to her at that time she would return to normal in every way.

In two hours' time, M.R. could walk again and was totally alert. We had successfully removed her conflict concerning disappointing her family and her friends, and we had resolved the Marine Corps' unhappiness of having a poorly performing recruit who was holding back her platoon. The Drill Instructor viewed her as having a behavior disorder. Later, this Emergency Room procedure was explained to M.R. in psychotherapy over the weeks following this event and prior to her being discharged from the Marine Corps. She was to follow up with a psychologist in her home town upon discharge.

These clinical vignettes show that behavior disorders come in a variety of forms, and require a wide array of clinical strategies.

Caveats

Behavior disorder is not a diagnostic term. It is a descriptive term that includes many diagnoses. It is defined by the setting and the experiential past of the person in authority who is viewing the behavior, an authority figures' tolerance for the behavior in a given setting, and the persistence of the behavior over time.

To effectively treat a patient presenting with a behavior disorder, it is imperative to gather an in-depth clinical assessment that determines what led the patient to come into treatment at that time, how the symptoms are benefiting the patient, and whether or not hypnotherapy is the treatment of choice in a given case. I do not utilize standardized tests of hypnotic responsivity to determine who will be a good hypnotherapy patient and who will not. I have gotten excellent results in hypnotherapy with persons who would not perform well on any of the Stanford Hypnotic Susceptibility Scales (Weitzenhoffer & Hilgard, 1962) the Harvard Scale of Hypnotic Susceptibility (Shor & Orne, 1962) or any other standardized scale of that type. While it is recognized that standardized measures are valuable for some research purposes, they have not been necessary in my work.

The cases presented here clearly show that in daily clinical practice, rarely is hypnosis used as the only intervention. The goal is to change behavior as quickly as possible without doing harm. This is generally best accomplished through the use of several different interventions specifically tailored for the individual patient.

The use of hypnotherapy in treating behavior disorders of children and adolescents clearly needs more empirical study. This, however, may prove to be a difficult task. The shear breadth of diagnoses that fall under this heading complicates and clouds the establishment of behavioral definitions. Alas, it appears we have some distance to travel before we can meet the criteria outlined by Milling and Costantino (2000) to be considered an empirically supported therapy (EST). The definition of hypnosis, however, has made great strides and technology now allows empirical studies to be carried out that clearly support hypnosis as a unique state of altered consciousness that can enhance therapeutic behavioral change. (Barabasz and Watkins, 2005).

References

Aman, L. A. (2001). Family systems multiple-group therapy for ADHD children and their families. *Dissertation Abstracts International: Section B: The Sciences and Engineering*, Vol. 61 (10-B), 5548.

American Psychiatric Association. (1968). *Diagnostic and statistical manual of mental disorders-II.* Washington, D.C.: Author.

American Psychiatric Association. (1980). *Diagnostic and statistical manual of mental disorders-III.* Washington, D.C.: Author.

American Psychiatric Association. (2000). *Diagnostic and statistical manual of mental disorders-IV-TR.* Washington, D.C.: Author.

Anbar, R. (2001). Automatic word processing: A new forum for hypnotic expression. *American Journal of Clinical Hypnosis*, 44, 27–36.

Araoz, D. L. (1979). *Hypno-counseling.* No. Ed. 182, 624). ERIC Document Reproduction Service. Available at: www.eric.ed.gov

Araoz, D. L. (1982). *Hypnosis and sex therapy.* New York: Brunner/Mazel.

Araoz, D. L. (1985). *The new hypnosis.* New York: Brunner/Mazel.

Bandura, A. (1969) *Principles of behavior modification.* New York: Holt, Rinehart and Winston.

Barabasz, A., & Watkins, J. G. (2005). *Hypnotherapeutic techniques 2E.* New York: Brunner-Routledge.

Barber, J. (1996a). Psychological evaluation of the patient with pain. In J. Barber (Ed.), *Hypnosis and suggestion in the treatment of pain* (pp. 50–66). New York: W.W. Norton.

Barber, J. (1996b). Hypnotic Analgesia: Clinical considerations. In J. Barber (Ed.), *Hypnosis and suggestion in the treatment of pain* (pp. 85–118). New York: W.W. Norton.

Barkley, R. A. (2002). Psychosocial treatments for Attention-Deficit/ Hyperactivity Disorder in children. *Journal of Clinical Psychiatry*, 63 (Suppl. 12), 36–43.

Basmajian, J. V. (1976). *Stedman's medical dictionary* (23rd ed.). Baltimore, MD: Williams & Wilkins.

Bates, M. D., & Johnson, D. J. (1972). *Group leadership: A manual for group counseling leaders*. Denver, CO: Love.

Baumann, F. (1970). Hypnosis and the adolescent drug abuser. *American Journal of Clinical Hypnosis*, 13, 17–21.

Bjornstad, G., & Montgomery, P. (2005). Family therapy for Attention-Deficit/Hyperactivity Activity Disorder in children and adolescents. *Cochrane Database Systems Review*, 18(2), CD005042.

Blanton, J., & Johnson, L. J. (1991). Using computer assisted biofeedback to help children with Attention-Deficit/Hyperactivity Disorder to gain self-control. *Journal of Special Education Technology*, 11(1), 49–56.

Bonica, J. J., & Loeser, D. L. (1996) Medical evaluation of the patient with pain. In J. Barber (Ed.). *Hypnosis and suggestion in the treatment of pain* (pp. 33–49). New York: W.W. Norton.

Bor, W., Sanders, M. R., & Markie-Dadds, C. (2002). The Effects of the triple p-positive parenting program on pre-school children with co-occurring disruptive behavior and Attention-Deficit/Hyperactivity difficulties. *Abnormal Child Psychology*, 30(6), 571–587.

Boris, N. W., & Zeanah, C. H. (2005). Practice parameters for the assessment and treatment of children and adolescents with Reactive Attachment Disorder of infancy and early childhood. *Journal of The American Academy of Child and Adolescent Psychiatry*. 44(11), 1206–1219.

Brown, D. P., & Fromm, E. (1987). *Hypnosis and behavioral medicine*. Hillsdale, NJ: Lawrence Erlbaum.

Calhoun, G., Jr., & Bolton, J. A. (1986). Hypnotherapy: A possible alternative for treating pupils affected with Attention Deficit Disorder. *Perceptual Motor Skills*, 63(3), 1191–1195.

Cautela, J. R. (1969). Behavior therapy and self-control. In C. M. Franks (Ed.), *Behavioral therapy appraisal and status* (pp. 323–340). New York: McGraw-Hill.

Coleman, M. C. (1986). *Behavior disorders: Theory and practice.* Englewood Cliffs, NJ: Prentice-Hall.

Coleman, M. C., & Gilliam, J. E. (1983). Disturbing behaviors in the classroom: A survey of teacher attitudes. *Journal of Special Education,* 17, 121–129.

Cooper, L., & Erickson, M. (1959). *Time distortion in hypnosis.* Baltimore: Williams & Wilkins.

Crasilneck, H., & Hall, J. (1985). *Clinical hypnosis: Principles and applications* (2nd ed.). Boston, MA: Allyn and Bacon.

Culbertson, F. M. (1989). A four-step hypnotherapy model for Gilles de la Tourette's syndrome. *American Journal of Clinical Hypnosis,* 31(4), 252–256.

Dinkmeyer, D., & McKay, G. (1976). *Parents handbook: Systematic training for effective parenting.* Circle Pines, MN: American Guidance Services.

Dunn, F. M., & Howell, R. J. (1982). Relaxation training and its relationship to hyperactive boys. *Journal of Clinical Psychology,* 38(1), 92–100.

English, H. B., & English, A. V. (1974). *A comprehensive dictionary of psychological and psychoanalytical terms* (3rd ed.). New York: David McKay.

Feindler, E. L. (1998). Adolescent anger management groups for violence reduction. In K.C. Stolber & T. R. Kratochwill (Eds.) *Handbook of group intervention with children and families* (pp. 100–119). Needham Heights, MA: Allyn and Bacon.

Frankel, F., Myatt, R., Cantell, D. P., & Feinberg, D. T. (1997). Parent-assisted transfer of children's social skills training: Effects on children with and without Attention-Deficit/Hyperactivity Disorder. *Journal of the American Academy of Child & Adolescent Psychiatry,* 36(8), 1056–1064.

Glasser, W. (1975). *Reality therapy: A new approach to psychiatry.* New York: Perennial Library, Harper and Row.

Goldbeck, I., & Schmid, K. (2003). Effectiveness of autogenic relaxation training on children and adolescents with behavioral and emotional problems. *Journal of the American Academy of Child and Adolescent Psychiatry*, 42(9), 1046–1054.

Goldenberg, I., & Goldenberg, H. (1985). *Family therapy: An overview* (pp. 183–203). Pacific Grove, CA: Brooks/Cole.

Guralnik, D. B., & Friend, J. H. (Eds.) (1968). *College Edition: Webster's New World Dictionary of the American Language*. New York: The World Publishing Company.

Guyer, C. G. (1991). Hypnosis in the treatment of behavior disorders. In W. C. Wester & D. J. O'Grady (Eds.), *Clinical hypnosis with children* (pp. 150–164). New York: Brunner/Mazel.

Guyer, C. G. (2000). Spouse abuse. In F. W. Kaslow (Ed.), *Handbook of Couple and Family Forensics: A Sourcebook for mental health and legal professions*, (pp. 206–234). New York: John Wiley and Sons.

Guyer, C. G., & Matthews, C. O. (1981). Nonverbal Warm-up exercises with adolescents: effects on group counseling. *Small Group Behavior*, 12(1), 55–67.

Guyer, C. G., & vanPatton, I. T. (1995). The treatment of incest offenders: A hypnotic approach: A brief communication. *International Journal of Clinical and Experimental Hypnosis*, 42(3), 266–273.

Guyer, N. P., & Guyer, C. G. (1984). Implementing relaxation in counseling emotionally healthy adolescents: A comparison of three modes. *American Mental Health Counselors Association Journal*, 6, 79–87.

Hammond, D. P., Garver, R. B., Mutter, C. B., Crasilneck, H. B., Frischholz, E., Gravitz, M. A., Hibler, N. S., Olson, J., Scheflin, A., Spiegel, H., & Wester, W. C. (1994). *Clinical hypnosis and memory: Guidelines for clinicians and for forensic hypnosis*. Des Plains, IL: American Society for Clinical Hypnosis.

Hansen, S. (2000). Kids together: A group play therapy model for children with ADHD symptomology. *Journal of Child and Adolescent Group Therapy*, 10(4), 191–211.

Helton, G. B., & Oakland, T. D. (1977). Teachers' attitudinal responses to differing characteristics of elementary school students. *Journal of Educational Psychology*, 64, 261–264.

Henley, D. R. (2000). Blessings in disguise: Idiomatic expression as a stimulus in group art therapy with children. *Art Therapy*, 17(4), 270–275.

Hilgard, E. (1977). *Divided consciousness: Multiple controls in human thought and action.* New York: John Wiley and Sons.

Hobbs, N. (1975). *The future of children: Categories, labels and their consequences.* San Francisco, CA: Jossey-Bass.

Houck, G. M., King, M. C., Tomlinson, B., Vrabel, A., & Weeks, J. (2002). Small group intervention for children with attention disorders. *Journal of School Nursing*, 18(4), 196–200.

Hunter, M.E. (1996). *Making peace with chronic pain.* New York: Brunner/Mazel.

Illovsky, J., & Fredman, N. (1976). Group suggestions in learning disabilities of primary grade children: A feasibility study. *International Journal of Clinical and Experimental Hypnosis*, 8, 269–274.

Jacobson, R. M., Swan, A., Adegbenro, A., Ludingten, S. L., Woolen, P. C., & Poland, G. A. (2001). Making vaccines more acceptable—Methods to prevent and minimize pain and other common adverse events associated with vaccines. *Vaccine*, 19(17–19), 2418–2427.

James, A. C., & Javaloyes, A. M. (2001). The treatment of Bipolar Disorder in children and adolescents. *Journal of Child Psychology and Psychiatry*, 42(4), 439–449.

Kroger, W. S., & Fezler, W. D. (1976). *Hypnosis and behavior modification— Imagery conditioning.* Philadelphia: J.B. Lippincott.

Kroger, W. S., & Freed, S. C. (1951). *Psychosomatic gynecology: Individual problems of obstetrical care.* Philadelphia: W. B. Saunders.

Lawlor, E. D. (1976). Hypnotic intervention with "school phobic" children. *International Journal of Experimental and Clinical Hypnosis*, 10, 79–92.

Lawlor, E. D. (1978). Hypnotic intervention with school phobic children. *International Journal of Social Psychiatry*, 24(1), 38–46.

Lipsitt, P. D., & Lipsitt, L. P. (2000). Delinquency and criminality. In F. W. Kaslow (Ed.), *Handbook of couple and family forensics: A sourcebook for mental health and legal professionals* (pp. 188–205). New York: John Wiley and Sons.

Littell, J. H., Popa, M., & Forsyth, B. (2005). Multisystemic therapy for social, emotional, and behavioral problems in youth aged 10–17. *Cochrane Database Systems Review*, July 20(3), CD004797.

Loo, S. K., & Barkley, R. A. (2005). Clinical utility of EEG in Attention-Deficit/Hyperactivity Disorder. *Applied Neuropsychology*, 12(2), 64–76.

McCary, J. L, & McCary, S. T. (1982). *McCary's human sexuality* (4th ed.). Belmont, CA: Wadsworth.

Mears, A. (1960). *A system of medical hypnosis*. Philadelphia: W. B. Saunders.

Miklowitz, D. J., George, E. L., Richards, J. A., Simoneau, T. L., & Suddath, R. L. (2003). A randomized study of family-focused psychoeducation and pharmacotherapy in the outpatient management of Bipolar Disorder. *Archives of General Psychiatry*, 60(9), 904–912.

Miklowitz, D. J., Simoneau, T. I., George, E. L., Richards, J. A., Kalbag, A., Sachs-Ericsson, N., & Suddath, R. (2000). Family-focused treatment of Bipolar Disorder: 1 year effects of a psychoeducational program in conjunction with pharmacotherapy. *Biological Psychiatry*, 48(6), 582–592.

Miklowitz, D. J., George, E. L., Axelson, D. A., Kim, E. Y., Birmaher, B., Schneck, C., Bersford, C., Craighead, W. E., & Brent, D. A. (2004). Family-focused treatment for adolescents with Bipolar Disorder. *Journal of Affective Disorders*, 82 (Suppl. 1)(5), 113–128.

Miklowitz, D. J. (2004). The role of family systems in severe and recurrent psychiatric disorders: A developmental psychopathology view. *Developmental Psychopathology*, 16(3), 667–688.

Miller, N. E. (1969). Learning of visceral and glandular responses. *Science*, 163, 434–445.

Milling, L. S., & Costantino, C. A. (2000), Clinical hypnosis with children: First steps toward empirical support. *International Journal Clinical & Experimental Hypnosis*, 48(2), 113–137.

Moene, F. C., Spinhoven, P., Hoogduin, K. A., & van Dyke, R. (2002). A randomized controlled clinical trial on the additional effect of hypnosis in a comprehensive treatment program for inpatients with Conversion Disorder of the motor type. *Psychotherapy Psychosomatic*, 71(2), 66–76.

Monastra, V. J., Lynn, S., Linden, M., Lubar, J. F., Gruzelier, J., & LaVaque, T. J. (2005). Electroencephalographic biofeedback in the treatment of Attention-Deficit/Hyperactivity Disorder. *Applied Psychophysiological Biofeedback*, 30(2), 95–114.

Morris, K. T., & Cinnamon, K. M. (1975). *A handbook of nonverbal group exercises*. Springfield, IL: Charles C. Thomas.

Murphy, K. (2005). Psychosocial treatments for ADHD in teens and adults: A practice friendly review. *Journal of Clinical Psychology*, 61(5), 607–619.

Murray, L. P. (2001). Treatment of Attention-Deficit/Hyperactivity Disorder. *Indian Journal of Psychiatry*, 68(1), 1–9.

Navaco, R. W. (1975). *Anger control: The development and evaluation of experimental treatment*. Lexington, MA: D.C. Heath.

Olness, K., & Kohen, D. P. (1996). *Hypnosis and hypnotherapy with children* (3rd ed.). New York: Guilford Press.

Orne, M. (1966). Hypnosis, motivation, and compliance. *American Journal of Psychiatry*, 122, 721–726.

Pelham, W. F., Wheeler, T., & Chronis, A. (1998). Empirically supported psychosocial treatments for Attention-Deficit/Hyperactivity Disorder. *Journal of Clinical Child Psychology*, 27(2), 190–205.

Pfiffner, L. J., & McBurnett, K. (1997). Social skills training with parent generalization: treatment effects for children with Attention-Deficit Disorder. *Journal of Consulting and Clinical Psychology*, 65(5), 749–757.

Relinger, H. (1986). Fabrication in hypnosis. In B. Zilbergeld, M. G. Edelstein & D. L. Araoz (Eds.), *Hypnosis questions and answers*. New York: W.W. Norton.

Robbins, C. A. (2005). ADHD couple and family relationships: Enhancing communication and understanding through image relationship therapy. *Journal of Clinical Psychology*, 61(5), 565–577.

Rossi, E. (2002). *The psychobiology of gene expression.* New York: John Wiley and Sons.

Salloum, A., Avery, L., & McClain, R. P. (2001). Group psychotherapy for adolescent survivors of homicide victims: A pilot study. *Journal of the Academy of Child and Adolescent Psychiatry*, 40(11), 1261–1267.

Schinke, S. P., Schilling, R. F., Barth, R. P., Gilchrist, L. D., & Maxwell, J. S. (1986). Stress management intervention to prevent family violence. *Journal of Family Violence*, 1(1) 13–26.

Shor, R. & Orne, E. (1962). Harvard group scale of hypnotic susceptibility. Available at: http://socrates.berkeley.edu/~kihlstrm/PDFfiles/Hypnotizability/HGSHSAScript.pdf

Skinner, B. F. (1953). *Science and human behavior.* New York: The Free Press.

Smith, E. P., Gorman-Smith, D., Quinn, W. H., Rabiner, D. L., Tolan, P. H., & Winn, D. M. (2004). Community-based multiple family groups to prevent and reduce violent and aggressive behavior: The great families program. *American Journal of Preventative Medicine*, 26(1–Suppl.), 39–47.

Sommers-Flanagan, J., & Sommers-Flanagan, R. (1996). The Wizard of Oz metaphor in hypnosis with treatment resistant children. *American Journal of Clinical Hypnosis*, 39(2), 105–114.

Spiegel, H., & Spiegel D. (2004). *Trance and treatment: Clinical uses of hypnosis* (2nd ed.). Arlington, VA: American Psychiatric Publishing.

Stacy, W. A., & Shupe, A. (1983). *The family secret: Family violence in America.* Boston: Beacon Press.

Stiefel, I., & Dossetor, D. (1998). The synergetic effects of stimulants and parental psychotherapy in the treatment of Attention-Deficit/Hyperactivity Disorder. *Journal of Pediatric and Child Health*, 34(4), 391–394.

Tansey, M. A. (1993). Ten year stability of EEG biofeedback results for a hyperactive boy who failed fourth grade perceptually impaired class. *Biofeedback and Self Regulation*, 18(4), 33-44.

Traven, S., Bluestone, H., Coleman, E., Culler, K., & Melella, J. (1986). Pedophilia: An update on theory and practice. *Psychiatric Quarterly*, 57(2), 89–103.

Traven, S., Bluestone, H., Coleman, E., & Melella, J. (1986). Pedophilia types and treatment perspectives. *Journal of Forensic Science*, 31(2), 614–620.

van de Wiel, N. M., van Goozen, S. H., Matthys, W., Snock, H., & van Engeland, H. (2004). Cortisol and treatment effects in children with disruptive behavior disorders: A preliminary study. *Journal of the American Academy of Child and Adolescent Psychiatry*, 43(8), 1011–1018.

Watkins, J., & Watkins, H. (1981). Ego-state therapy. In R. J. Corsini (Ed.), *Handbook of innovative psychotherapies*, (pp. 252–270). New York: John Wiley and Sons.

Watkins, J., & Watkins H. (1997). *Ego states: Theory & therapy*. New York: W.W. Norton.

Weitzenhoffer, A., & Hilgard, E. (1962). *Stanford hypnotic susceptibility scale, form C*. Palo Alto, CA: Consulting Psychologists Press.

Wester, W. C. (2006). *Questions and answers about clinical hypnosis* (revised edition). Columbus, OH: Ohio Psychology Publications.

Williams, D. T., & Snigh, M. (1976). Hypnosis as a facilitating adjunct to child psychiatry. *Journal of the American Academy of Child Psychiatry*, 15, 326–342.

Williams, D. T. (1979). Hypnosis as a therapeutic adjunct. In J. D. Noshpitz (Ed.), *Basic handbook of child psychiatry – Vol. 3*, (pp. 108). New York: Basic Books.

Yapko, M. D. (1992). *Hypnosis and the treatment of depressions: Strategies for change*. New York: Brunner/Mazel.

Yapko, M. D. (1997). *Breaking the patterns of depression*. New York: Doubleday.

Zarren, J. I., & Eimer, B. N. (2002). *Brief cognitive hypnosis*. New York: Springer.

Zimbardo, P. G., Weber, A. L., & Johnson, R. L. (2003). *Psychology core concepts*. (4th ed.). New York: Allyn and Bacon.

Chapter Thirteen

Family Therapy as Hypnotic Conversation

Andrew E. Roffman, LCSW

> *There is really no such thing as hypnotherapy. There is therapy wherein you use hypnotic modalities, hypnotic understanding; but hypnosis in itself is not a therapy. Hypnosis is a means of establishing a more adequate contact with your patient and a more favorable environment in which your patient can seek to understand the total situation.*
>
> Milton H. Erickson*

Therapy with children and adolescents always occurs within the context of their family, whether or not the family is in the room. Family therapy makes deliberate use of that context to facilitate change. How does hypnosis play a role in family therapy? How can family therapy be seen as a context for hypnotic interaction? Hypnosis, through the work of Milton H. Erickson, has been influential in the development of family therapy (Beels, 2002; Nichols & Schwartz, 2005). This chapter presents a description of how hypnosis can serve as a contextual framework for family therapy process such that family therapy is conducted as a "hypnotic conversation" (Teleska & Roffman, 2004). This is not hypnosis as a method within the context of family therapy or trance as a model for family process. Rather, this chapter shows how the frame of the hypnotic conversation can organize the wonderfully fertile context created when family and therapist join together. This framework makes possible a variety of ways of interacting therapeutically with families, including the utilization of hypnotic principles and techniques. Family therapy in this sense is a systemic hypnotic

---

* M. Erickson (1992). *Creative Choice in Hypnosis*. E. Rossi & M. Ryan (Eds). New York: Irvington, p. 126.

interaction that utilizes the family as a primary resource for change.

Family therapists are a diverse group; and a variety of models of family therapy abound, each with its array of constructs and techniques (Nichols & Schwartz, 2005). Most are united under the capacious umbrella of systems theory that views all phenomena as relational and contextual. The hypnotic conversation framework in this chapter binds itself closely to systems theory, particularly the work of Bateson (1972; 1979), Maturana and Varela (1987), and Maturana and Poerksen (2004). Family therapists and hypnotherapists will find common ground in the following clinical vignettes.

Frieda

Frieda, a 14-year-old girl, had been seen with her parents in family therapy for several months before the case was transferred to my treatment team, a training group in family therapy that utilizes a one-way mirror set-up. I saw the family with a co-therapist (a resident training in psychiatry). We had struggled through several sessions in which Frieda typically worked herself up into a frothing rage within the first 15 minutes, rendering the remainder of the session unproductive. We tried a variety of means of addressing this pattern and failed.[1] I decided that in the next session, I would head her off at the pass. At the very beginning of the session I said to Frieda, "I'm pretty certain you're going to get really angry at your parents in this session. How soon do you think you're going to get really angry at your mother or father?" Frieda and her parents found this very amusing. Later in the session, as she started to show signs of emotional arousal, I said, "Now looks like it would be a pretty good time to get really mad at your mother, don't you think so?" And still later [*Frieda had, by now, broken a record in family session by not having had an explosion*] I said, "I'm starting to get a little concerned—you haven't gotten really

---

[1] My co-therapist attempted a variety of cognitive-behavioral techniques for getting Frieda to calm down, including deep breathing, distraction, and guided imagery.

angry yet—when do you think it will be? Are you getting ready? Would now be too soon?" These questions conveyed a deliberate ambiguity of intent: Was I being serious? Was I joking? Did I really want her to get angry? The interaction with Frieda was also indirectly intended for her parents, whose behavior I closely monitored. Anytime either gave what had by now become a familiar trigger (conscious or unconscious) for their daughter's explosive anger, I jumped in with my queries about whether or not it would be a good time to get very angry. By the end of the session, we had accomplished a great deal more than in any previous session.

The hypnotic elements embedded in this encounter with Frieda and her family will surface as this chapter unfolds. Frieda and her family will return later for another illustration. First, some basic definitions and concepts will lay the groundwork for rest of this chapter.

Family Therapy as a Hypnotic Interaction

Family Therapy

The first basic premise of family therapy is that *family members are connected to one another in a web of significant relationships.* Optimally, that web supports and sustains the growth, development, and well-being of each individual, especially children for whom it is arguably the central context. The second basic premise is that *therapists need to see those relationships as integral to the change process.* Relationships are comprised of patterns of mutually influencing behavior, ideas, and beliefs held together by strong emotional glue. The third basic premise is one that family therapy shares with hypnosis: both build upon the belief that *individuals are inherently resourceful.* Family therapy goes one step further to assert that family relationships are vital for the emergence of that resourcefulness.

Family therapy's primary framework is systems theory, a conceptual domain that spans a variety of disciplines. A full description of systems theory's relevance to family therapy is beyond the scope of this chapter.[2] However, each living system, whether a cell, a multicellular entity (such as a human being), or a social unit (such as a family), shares formal qualities. All living systems are, in Maturana's (2004) terms, "structure determined." That is, their response to *perturbations* is determined not by "input," but by the structure of the system at that point in time. A perturbation is any stimulus that a system must respond to. Bateson (1979) gives the example of the difference between kicking a stone and kicking a dog. While the effect on a stone is relatively predictable (based on Newtonian physics), a dog's reaction will be determined largely by its interpretation of the kick.[3] The dog will interpret it as a communication about the relationship with the kicker: Was the kick an act of aggression? An invitation to play? How the dog responds will be determined by his structure in the moment. Family therapy, and arguably hypnosis, is more like kicking the dog than the stone.

Families are complex and dynamic. Parents influence each other and their children who, in turn, influence each other and their parents in an ongoing reciprocal process. Add on grandparents, uncles and aunts, cousins, significant friends and one has an increasingly rich domain. When a therapist enters that web of relationships he or she becomes a part of this responsive system, his or her presence adding to the richness and "requisite variety" (Ashby, 1965) that makes growth and change possible. The

---

[2] Systems theory is a broad category, encompassing cybernetics (both first- and second-order), general systems theory, and Maturana and Varela's (1987) concept of *autopoeisis*. A simplified mapping of these ideas onto families might go as follows: Like a cell whose cell bodies produce the membrane that allows for the integrity of the cell as whole, the individual members of a family compose the larger third-order unity that is a family, which as a network of interdependence, allows for the growth and well-being of the members. Though the notion of family is a social construction, so, in turn, is the notion of "the individual" (Gergen, 1991). It is largely our Western beliefs that see individuals as such. On one level of description, an individual as an autonomous entity is a third-order unity in relation to its billions of cells—we are multicellular creatures—and we are habitats for a tremendous array of microbial life.

[3] ...leaving aside the case of a large man kicking a very small dog, where Newtonian physics may be quite applicable.

therapist's role is much like an enzyme's in providing the perturbations that evoke responses in the direction of the therapeutic goals.

As children are born and grow up, as family members age and die, as a variety of other changes arise from within (development and the family life cycle) or without (environment and circumstance) most families retain a sense of identity, a sense of "this is who we are, the X family." Even in the face of often devastating circumstances, families preserve their organization, their basic *being-as-a-family*. Each family is a microculture embedded within political, religious, ethnic, and other large networks of meaning and influence. It is within this microculture, this tightly interwoven web of meaningful relationships, that an individual comes to know himself or herself and the world. When a therapist gains access to this microculture, he or she has the opportunity to set off new chains of responses that resonate through the whole web, breaking up old patterns and facilitating new ones.

There are a wide variety of viable family compositions, but perhaps the common denominator is that the individual members have a basic sense of belonging to one another. Indeed, families are the primary context for the kinds of attachment relationships that are considered basic to emotional health (Akister & Reibstein, 2004; Hill, Fonagy, Safier & Sargent, 2003; Byng-Hall, 1995; Donley, 1993). Family therapy has shown itself to be effective with a wide variety of psychiatric and biobehavioral (Liddle & Rowe, 2005) conditions. While family therapy is a diverse field, most effective family therapy works from shared premises such as those outlined above.

Therapeutic Conversation

A *therapeutic conversation* occurs when therapist and family establish a context of mutual interest, mutual influence, and mutual responsiveness. It is an interactional process that embodies the interests of all participants towards some direction of mutual benefit, includes *all* forms of communication, and optimally leads to enriched and expanded possibilities for the family and therapist.

Hypnosis

Writers such as Ritterman (1983), Whitaker (1982), and Araoz (1988) have variously used the constructs of hypnosis and trance as models of family process such that there is a kind of family trance in which positive and negative suggestions abound, structuring how members think, feel, and interact. Theoretically, the question of whether hypnosis or trance is or is not an apt metaphor for family process—especially regarding the communication of such things as rules, norms, world views or any other such enacted cognitive domain—is interesting but irresolvable. Communication goes on all the time in families, much of it under the radar of both sender and receiver such that we can safely call it "unconscious." I will reserve *hypnosis* not for what family members do consciously or unconsciously in relation to one another, but for what a therapist does deliberately in an interactional framework on the client/family's behalf.

It is important to remember, as Fourie (1991) notes, that words such as hypnosis and trance are descriptions we use as observers rather than explanations of "what is really going on." To interact hypnotically with a family is an intention the therapist may hold that organizes his or her behavior. Whether or not this is "truly hypnosis" begs the question as to what hypnosis truly is. Such questions, as Rorty (1991) points out, lead not to transcendent, foundational answers but to consensus arrived at by a community of like-minded thinkers. When it was published, the *2003 American Psychological Association's Division 30 Definition of Hypnosis* (Green, Barabasz, Barrett,& Montgomery, 2005) evoked 11 articles in the *American Journal of Clinical Hypnosis* (*AJCH*, 48 (2–3)) seeking to interpret, expand, and hold open the APA's definition. As evidenced by the ongoing discussion on this topic, consensus continues to be elusive.

Hypnotic Conversation

A *hypnotic conversation* is a therapeutic conversation that utilizes the principles and practices of hypnosis in order to thicken, deepen, and broaden the therapy process. *In essence, family therapy is an opportunity for hypnotic conversation with a group of individuals whose lives are importantly intertwined.* The work has resonance with a system of relationships that goes beyond the boundaries of each individual. Hypnotic conversation on this systemic level is targeted at expanding each family member's construction of him or herself, the other family members, and of their relationships. These new constructions of self and other allow for more possibilities for thinking, feeling, and doing. In this way, the individual and the web are affected: the parts influence the whole and the whole influences the parts.

The Framework of Hypnotic Conversation

To do therapy well one needs to know what one is doing. Faced with family members who are heatedly arguing or, at the other extreme, are sitting in anxious silence, a therapist must have some set of principles, a framework, to guide his or her actions. The hypnotic conversation framework gives the therapist a means of steering the complex flow of therapist-family interaction in a useful direction. Below are six therapy strategies[4], adapted from P. Lounsbury and N. Winston (personal communication, April 2006) and Erickson and Rossi (1979). Each strategy is closely linked to every other, not as a series of linear stages (though often one follows from another), but as a set of mutually supporting sets of actions.

1. Establishing and maintaining a viable frame
2. Gathering and focusing attention
3. Depotentiating conscious/habitual ways of making sense
4. Accessing resources
5. Breaking up experience
6. Linking resources to new contexts

First and foremost, the hypnotic conversation is a way of being in relationship to a family. As the "common factors" research has

---

[4] The word *strategy* is used in the sense that Weakland (1993) portrays as the therapist's intentional choice of action. Despite the word's unfortunate associations to competitive games and war, it aptly and honestly describes the fact that therapists are interested in promoting change and, whether they can accomplish it or not, try to influence their clients in that direction.

shown (Sprenkle & Blow, 2004), the *quality* of the therapeutic relationship influences outcome more than the type of therapy or
kinds of techniques. While technical skill is a prerequisite for interacting effectively, it has little or no value in the absence of a strong
relationship. Erickson, in his usual cutting to the heart of the matter, said, "You go along with them and they will go along with
you" (P. Lounsbury, personal communication, October 2000).

Establishing and Maintaining a Viable Frame

In their model of hypnotic work, P. Lounsbury and N. Winston
emphasize the necessity of creating and maintaining a frame that
organizes and directs the spontaneous flow of the hypnotic interaction (personal communication, April 2006). Goffman (1974)
defines frame in this way:

> I assume that when individuals attend to any current situation
> they face the question: "What is it that's going on here?" Whether
> asked explicitly, as in times of confusion and doubt, or tacitly, dur-
> ing occasions of usual certitude, the question is put and the answer
> to it is presumed by the way the individuals then proceed to get on
> with the affairs at hand. (p. 8)

The therapist and family must have some agreement about the
answer to Goffman's question. They must agree that "What is
going on here" is *therapy*, and come to some reasonable consensus
about what it is for. Reaching agreement on this is a prerequisite in
most cases to effective therapy. Establishing and maintaining a
viable frame is a process that continues as the therapy proceeds
such that the frame evolves with the therapy. Goals and interests
change over the course of therapy as family members come to new
understandings of themselves and their relationships with each
other.

Gathering and Focusing Attention

In order to establish a frame the therapist must be able to connect
with family members and gather and focus their attention.

Imagine being confronted with a father who impatiently looks at his watch, a mother who seems ready for an argument, a teenager who slumps in his chair and pretends to be asleep, and a 5-year-old who rolls around on the floor. The family therapist has to connect with each member according to where that member is in the moment. Additionally, the therapist has to think about gathering and focusing the attention of the family as a whole. "The family as a whole" in this sense is a kind of abstraction. While a family is greater than the sum of its parts, treating it as an entity requires a finessed balancing of the literal and metaphoric. A therapist can speak to a family *as a family* with such questions as, "Is this a family that doesn't show closeness?"; "Is this a family that's got a problem with anger?" Questions such as these, addressed to no individual member in particular, have a galvanizing effect on all the members. Implicit in these questions is a fundamental presupposition: they *are* integrally connected to one another in spite of the conflicts and painful emotions that may seem to divide them.

Minuchin (1974) has described this gathering and focusing of attention as *joining*: a means of creating rapport with families. Joining is typically a process of helping family members feel welcome and compellingly engaged. In most cases, this is accomplished by the therapist's genuine interest and concern. However, there are times, as shown in the vignette about "Tom" below, where that interest and concern are demonstrated in unusual ways.

Depotentiating Conscious/Habitual Ways of Making Sense

One reason families come to therapy is that they have gotten stuck in their habitual ways of doing things. Yet they do not know what else to do and commit the error of "if it's not working, do more of it." Some families respond to direct advice: "Stop doing that! Do this instead." However, as Haley (1996) says, telling families what they are doing wrong rarely helps them to change. A central task, then, in family therapy is to help a family get *un*stuck from how they are responding to each other and the context of the problem. Erickson and Rossi (1979) describe this process as "depotentiating habitual frameworks and belief systems" (p. 4). Erickson's strategy of creating an acceptable context of "not-knowing" is particularly effective in this regard. The state of not-knowing can evoke a powerful responsiveness on the part of family members. For example, in front of his parents a child might be asked:

> You really don't know how you're going to get along better with your parents do you? And they don't know yet how they're going to help you feel better, do they?

It can be both a relief to not know (or not have to know) and a motivation to learn. "Not-knowing" is a way to destabilize beliefs, encourage comfort with uncertainty and doubt, and increase expectancy (Council, 1999; Kirsch, 1999; Weinberger & Eig, 1999).

Accessing Resources

Family therapy has long been associated with a "strengths and resource" orientation. A seminal example can be seen in the last chapter of Haley's *Problem Solving Therapy* (1976), "A Modern 'Little Hans.'" In this case a family comes to therapy because of the 8-year-old son's dog phobia. The therapy team makes use of father's authority on dogs—he is a postman who deals with dogs on his daily route—to accomplish two connected tasks: strengthening the father-son relationship and helping the boy overcome his fears. Until the point when the therapist mobilizes this interaction, the father is rather disengaged both in session and in the boy's life.

As in hypnotherapy, family therapy actively searches for the inherent and often latent resources in the family that can be utilized on the family's behalf. Erickson's work provides a rich source of how he accomplished this using both formal and informal hypnotic methods (Haley, 1973; 1985). A family presents an expanded version of what is available in an individual therapy context—there are always more resources than are immediately evident or that the person/family manifests. Therapists must believe that a family is a primary resource for its individual members; and conversely, that individual members are a resource for each other and the family as a whole.

Breaking Up Experience

A child who takes apart a radio to find out how it works soon learns that it is much harder to put it back together again. Yet he can find many interesting uses for the parts strewn out on the table. Breaking up experience occurs when a therapist takes, for example, a mother's statement such as "Johnny doesn't know how to listen!" and does some variation on the following:

> Doesn't *listen* or doesn't know *how* to listen?

> How do you know he doesn't know *how* to listen?

> Doesn't listen or know how to listen to whom, when, where?

> Johnny, can you hear me now? Yes? Does that mean you know how to listen?

> Do you know how to *not* listen? Can you show me how to not listen to your mother right now?

Breaking up experience is a form of pattern disruption. In systems theory, all phenomena maintain coherence through patterning; that includes behavior, thought, emotion, belief and so forth. Hypnotic work is often focused on breaking up pre-existing patterns of experience thus enabling change to occur.

Linking Resources to New Contexts

A basic principle of hypnotherapy is that each individual has more resources than are consciously known and actively employed (*see* Chapter Four). Hypnotherapy is very often a matter of taking an accessed resource (e.g., not listening) and linking it (O'Hanlon, 1987) to some new context (e.g., being teased by a classmate). Family therapy has a history of seeing family members, both present in the session as well as in the extended system, as resources that can be utilized both for the individual and the family relationships. Taking the example above ("Johnny doesn't know how to listen!") one step further might go as follows:

283

> You know *how to listen* and how to *not* listen. That's terrific. How do you decide when to do one or the other? Is it difficult to figure out? Can you teach me how to do that? I have an awfully hard time not listening to people who talk on their cell phones next to me on the train. I'd like to learn how to not listen. Can you not listen to that kid in your class you told me about? The one who tries to get you to act silly?

Linking resources to new contexts is a matter of taking those parts that have been freed up—the radio pieces—and applying them in some novel ways that allow for further growth. It is, as Gilligan (1987) points out, a generative process.

Clinical Vignettes

Each of the following examples highlights one of the six strategies. Instances of the other five are described in the text or indicated by brackets and italics as they occur in each example.

Establishing and Maintaining a Viable Frame

Tom

This family was strongly urged to come to see me. The "identified patient," Tom, a 17-year-old boy with the diagnosis of major depression, made it quite clear he had no interest in participating. When I spoke with his mother on the phone I insisted she and her husband be present at the first session. She told me it would be difficult to get either son or husband to come but that she would do her best. I suggested that she use her power as a wife and mother to make it happen [*accessing and linking resources*]. The family showed up: mother, a teacher's aide, father (a construction worker unemployed since the family's recent move back to New York City from Florida), and Tom (a large, scowling teen half hidden in a hooded sweatshirt, oversized t-shirt and jeans). It was clear from this initial contact that I would have to move quickly to establish a frame that would include each individual member's attitude about therapy. In this, as in most cases, establishing the frame overlaps considerably with gathering and focusing attention.

As soon as the session started Tom spoke up.

Tom: No offense, but I don't want to be here and I think therapy is a waste of time and therapists are all full of it.

A. Roffman [AR]: No offense taken. I happen to agree with you. [*This seemed both to get his attention and to throw him off guard—depotentiation*].

Tom: Really, I hate therapy. It doesn't do anything. Nothing helps except the medication. That's all I want, the medication. The rest is a waste and I ain't coming to therapy.

AR [*leaning forward in my chair*]: You came here today, I'm not sure how or why. Maybe it's because you respect your parents [*breaking up experience*]. You think therapy is a waste and therapists are full of it. The only thing you want is your medication and you're not gonna do anything else, is that right? [*I said all this slowly and with emphasis—gathering and focusing*].

Tom: Yeah [*with some hesitation*].

AR: Then I want you to just sit there and keep your mouth shut while I talk to your parents. And no matter what I say or they say you'll just sit right there keeping your mouth shut.

My response to Tom both captured his attention and served to depotentiate his conscious expectations of meeting with a therapist who was "full of it." My pacing of his initial comments was followed by the seemingly antagonistic command of "keep your mouth shut!" My injunction to Tom was a variation of the bind, "cooperate with me by not cooperating with me." I then quickly turned to the parents and switching tones of voice talked with them about their situation. I learned that they were having trouble in the marriage because the mother was working a low-paying full time job and doing all the housework while the father, depressed and demoralized because of the failure of a business venture in Florida, stayed home and neither looked for a job nor helped around the house. The mother told me how Tom and her husband had become alarmingly depressed while in Florida and that this prompted their leaving. She and their younger daughter, not present in this session, had not wanted to leave.

During the course of this conversation Tom tried several times to speak. Each time I told him he was not permitted to talk, that I would tell him when he could talk and until then he was to keep his mouth shut. He obeyed my injunction but looked increasingly agitated. Finally, when I finished speaking with his parents I turned to him and said,

> AR: Tom, your family's in bad shape [*establishing frame, gathering and focusing*]. It was in bad shape in Florida and it's in bad shape now. Your parents have botched things up and need a lot of help to straighten it out. So I want you to come back to see me in a month to report on their progress in fixing things up in the family. I want to see you in a month and no sooner [*depotentiation*].

I then repeated to the father what I knew about him [*gathering and focusing*]: that he was depressed, demoralized, unemployed, and nervous; that he would spend the day sitting around and in the afternoon would pace or stand by the window watching for his wife to come home—behaviors that infuriated her. I then suggested that if he was going to pace, he could do so with the vacuum cleaner in his hand; if he were to stand by the window, he could hold some Windex and paper towels and clean the windows [*breaking up, linking to new context*]. Father looked initially confused and then very irritated as I said this [*depotentiation*]. Mother smiled, and Tom looked perplexed. I ended by saying I would meet them in two weeks (without Tom) to hear how it is going. By the next session, the father had a job. In the third session, the teenager attended and was less angry, more cooperative, and doing better in school.

Once the frame was set—that I would work with Tom's parents to straighten things out and that he would report on their progress—I intervened in the parents' relationship by breaking up the context of father's depression and anxiety and linking his compulsive behavior to a new context such that it could be helpful to her. This is an example of the kind of reframing (Watzlawick, Weakland, & Fisch, 1974) that Whitaker described as "contamination" (Whitaker & Bumberry, 1988): the old meaning for a behavior can no longer stand.

Gathering and Focusing Attention

Frieda

Frieda's family, as mentioned earlier, had been in therapy for several months prior to starting with me and my co-therapist. The therapy had focused on Frieda's overeating, obesity, and on her behavior at home where she was both highly reactive and oppositional to her parents' conflict. From watching a few of these previous sessions from behind the one-way mirror and sitting in on several discussions of the case, I knew this family to be a volatile one. Their previous therapist had great difficulty maintaining control and direction. Consequently, I took time to formulate a framework for the first session. I began by declaring the following [*establishing frame*]:

> **AR**: We need your permission to be tough with you—to be tough on Frieda's behalf and on your behalf. Do we have your permission to be tough with you?
>
> We need your permission to interrupt—to do so in ways that may be very frustrating, but to do so when we believe it's important to interrupt. Do we have your permission—even if at times it seems rude?
>
> We need your permission to be "traffic policemen," directing who says what and when, to prevent gridlock and accidents so we can get where we need to go together.
>
> And we also need your permission to care about you and be concerned.

This was an intriguing frame for them that effectively gathered and focused their attention. After securing their explicit permission I proceeded immediately to interrupt, frustrate, and redirect such that the family members became increasingly expectant and curious as to what would happen next [*gathering and focusing, depotentiation*]. This freed them, at least for the hour, from the compelling pulls of their typical patterns. My interrupting and invoking the frame also broke up their experience of each other and the therapy. Moments of anger shifted to sadness or laughter, criticism changed to care and concern, disgust to frustration and desire. They walked out of the session smiling, shaking my hand and saying, "We don't know what we accomplished today but it felt very helpful." In subsequent sessions I invoked this frame and the permission granted to intervene aggressively. My co-therapist, team, and I also found that the permission to care had a powerful effect, helping us to "hang in there" with this family when things seemed hopeless.

Depotentiating Conscious/Habitual Ways of Making Sense

Donald

Donald, 14 years old, and his mother, a single working parent, had been coming to see me for several weeks for a variety of issues. Donald was in a school for children with behavioral and learning disabilities. He was, by his description, "the angriest teenager alive." He was doing poorly in school, not for lack of ability, but because of the bind he had gotten into. The bind was this: if he does well he is "sucking up to the idiot teachers"; if he doesn't do well, he is disappointing his mother and confirming the teachers' negative opinions of him. In one session the mother was complaining about how she would come home from work to find Donald on the couch playing video games, junk food wrappers strewn around him, the dog not walked, and homework left untouched. "I'm tired of screaming at him," she said. "It doesn't work—he feels bad, I feel bad, we both cry, but it doesn't change things."

Donald and his mother were stuck in a negative pattern of responding to one another. Mother felt she had "tried everything" from star charts to guilt and remonstrance, all to no avail. Given this "stuckness" and sense of hopelessness I moved in to depotentiate and at the same time break up their experience.

I told Donald and his mother that this was indeed a stuck situation and I had a solution that would sound crazy to them. I took some time before disclosing what it was, building up their interest and expectancy [*gathering and focusing*], and then told them:

> **AR**: The next time you come home and Donald is sitting on the couch like that, you give him a quarter for every chore he's supposed to have done but didn't do.

> [*His mother's response was predictable.*]

> **Mother**: What?! Reward him for not doing his chores? That *is* crazy! Why would I do that?

> [*Donald's response was also predictable.*]

> **Donald**: Yeah! That sounds great!

I reassured Mother that there was a very good reason for this but I would not tell them until after they had done it.

Circumstances were such that I was unable to see them for three weeks. When they returned, mother smiled at me and said to Donald, "You tell him." Donald then went on to describe his initial delight at getting paid not to do his chores. "But then I started to feel guilty," he said, and spontaneously cleaned the whole house. However, the big news was that he decided he could think about school as a job and getting good grades as something he could get paid for. He and his mother worked out reasonable terms for this, but soon Mother found out that she could not afford it because he was bringing home too many A's. When I asked Donald about this he told me,

> **Donald**: I figured if I was getting paid to get good grades, then it was just doing a job and not sucking up.

In no way did I specify an outcome for my intervention. Donald and his mother responded to my "crazy solution" by accessing resources and linking them to a new context, that of school. When a family becomes unstuck they often rediscover their resourcefulness without needing a therapist to show them how to use it.

Accessing Resources

The K family

The K family, consisting of parents and four young adult children, all in their 20s, came to see me at the recommendation of the youngest son's individual therapist. This son, Joey, described the family as a "giant boil that needed the pus drained from it" and encouraged me to be the one to wield the scalpel. I accepted his invitation and engaged in a few sessions of highly productive pus draining in a family that had no trouble bringing their conflict to my office. In the fifth session Joey had been heatedly describing his problems with his mother and father. I abruptly asked him,

> **AR** [*to Joey*]: Who in the family is going to have the most insight into what you just said about your relationship with your parents? [*gathering and focusing. Before Joey could answer I said,*] I think it will be your brother, [*depotentiation—and I turned to face Kevin, his older brother, who in the "family story," functions at the lowest level in the family*].

> **Kevin** [*initially demurred*]: I don't have anything to say.

> **AR** [*holding my position*]: Sure you do and you know it.

> [*Kevin then came out with an insight that startled the whole family.*]

> **Joey** [*looking at Kevin dumbfounded*]: Oh my God, he just nailed it!

By utilizing Kevin as a resource for Joey and the family I accomplished two tasks. First I accessed Kevin's undervalued knowledge and understanding of the family. And second, by challenging and undermining the beliefs about Kevin as the least functional, most problematic member of the family, I broke up the family's experience of him and, by consequence, of each other.

Kevin's relationship with his mother was described as the most distant in the family. In another moment of startling (to his family) clarity Kevin had expressed his anger with his mother over the negative things she had repeatedly said to him when, as a young boy, he had struggled with his homework. In one session where, unplanned, I met with just Kevin and his parents, I had an image in my mind of mother and Kevin playing a game of cards. I interrupted what was being discussed and said,

> **AR**: I just had this crazy image I wanted to share with you [*depotentiation*].
>
> **Mother**: Yes?
>
> **AR**: I was sitting here listening when all of a sudden I had this crystal clear image of you and Kevin playing cards together.
>
> **Father**: [*laughing*] *That* will never happen.
>
> **AR**: [*I pressed on*] Really, and why not? Don't you think your wife and son are entitled, after so many hard years, to enjoy each other's company?
>
> **Mother**: He'd never play cards with me.
>
> **Kevin**: [*sitting forward in his chair*] Not cards, Monopoly.

In the next session with the whole family present I asked about the Monopoly game. Mother reported, to the amazement of her other kids, that she and Kevin had played multiple games of Monopoly.

> **Kevin** [*added with relish*]: And I beat her!

If this relationship can change, by implication, how many other "impossible" matters can change in the family?

The K family, to paraphrase Bateson (1972), was not simply learning, they were learning to learn, and learning about their ability *to learn*.

Kevin's resource (manifested in his newly awoken "voice") and the family's resource (their demonstrated ability to be startled by, and receptive to, new behavior) were linked to this new context: that of playful interaction between Kevin and his mother, and by association, between any other dyad in the family.

Breaking Up Experience

Barry

Sowing the seeds of not knowing is an effective means of both depotentiating and breaking up experience. Sometimes breaking up is a matter of opening a slight crack and sticking a wedge in it.

In a family with Barry, a 12-year-old boy whose oppositional behavior so frustrated his parents that they were ready to send him to boarding school, I spent the second half of the first session laying the ground for not knowing. After commiserating with them over the family state of affairs, I suggested to the parents that perhaps they did not know Barry as well as they thought they did.

AR: Would it be OK if Barry were to surprise you in some way? [*establishing a frame. This question immediately focused their attention*].

Father: Well, it depends what kind of surprise....

Mother: [*looking at me with a mixture of irritation and confusion*] I don't know what you mean.

[*Rather than answer them directly I turned to Barry and asked,*]

AR: They really don't know what you're capable of, do they? [*This got his attention. It was deliberately ambiguous as a statement, thus hard to contradict.*] And wouldn't it be nice to surprise them because they really don't know you as well as they think they do, do they? And maybe you don't know yourself as well as you think you do? Maybe you don't know them as well as you think you do?

Barry: [*looking at me*] Maybe.

AR: It's OK not to know: for them to not know you so well and for you to not know them so well. People often get stuck in what they think they know about each other. [*Barry and his parents stared at me expectantly.*] You really don't know how much fun you could have surprising them—[*accessing resource*] the look on your mother's face, your father's face. Maybe it will be more enjoyable than you think it will be? So the next time your mother asks you to do something, you surprise the hell out of her, out of your father, by just doing it, and you look at their faces and take a devilish, secret enjoyment out of the look you see! Just see what that look looks like, OK?

Barry and his parents' experience of each other had grown static; their expectations were fixed and predictably fulfilled. Once they accepted the premise that they could be surprised—the wedge in the crack—I spent the remainder of the hour recounting some of the situations they had described as problematic and recasting these as intriguing possibilities for something surprising to happen. The ability to surprise and be surprised served as resources to be accessed and linked to a new context, one that would be enjoyable to each according to their needs.

In the second session, the parents said that Barry had surprised them by being much more cooperative. I then shifted attention away from his behavior to the quality of relationship that each parent had with him and with each other [*establishing frame*]. Not surprisingly, both parents were taken aback by how little they knew about what Barry had been thinking and feeling.

Linking Resources to New Contexts

Jimmy

A supervisee asked me to sit in as a consultant on a family session with a mother, father, and their 8-year-old son, Jimmy, who had been urinating in his sleep his whole life. The parents were fed up having tried medication, the bell and pad, and such old fashioned methods as yelling, bribery, punishment, and humiliation. My supervisee had described the parents as nice, well-meaning people, neither of whom had graduated from high school, who wanted their son to do well in the world.

After the first 15 minutes getting to know them and building rapport without talking at all about the problem, I shifted to Jimmy and began to ask him questions about himself [*gathering and focusing*]. How tall is he? How did he manage to get that tall in just 8 years? How strong is he? Could he really do 10 pushups without touching his chest to the ground? How high can he jump? And can he show me? We proceeded in this fashion for at least 20 minutes, with my showing appreciation for each of his described or demonstrated achievements. Finally I looked at him with intensity as he stood in front of me and said slowly,

> **AR**: Jimmy, with all these abilities, how quickly do you think you will start keeping the bed dry? [*breaking up, linking to new contexts*].

> [*Pumped up as he was, he answered immediately*],

> **Jimmy**: No problem, right away!

> [*His parents both scoffed at this, so I turned to him and said,*]

> **AR**: They don't believe you can do it. They know you're 8 years old, you've grown this tall, you can do 10 pushups without touching your chest to the floor, [*and so forth, recounting all that he'd demonstrated in session*], but your parents don't know *yet* that you are big and strong enough to start having dry beds at night, do they? [*gathering and focusing, accessing resources, linking to new contexts. He seemed to enjoy this so I continued,*] Every kid likes to show his parents that they are wrong sometimes, and every parent can enjoy being surprised and delighted at their child's growth [*establishing frame*].

I then suggested he decide what night would be his first dry night, but that he keep it a secret from his parents so he could enjoy showing them up and they could enjoy being surprised. I then asked him to tell me who would notice first, and so forth.

A week later my supervisee told me Jimmy had kept his bed dry since that session. She continued with the frame I had set up in the consultation, and employed it to foster development in other areas of his life.

All eyes and ears were focused on my interaction with Jimmy as he answered my questions and showed me his abilities. This dialogue also served to break up the parents' (and therapist's) experience of the boy as it shifted the emphasis away from his night time bladder control to the host of abilities he possessed. The important moment occurred when Jimmy accepted the suggestion, embedded in a question, that with all those resources he could quickly overcome his problem. Perhaps the essential accessed resource that got linked to the context of keeping the bed dry was Jimmy's inherent striving for and satisfaction in the experience of mastery. I broke up the parents' doubts by accessing their high hopes for their child (another resource) and linking these to the anticipation of being surprised and delighted by his development.

Summary

The principles and techniques of hypnosis employed in the context of family therapy serve to evoke and utilize the kinds of abilities Teleska and Sugarman describe in Chapter Four. The hypnotic conversation format can be used deliberately to elicit trance phenomena as well as utilize those phenomena that arise spontaneously (Kane & Olness, 2004). This format allows the therapist to structure a family therapy session as a hypnotic interaction, making use of the six strategies given above. Family therapy, construed as a form of hypnotic conversation, can look to an observer like formal hypnosis, informal hypnosis, or only remotely like hypnosis. In Chapter One, Sugarman and Wester quote James Maddox, writing "While all hypnosis is not therapy, all therapy is hypnosis." In the same way, family therapy can be hypnotic in and of itself, but is that much more so when the therapist intentionally utilizes the framework presented in this chapter to organize and shape the therapy context.

References

Akister, J., & Reibstein, J. (2004). Links between attachment theory and systemic practice: Some proposals. *Journal of Family Therapy*, 26, 2–16.

Araoz, D., & Negley-Parker, E. (1988). *The new hypnosis in family therapy.* New York: Brunner-Mazel.

Ashby, W. R. (1965). *An introduction to cybernetics.* New York: John Wiley and Sons.

Bateson, G. (1972). *Steps to an ecology of mind.* New York: Dutton.

Bateson, G. (1979). *Mind and nature: A necessary unity.* New York: Dutton.

Beels, C. (2002). Notes for a cultural history of family therapy. *Family Process*, 41, 67–82.

Byng-Hall, J. (1995). Creating a secure base: Some implications of attachment theory for family therapy. *Family Process*, 34, 45–58.

Council, J. (1999). Hypnosis and response expectancies. In I. Kirsch (Ed.), *How Expectancies Shape Experience* (pp. 383–401). Washington, D.C.: American Psychological Association.

Donley, M. (1993). Attachment and the emotional unit. *Family Process*, 32, 3–30.

Erickson, M., & Rossi, R. (1979). *Hypnotherapy: An exploratory casebook.* New York: Irvington.

Erickson, M. (1992). *Creative choice in hypnosis.* E. Rossi & M. Ryan (Eds). New York: Irvington.

Fourie, D. (1991). Family hypnotherapy: Erickson or systems? *Journal of Family Therapy*, 13, 53–71.

Gergen, K. (1991). *Realities and relationships: Soundings in social construction.* Cambridge, MA: Harvard University Press.

Gilligan, S. (1987). *Therapeutic trances: The cooperation principle in Ericksonian hypnotherapy.* New York: Brunner/Mazel.

Goffman, E. (1974). *Frame analysis: An essay on the organization of experience.* Boston: Northeastern University Press.

Green, J., Barabasz, A., Barrett, D., & Montgomery, G. (2005). The 2003 APA division 30 definition of hypnosis. *Journal of Clinical and Experimental Hypnosis,* 53(3): 262–264.

Haley, J. (1973). *Uncommon therapy: The psychiatric techniques of Milton H. Erickson, M.D.* New York: W.W. Norton.

Haley, J. (1976). *Problem-solving therapy.* New York: Harper & Row.

Haley, J. (1985). *Conversations with Milton H. Erickson, M.D. Volume III: Changing children and families.* New York: Triangle.

Haley, J. (1996). *Learning & teaching therapy.* New York: Guilford Press.

Hill, J., Fonagy, P., Safier, E., & Sargent, J. (2003). The ecology of attachment in the family. *Family Process,* 42, 205–221.

Kane, S., & Olness, K. (2004). *The art of therapeutic communication: The collected works of Kay F. Thompson.* Carmarthen, Wales, U.K.: Crown House.

Kirsch, I. (1999). Response expectancy: An introduction. In I. Kirsch (Ed.), *How expectancies shape experience* (pp. 3–13). Washington, D.C.: American Psychological Association.

Lebow, J. (2000). What does research tell us about couple and family therapies? *Journal of Clinical Psychology,* 56, 1083–1094.

Liddle, H., & Rowe, C. (2005). Advances in family therapy research. In M. Nichols & R. Schwartz, *The Essentials of Family Therapy,* (pp. 298–328). Boston: Pearson.

Maturana, H. & Poerksen, B. (2004). *From being to doing: The origins of the biology of cognition.* Heidelberg: Carl-Auer.

Maturana, H., & Varela, F. (1987). *The tree of knowledge.* Boston: Shambhala.

Minuchin, S. (1974). *Families & family therapy.* Cambridge: Harvard University Press.

Nichols, M., & Schwartz, R. (2005). *The essentials of family therapy (2nd edition).* Boston: Pearson.

O'Hanlon, W. (1987). *Taproots: Underlying principles of Milton Erickson's therapy and hypnosis.* New York: W.W. Norton.

Ritterman, M. (1983). *Using hypnosis in family therapy.* San Francisco: Jossey-Bass.

Rorty, R. (1991). *Objectivity, relativism, and truth.* Cambridge: Cambridge University Press.

Sprenkle, D., & Blow, A. (2004). Common factors and our sacred models. *Journal of Marital & Family Therapy,* 30, 113–130.

Teleska, J., & Roffman, A. (2004). A continuum of hypnotherapeutic interactions: From formal hypnosis to hypnotic conversation. *American Journal of Clinical Hypnosis,* 47, 103–115.

Watzlawick, P., Weakland, J., & Fisch, R. (1974). *Change: Principles of problem formation and problem resolution.* New York: W.W. Norton.

Weakland, J. (1993). Commentary. In S. Gilligan & R. Price (Eds.), *Therapeutic conversations.* New York: W.W. Norton.

Weinberger, J. & Eig, A. (1999). Expectancies: The ignored common factor in psychotherapy. In I. Kirsch (Ed.), *How expectancies shape experience* (pp. 357–382). Washington, D.C.: American Psychological Association.

Whitaker, C. (1982). Hypnosis and family depth therapy. In J. Zeig (Ed.). *Ericksonian approaches to hypnosis and psychotherapy* (pp. 491–504). New York: Brunner-Mazel.

Whitaker, C., & Bumberry, W. (1988). *Dancing with the family: A symbolic-experiential approach.* New York: Brunner-Mazel.

Part III

Medical Implications

Chapter Fourteen

Integrating Hypnosis in Acute Care Settings

Laurence I. Sugarman, MD, FAAP, ABMH
Daniel P. Kohen, MD, ABMH

It was a typically busy day in the pediatric office. The schedule was full with kids needing camp physicals, having fevers, stomachaches, and sore throats. Unscheduled, a mother rushed in with her 7-year-old daughter who had just fallen at the nearby playground. The girl had a laceration of her chin that required sutures. The pediatrician looked forward to these unexpected opportunities to use hypnosis. While he washed the wound he asked her what she did best at the playground, "Sliding, climbing, swinging, running fast?"

Engaged, and a bit surprised, she replied that she could "Swing real high."

The pediatrician suggested, "You go back to the playground and leave your chin here where it will rest and be comfortable and have some stitches to help it heal up." Lying on the examination table, she gazed up at the ceiling where engaging stickers of cartoon characters, action heroes, and outdoor scenes were placed strategically. He carefully sutured her laceration while asking her how much fun she was having swinging back and forth, feeling the wind through her hair, seeing everything from way up high, breathing the fresh outside air, and feeling the warm sun.

When he was done, she asked, "Was that it?" The pediatrician replied, "You sure did a good job playing at the playground and letting me sew up your chin. It must be good to know that you can help yourself by using your mind that way. When you come back to have the stitches removed you can do it again."

Later that week the pediatrician received a card in the mail from the girl's mother. She thanked him for taking unscheduled time out of his busy day to help her daughter. The mother noted that her daughter was particularly proud of herself, "I have to tell you, when we left, just as we were walking out, she said to me, 'This is the best day of my life!'"

General Principles of Integrating Hypnosis in Acute Care Settings

The clinician who works with children and adolescents in an emergency department (Kohen, 1986; Brunnquell & Kohen, 1991), clinic, or at a hospital bedside (Barnes & Kohen, 2006) has an opportunity to use hypnosis creatively. Young people are entranced by these circumstances. Their attention is intensified and narrowed by the conditions of illness, injury, environment, and expectation (Sugarman, 2006). Due to this heightened sensitivity, they may be exquisitely responsive to the language and intention of those around them. Perhaps the situation is novel and intensifies their curiosity. Maybe it is familiar and influenced positively or negatively by the memory of previous experiences. In either case, the clinician does not really inject hypnosis into the situation as much as recognize those hypnotic elements that are already present and then utilize them. This is about finding the hypnosis in the encounter. In this chapter, we take a "guided tour" through a variety of clinical interactions common to the daily routine of acute pediatric care in order to explore the trances inherent in them and how they may be engaged and developed in therapy.

Most clinicians who work in acute care settings learn by experience to use some form of distraction or playfulness when working with children and adolescents. Such techniques can include imaginative involvement on the part of the child, such as when the practitioner claims to see little animals in the child's ear during an examination or suddenly exclaims, "Look at that bear over there!" just as she gives the child an injection in the arm. The clinician can even place his hand in a puppet and use that animated creature to examine the child's abdomen. There are countless approaches, as many as there are clinicians and children. The purpose of these strategies is to guide the patient's attention away from the intravenous line insertion, the examination of a painful area, or simply to defuse anxiety. To the extent that such methods shift attentional focus, intensify it, and evoke imagination, they include hypnotic elements. We have identified the acute clinical setting as being trance-inducing at some level. So what is the difference between these methods and "hypnosis?"

To the extent that such interactions, occurring spontaneously or purposefully, contain hypnotic elements, they are hypnotic. But hypnotic techniques alone are not hypnosis or hypnotherapy. Integrating hypnosis in acute care settings with children and adolescents can and, we believe, should serve a deeper therapeutic purpose than temporary comfort, increasing efficiency or decreasing resistance to a procedure. If, as is proposed in Chapter One, clinical hypnosis with children and adolescents can be conceived of as an effort to promote adaptive psychophysiological responses, and, at a neurocellular level, to stimulate brain plasticity, then we must shift our perspective on these practices from a simple, playful distraction directed by the clinician to more evocative, child-centered, and reflective exchanges founded on the empathic awareness of rapport. This distinction will be illustrated and highlighted in the clinical vignettes that follow.

Essentially, we can frame the integration of hypnosis in acute care settings as situation-induced episodes of trance that create opportunities for utilization of the young person's subconscious resources to accumulate coping skills for his or her future. Within this context we can list four guidelines for making use of hypnotherapy in acute care settings.

1. *Utilize what the patient gives you.* Utilization begins with the clinician understanding that whatever the child says or does, with rare exception, is not only acceptable but meaningful and instructive. This may involve asking children what they have done before to cope with such a situation, as in, "How have you helped yourself before?" or "What do you do to calm yourself when you are worried?" On the other hand, if a child is screaming with pain or anxiety as you enter the room,

utilization may mean asking the child to scream louder or longer, "… until you have screamed enough to help yourself become comfortable," or "Please keep crying until you tell yourself it's okay to stop."

2. *Join the patient's trance.* Start empathizing with the patient's situation before suggesting ways to change it. With a child experiencing acute abdominal pain due to appendicitis, the clinician might simply observe, "You look uncomfortable. I bet you would rather be some place other than here. While you're lying here, go ahead and go there … so you can begin to feel more comfortable." Or perhaps say, "I'm sorry you're unhappy and uncomfortable. I'm glad you came over … that was smart because now you can start to feel better. While I do the [procedure, examination, etc.] you can imagine you're not even here." Contrast this with attempting to direct a hypnotic induction with a patient who is already entranced by circumstances, or, worse, beginning to describe the details of some hypnotic technique you are about to perform while he or she is focused on his or her pain.

3. *Embed ego-strengthening, affirming suggestions.* As the patient responds to suggestions for comfort, self-control, relaxation, dissociation, and other recommendations, the clinician has the opportunity to help him or her take credit for, appreciate, and own the process. Ego-strengthening suggestions such as, "It's good to know that you're doing this just right … ," or "You are really very good at helping yourself become more and more comfortable." This language affirms that the child is not being hypnotized or controlled. He or she is doing this with his or her own ability.

4. *Generalize the experience.* The realization of increased self-control and comfort in the face of potential anxiety and pain ratifies the hypnotic experience. At that moment, to generalize what has just been practiced constitutes a post-hypnotic suggestion that reinforces learning. For example, immediately after a 5-year-old boy has successfully received his immunizations without crying or anxiety by focusing his breathing on a spinning pinwheel, the nurse says, "Now you know what to

do when something worries you," adding, "And you know Mommy is very proud of you, too." This is not simply ego-strengthening reinforcement for the child, but also modeling and teaching the parents how they can reinforce this learning. This success can be referenced at future visits.

A Shift in Perspective

The integration of hypnosis into practice can be a paradigm change for the clinician. In daily practice on the hospital ward, the emergency department, or the outpatient clinic, the practitioner tends to fall into the common trap of routine, the comfort of doing things the same way. This can blur the differences between children and their problems. It tends to cause us to treat each child in the same way, from the questions we ask to the order of the examination. But when we add hypnosis as a lens through which to view each encounter, there is new depth and value each time. Each new child with an ear infection or sore throat comes with a different set of anxieties, coping skills, and expectations conditioned by previous experiences. The intriguing challenge becomes, "How do I diagnose this particular child's pharyngitis, fractured radius, or appendicitis in a way that helps him or her develop a sense of improved self-control and mastery?" In order to do this, the clinician must listen and watch the patient carefully, paying attention to the minimal cues that the child always brings to the encounter. Because this child is frightened of having his or her ears looked at, the clinician examines his or her doll's ears first. Because that child seems scared of having his or her throat swabbed, the clinician takes time to address that fear before taking a history, and then make a plan to "work on that in the future." In each case, the anxiety, originating from pain, an expected procedure, or bad news, dictates the trance of the encounter, thereby presenting the opportunity for therapeutic suggestions.

Milton Erickson, the father of modern clinical hypnosis, did not say "lead the child," "take the child," or "tell the child," he said, "...work primarily *with*, and not on, [italics added] the child" (Erickson, 1958, p. 26). This recurrent "...pacing then leading then pacing then leading" approach to clinical encounters with children stands in contrast to the routine of collecting a history, doing an exam, making a diagnosis, and prescribing treatment. While those steps are necessary, and may treat the presenting problem, they alone do not invest in the child's ability to cope. As such, they may be counterproductive and risk perpetuating dependency and negative expectations.

Pediatric clinicians in acute care settings are usually pressed for time. When first introduced to the idea, many express concern that "adding hypnosis" will take more time from an already burdensome schedule. Our experience is that integrating hypnotic skills into clinical encounters actually saves time and increases efficiency (Reaney, Sugarman, & Olness 1998; Sugarman, 1996a; 1996b; 2006). The hypnotic realm is already there, waiting to be engaged. Children who learn to calm themselves during procedures will bring that learning with them, if needed, for other procedures. The skills used for one problem (e.g., breathing and dissociative imagery while having a wound sutured) can be called up efficiently and then applied for another problem (anxiety, headaches, or habit change) in the future. This is especially true if the clinician includes suggestions for the generalization of this learning every time (*see* "4. Generalize the experience," above).

Intriguing research questions emerge when one considers the implications of integration of hypnosis in the continuum of pediatric care. Do children who routinely learn self-regulation as a part of their healthcare catch fewer infectious diseases (Hewson-Bower & Drummond, 1996); have fewer headaches (Olness, McDonald, & Uden, 1987); shorter postoperative hospital stays (Lambert, 1996); and use fewer medications (Jacknow, Tschann, Link, & Boyce, 1994; Olness, McDonald, & Uden, 1987)? The cited research indicates that the answer will be affirmative. How cost effective can that be?

Finding Hypnosis in Acute Care Encounters

The following clinical vignettes exemplify the principles discussed in this introduction. They are not intended to be prescriptive. Rather, they are examples of creative, hypnotic exchanges in which a clinician utilizes the unique cues that the child or adolescent brings to the encounter.

Procedural Pain and Anxiety

Along with abandonment, fear of being kidnapped, and fear of death, getting "a shot" at the doctor's office is a major primary fear of children (French, Painter, & Coury, 1994). The actual tissue damage that triggers nerve fibers carrying the message of pain up the spinal cord to the brain after an injection, the so-called nociceptive component of pain, is small (*see* Chapter Eighteen) There is less tissue damage and subsequent pain signals from the injection of 0.5 milliliters of neutral pH liquid through a 25-gauge needle into the muscle than, say, stubbing one's toe, falling on one's knees, or bumping one's head under the table. Children do these things all the time without as much as a whimper. But even many adolescents will carry with them into the doctor's office a conditioned fear of getting an injection. They often will ask about "needing a shot" and then visibly relax when they learn that no immunizations or blood tests are needed at this visit.

Of course the fear of needles is not about the pain. It is the anxiety that colors and shapes the perception of discomfort, and, with its intensity, helps encode the psychophysiological response that is fear, sympathetic nervous system arousal, withdrawal, and self-protection. This reflex anxiety is conditioned early because we begin immunizations in early infancy, when internal coping strategies are primitive and formative. Such early conditioning can lay down the template of intensified awareness, heightened expectancy, and sensitivity to cues, language, and suggestion that is the trance of coming to the pediatrician.

The reader may begin to think that it is unimportant to focus on the relatively minimal procedure of an immunization, compared to surgery, cancer chemotherapy, or serious physical trauma. Certainly these other experiences seem to be more significant challenges. But these are not as universal and, consequently, not as influential and defining in the child's early life as are injections. Furthermore, this discounting of the fear of needles in the doctor's office may indeed be part of the problem. Despite obvious anxiety, parents, nurses, and physicians commonly tell children who are receiving injections that "It's not that bad," or "This is just a little poke." During a prospective study in which children were taught to "blow away shot pain," French et al. (1994) reported that clinicians in the clinic at which the study was being performed made comments dismissing the importance of teaching children to cope with injections. Of course, minimizing the significance of a child's fear builds alienation, not rapport. Once again, we are asked to remember the significance of Erickson's advice to "work with the child." If the child's trance of anxiety indicates that this is an important opportunity to invest in his or her resilience, then that is exactly where the clinician ought to go.

The following clinical vignette represents an actual encounter in which 5-year-old Emily (name changed) receives her immunizations. The inserted commentary explores meanings and strategic implications of the dialog.

Emily

Emily and her mother are waiting in the examination room as the clinician enters. Upon seeing the physician,

> **Emily**: [*screams*] I'M NOT GETTING ANY SHOTS!

> **Mother**: Emily! [*To the clinician*] I'm so sorry. This is all she has been talking about.

What does this mean? It means that Emily is willful and does not keep her opinions to herself. We can assume that she is in a sort of negatively expectant trance. She expects a shot and she thinks she can make it go away. This behavior has worked for her at home or other places and her mother would like some help with her. Mostly, it means that Emily does not want a "shot."

> **L. Sugarman [LS]**: [*Starting loudly then softening my voice*] I'M DR. SUGARMAN AND I CAN TELL YOU DON'T WANT ANY SHOTS, RIGHT? Would it be okay if the needle poke bothered you less?

Here the doctor first attempts to entrain anxiety by matching the volume and tone of the patient, while building rapport by making a connection with his name and by empathizing with Emily's plight. After this "pacing" he immediately, but subtly, leads by changing the language. While Emily insists she is not getting any shots, the doctor says she does not "want any shots." Then he calls it a "needle poke" that bothers (not "hurts").

Emily: BUT IT WILL!

LS: [*Softly*] You want it to?

Emily: [*Shakes head "No," appears curious*]

LS: Good. Your Mom and I don't want it to hurt you either. You can make it better and your Mom and I will help you. Would that be okay?

Here, Emily makes an implicit statement that what she says or thinks is going to happen, will happen. With his simple question, the doctor suggests that if Emily changes how she thinks, she can change how she feels. This is about changing negative expectancy. The clinician also evokes curiosity. This invites Emily to narrow her attention and listen more carefully. It makes a connection. Then there is more leading, with an invitation to let us help her make it "better."

Emily: Okay. But I don't want a shot.

Emily has shifted her frame of reference. Instead of not "getting" a shot, she does not "want" a shot. "Okay" is utilized by the doctor as the beginning of a "yes set"—a series of affirmative responses elicited to encourage cooperation—that follows. In this case the "yes set" is ego-strengthening and empathetic.

LS: I know, and that's really smart because you don't want anything to bother you, right?

[*To mother*] It would be okay if Emily sat on your lap and got hugged, right?

[*To Emily*] Okay?

[All agree and Emily sits on Mother's lap] Great! Now that you are more comfortable, would you like to know something that feels good? Do you know how to blow your breath OUT? Like when you blow out birthday candles?

Emily: *[She nods]*

LS: Will you show me how you do it?

Emily: *[She blows]*

LS: That's right! You know you are good at that, aren't you? Do it again and keep blowing so you can blow away that worry about the shot bothering you. Here *[handing her a penlight]*, this can be your birthday candle. Your Mom can be surprised at how well you will make it work. Are you ready to be done with the shot?

Emily: *[Nods "Yes" while blowing on imaginary candle/penlight]*

Emily has gone along with this series of suggestions not because she is under the clinician's control but because the clinician has quickly guided her to focus on her own control with positive associations. The metaphor of the birthday candles reinforces these links. Blowing out birthday candles is something that she has probably done well recently or will do again soon because most parents schedule such health supervision visits around their child's birthday. Blowing out candles is an accomplishment attached to affirmation, wish fulfillment, and magical thinking. Everybody watches and claps when the child blows out those candles. The clinician has moved quickly to suspend logical judgment and thinking by Emily to allow those less conscious memories and experiences to overtake the threat of the shot.

Mother, who we can assume is in her own trance (informed by her daughter's fears, discomfort, and expectancy and her own attachment and sense of responsibility), has a role that at once lessens her own anxiety and provides the comfort and support that only mothers can give. Because the anxiety between parent and child is like a harmonic resonance, mother's cooperation is critical.

Finally, the clinician utilizes the elemental power of breathing as a coping method. Each breath out is fundamental to relaxation.

The injection is given. Emily winces and keeps blowing.

LS: There. You did it. How did you do?

Emily: [*Surprised*] That was the shot... ?

LS: Uh huh. It is all done.

Emily: I did good!

LS: You would know ... and you surprised your Mom, too! You can be proud about how you did. Well, now you know another way to keep things from bothering you, don't you?

Emily: Uh huh! [*She blows some more and laughs*]

LS: You deserve a sticker, right? I'll trade you the sticker for your "candle." Pick one out.

After the injection, the experience is *ratified* by Emily's recognition that "that was the shot" and that it was differently experienced, hence her surprise. The clinician's response continues to *reinforce Emily's ownership of the change* by asking her how she did, rather than telling her that she did well, and with the phrase, "You would know." Then he suggests *generalization*, " ... you know another way to keep things from bothering you" while implying respectfully, that she has some coping strategies. Finally, he *validates the value of her learning* and accomplishment with a sticker, another choice.

In addition to imaginary birthday candles, pinwheels, bubbles, hypnotic suggestions for—selective hand warming, cold sensations, turning down "pain switches," the application of magic gloves and Band-Aids can all be employed, alone or in varying combinations of one another, tailored to the needs of individual children (Kuttner, 1986; 1999; Olness & Kohen, 1996). The clinician can keep a large basket of all sorts of items for redirection of focus and bring this basket into the exam room so that the child can choose what he or she finds best to use. A variety of approaches to immunization injections as well as other procedures is demonstrated in the video documentary "Hypnosis in Pediatric Practice: Imaginative Medicine in Action" (Sugarman, 2006).

Nor does the passive cooperation of the child constitute the only evidence of success.

I entered the examination room to see a 4-year-old boy sitting on his mother's lap screaming, "No stitches! No stitches! No stitches!" He had sustained a laceration to his forehead that required closure. His mother held an antiseptic-soaked sponge to his forehead. The contents of the basket used in the office to offer children comfort and distraction during procedures were strewn about the room. This boy was angry, frightened, tense, and very still while sitting on his mother's lap. He remained still and screaming while the doctor cleaned the wound, injected lidocaine, and sutured it closed.

While applying a sterile dressing, the pediatrician whispered quietly, "All done."

The boy abruptly stopped screaming, wiped his tears, and said, "I did really good! Can I get a sticker?"

In this example, the boy's trance involved screaming, but not really crying, presumably as an expression of his anger and autonomy. The doctor noted that while in the trance of screaming the boy was relatively cataleptic. This was utilized successfully. Had the clinician attempted to make the boy quiet and passive by being directive or starting to induce another trance he would have been working against the boy's strong protective reflexes, perhaps less successfully, and far less efficiently. In the end, the boy's ego and autonomy remained intact.

When an acute procedure such as suturing a wound, draining a superficial abscess, or dressing a burn involves bleeding, risk of infection, and time to heal, suggestions to maximize those protective physiological responses can be incorporated into hypnotic suggestions for comfort. It has long been observed that, mediated by some unknown mechanisms, hypnotic suggestions can help patients stop bleeding. Similarly, there is no harm in suggesting that the child's immune system can do a great job keeping infection away from the wound and that his or her skin and soft tissues can feel nourished and grow quickly to heal the wound. While the child may not consciously select how he or she controls these physiologic responses, the fact is that he or she *does* control them, and therefore such suggestions constitute statements of faith and education.

The Trance of the Exam: Utilizing Reflexes

In acute medical settings the physical examination can be utilized to help children not only appreciate mind-body reflexes but also use them to provide comfort and self-control. When, once again, we decide to frame as a trance the novel and vulnerable interaction that is a physical examination, perhaps intensified when a child feels ill, then the various parts of this interaction can be offered and understood as hypnotherapeutic suggestions. Consider the following set of italicized hypnotic suggestions embedded into this physical examination. Note that the words "the," "these" and "those" are used to enhance dissociation. Instead of directive statements, the clinician asks the child to demonstrate his ability to be the "boss of his body":

"Because you're covering those ears with those hands, I can tell that they are worried about being examined. Which one will *you want to let go first*. Good. Keep that ear *nice and still* while this warm light shines in it and make sure it doesn't *tickle* too much. Now let's give the other ear a turn. Great. I wonder how wide your mouth can open while your tongue sticks out. That's really great! That lets me see all the way back. Thank you. Now as you *focus your eyes* wide on that picture over there, notice how this *light doesn't bother* them and they *stay comfortable*. Do you know where your heart is? That's right. Can you feel it beating by paying a lot of attention to it? That's great. Would you like to listen yourself? Good. Notice how it changes as

---

you breathe in and out. Now I'd like to listen to what your back sounds like when you breathe normally. Just *pay attention to your breathing* while I listen. Those are *nice, comfortable, deep breaths*. I wonder what your belly does when you let a nice big breath out. That's really cool! When you do that you make your belly *soft and comfortable*. Isn't that interesting? Can you do it again? Can you make it just *as comfortable* over here? How about over here? Can you *spread that relaxation and comfort* down these legs so I can examine them too? It must *feel really good* to know that *you can help your body* feel this comfortable when you *pay attention to it*. You're the *boss of your body*."

The normal physical finding of deep tendon reflexes can be used as a metaphorical example for psychophysiological reflexes.

"What happens with your leg when I tap this tendon here below your kneecap?[*Clinician elicits patellar reflex*]....That's interesting isn't it? Now, when I do this again, don't let your leg move....[*Clinician taps the patellar tendon again. Because the patient has tightened his quadriceps, the reflex is more pronounced*]....OK. Your leg moved more. This time do something different and keep it from moving. [*Clinician taps the patellar tendon. Again the reflex is brisk*]....Well, that didn't work the way you expected it to, did it? I suppose that if we kept at this for quite awhile eventually you would learn how to not let that leg move when I tap that tendon. Eventually, you would learn to change that reflex. You may not be able to explain to me how you do it. What is important is that you know that you can do it. Sometimes you just work at something that's important to you and you figure it out. Do you think that the [*headaches, abdominal pain, anxiety episodes, etc.*] would be a worthwhile reflex to learn to control?"

Following this cognitive reframing, with attention focused on subconscious somatic change, the patient can participate in a hypnotic induction that leads to exploring how to change the presenting problem.

Hypnosis and the Pelvic Examination

A pre-adolescent or adolescent young woman's first pelvic examination may be indicated because she is becoming sexually active, has gynecologic symptoms or questions, or is concerned about possible pregnancy. Regardless of the indication, when, in the context of rapport and history, it becomes clear that a pelvic examination should be part of the visit's agenda the clinician is presented with a "teachable moment" of spontaneous trance behavior. The young woman is predictably anxious, worried, probably physically tense, and self-conscious about her vulnerability during the imminent examination. The clinician is challenged to answer questions, shift negative expectancies to positive, provide comfort, and empower the patient to learn and understand that she has the capacity to make the experience a positive one (Kohen, 1980).

As part of the medical history, it is essential to ascertain if the patient has ever had a pelvic examination. Assuming that prior examination experiences have been negative is as much of a mistake as not thinking about or discussing it at all. Whether past experiences have been positive or negative, it allows the clinician to ask appropriately, "Would you please help me understand what I can do to make this even easier and more comfortable?" One may need to be very direct and explicit, even while setting the tone of positive expectations for a positive experience and outcome: "What did the other doctor or nurse do or say that you didn't like, and what would you like me to say or do to help?" The fact of asking, of course, offers the powerful and important message (a hypnotic suggestion) that says to the patient's subconscious mind "This is collaboration. Your opinion and needs are most important. My goal is to help you."

If this is an initial visit with a patient and this is her first ever pelvic examination, she may not be able or willing to articulate her fears. Instead, she is probably simply anxious, frightened, and saying things such as, "I know I have to have it and I should have it and it's the right thing to do, but I'm just really scared … ," and may even add, "and I don't know why … ." One reasonable response might be:

"Thanks for telling me. I know what you mean ... it's hard to go someplace new where you never met the doctor before and think about talking about personal stuff, and getting undressed, but also about having a check-up you never had. I guess I'd be surprised and worried about you if you weren't nervous about it. Most young women who I've met come in feeling pretty much the same, and usually they're quite surprised by how much easier it is than they thought."

Like most encounters that "work," this interaction reflects "joining" with the patient; i.e., acknowledging the anxiety, reframing it from "scared" to "nervous," and normalizing it by explaining that it is really "expected." The young woman learns that you have seen this before, and that most others have been reassured by their success.

Then, in order to move forward with the experience, the doctor might say:

"So, here's what we'll do. I'll go out while you get ready for the examination, when you get undressed, put on this gown over your underwear. Then, when I come back in we'll go through the examination. You've had most of the check-up before, right? So you know that I'll check your eyes, ears, throat, listen to your heart and lungs, check your vagina, and do the internal check-up, feel your belly, check your reflexes, check your breasts, and check your balance."

The mention of key features of the examination provides clear expectation of what will happen while establishing that the clinician will tell the young woman what will happen. In order to continue to defuse anxiety, the vaginal and internal examinations are explained in the context of the more familiar parts of the process.

Given that women often feel vulnerable with their legs up and spread apart while the doctor sits at the end of the table, it behooves the clinician to address this discomfort as well. This is often easily accomplished by first conducting most of the general physical examination with the patient sitting and the clinician standing alongside the exam table instead of at the end, before the abdominal and pelvic portions of the examination. This also affords the clinician the opportunity to provide positive and spontaneously hypnotic suggestions for comfort during the exam. For example, while examining the lungs, I [DK] commonly say:

> "Please take a deep breath in through your nose and out through your mouth. Great. Now, the next breath, do it the same way and just notice what happens to your shoulders as you breathe out. Right. What happened? Right, they go down, don't they? The coolest thing about that is that it's natural and kind of AUTOMATIC. So, as we breathe in, it's natural for the body to RELAX as we breathe out. So, now, take another breath, and as you let it out … right … as you let it out, NOW let that relaxing feeling from your shoulders move down into your arms … right. While I continue checking your breathing and your heart, just kind of experiment with yourself so that with each next breath out that relaxing feeling can continue moving down your body just right for you, down from your shoulders, to the upper arms, right … and then down your arms to your hands and fingers … and then down your chest … and to your belly, and you can let it keep going down like to your lower belly muscles and your thighs and your vagina muscles can get loose and soft and relaxed, too … so that in a few moments when it's time to do the check of the vagina and pelvic internal examination, the loose muscles will make it even easier to do the exam for me and for you … . So, it's really good to know how to do this as a way to help yourself be really comfortable during the whole check-up… ."

Finally, as the vaginal and internal examinations are completed, the clinician can affirm the young woman's coping and suggest that she reflect on how she has learned to have a pelvic examination differently. Perhaps most importantly, the clinician can finish the encounter by sitting with the patient, now clothed, and asking her for feedback. "How well did I do explaining what was happening and making certain that you were comfortable? What would you want me or another examiner to do better next time?" Even if the patient has no criticism, these important questions convey respect for the young woman who has placed herself in this vulnerable situation.

Hypnosis and Asthma

Asthma is one of those many chronic illnesses that children and adults often think of as something that "has them" and not only that "they have." This is evident from the emergence in our social language of the "-ic" words that essentially label people with the name of an illness that they "have," but that, in fact, only bothers them sometimes. Thus, we hear of *asthmatic*, and of *epileptic*, *leukemic*, *diabetic*. But, children are not an illness. With a clear intention of being therapeutic, when children (or their parents) say that they (or their child) is *"asthmatic,"* we tell them we have never met someone who is asthmatic—even though we know a lot of kids whose asthma used to bother them a lot and who "have" asthma sometimes—we don't know anyone who IS *asthmatic*. This begins to set the tone for thinking and talking perhaps differently about asthma. As with any illness or problem, we will wonder with the child in what way his or her asthma bothers him or her or gets in the way of his or her life; and more important, we ask what he or she will do differently when the asthma is not bothering them as much as it used to. This is a hypnotic way of talking, without any official ceremony of hypnotic induction, and necessarily without any discussion about hypnosis per se. It focuses attention because it is positive and because by implication it suggests that things could be different. Because the approach is different, it stimulates curiosity.

In response to these questions about what will be different, children say typically that they will be able to play more, run around more, sleep the whole night without coughing, participate better in a sport, or keep up with the other kids. Next, we ask what they already do to help themselves when they are having problems breathing. In this way, we focus on empowering the child and his or her recognition that he or she already has skills to help himself or herself. This contrasts with the typical medical interview that focuses primarily on symptom severity and medication use. We intend to help the child understand that his or her capacities to help himself or herself may be as, if not more, important and powerful than the valuable medications we prescribe.

"Did you know that your brain is the boss of your breathing? That's how, even when you're sleeping, your brain tells your lungs how to breathe just right ... , and the more your lungs learn the better they get. Did you know that you have muscles around each of your breathing tubes? Well, you do. Do you know how to make muscles tight and then relax them... ? That's right ... ."

Education about how the body works is an essential ingredient in helping any child understand, manage, and promote his or her health. Therefore, we discuss the two main ingredients in episodes of asthma: (1) the inflammatory response of the lining of the airways and hypersecretion of mucus there, and; (2) the spasm, tightening of muscles surround the airway (bronchospasm). Further, we explain that both of these processes lead to narrowing of the airway and to the familiar "wheezing" sound that signals difficulty in exhaling and the emergence of respiratory distress (dyspnea). Few experiences are as frightening as the inability to "catch one's breath" so that, with narrowing of the airway, coughing, and wheezing, there is also anxiety and more distress, which in turn contributes to even more wheezing and fear, reinforcing an intensifying spiral of dyspnea and anxiety. Most young people with asthma nod in agreement as this is explained to them and are comforted in knowing that we know.

By contrast, children can learn through self-hypnosis that, with very careful attention, they can detect the earliest "wheeze," cough, or "a little tightness" in their airways. That subtle change in breathing can be their body's signal to do self-hypnosis, interrupting the negative cycle, and making it one of comfort and control. (Olness & Kohen, 1996; Kohen, 1986; 1995; 1997; 2000). So, when a child says he is having trouble with his breathing acutely, we ask:

D. Kohen [DK]: How would you like it to be doing when you leave the office in a little while?

Child: Better.

DK: Great, want to learn how to get it better?

Child: Sure.

DK: Great, let your eyes close then pretend you're not here…Just imagine or daydream that you're at the park, and riding your bike, and let your head nod when you can feel like you're there … great. Now notice as you come around a turn, that you take a big breath in and let it out very slowly … great! [*the breathing rate will slow down*] … now let your breathing be even slower, kind of automatically while you keep riding … and every turn you make, it gets easier to breathe that fresh air, in … and … out … right. Look around in your mind and picture a video that lets you look inside your body and while you're riding your bike in one part of your mind, in another part just notice those breathing tubes getting wider and wider so all the air you want can go in … and … out … and notice how loose and floppy the muscles are around those breathing tubes … just like how relaxed your outside muscles are getting here even in the few moments that you've been doing your imagining. So, keep enjoying that until your breathing is right where you want it, and then bring the good feelings of easy breathing and little or no wheezing back with you when you finish your imagining and come back to this room.

A few moments of debriefing this spontaneous experience commonly includes a "waking suggestion" to:

"Practice this each night before bed, just like you just did, because the more you do it, the better you'll get, and before you fall asleep you could even just give your brain instructions to tell the breathing tubes to 'Stay wide open all night so I can sleep easily and wake up feeling great in the morning'; and then fall asleep and have a great dream."

Once again, the trance of the moment becomes an opportunity to suggest a change in a psychophysiological reflex. The child can learn to cope with the potent stimulus of dyspnea by responding not with sympathetic nervous system arousal (the fight or flight response) but with comfort and self-control.

Hypnosis and Hospital Care

The admission to a hospital is indeed an entry into trance, albeit often an unpleasant one. For a child becoming an "inpatient" is commonly a mysterious, confusing, bewildering, and frightening experience. As such, it has all of the ingredients of a spontaneous hypnotic event in which the child and family are often narrowly focused, concentrating intensely on the injured or ill parts of the body and physiologically vigilant. The child with an acute episode of asthma has trouble breathing and is focused on her hunger for air, worried about where the next breath will come from, and what will happen next. The child who is dehydrated may well have a disturbed sensorium as a result of water and electrolyte imbalance, and in addition to his trance behavior may not be thinking clearly amidst vomiting and/or diarrhea.

Regardless of the reason for hospitalization, invariably the child and family meet many, many new people in a short period of time, including the clerk in the Emergency Department, the Emergency Department nurse, the examining Emergency Department physician (and, at a teaching hospital, student and resident), the laboratory technician, the radiology technician, the admissions clerk, the transport person who accompanies their wheelchair or stretcher to the inpatient unit. There, an additional nursing assistant and nurse greet the patient and family and assist them in getting oriented to yet another new environment: bed, nightstand, "call button," and, thankfully, the remote control for the television. Moments later the nurse arrives to again check the temperature, blood pressure, pulse, respiration, and then explains that the resident physician will be in shortly to talk and examine the child ... again. During this time, children (and adults) commonly remain in their uncomfortable, environmentally and situation-induced hypnotic states ... frightened by the uncertainty of what is happening, by the newness of feelings of pain, or difficulty breathing, or vomiting; by the helplessness—and perhaps hopelessness of the moment—of things not improving from minute to minute, or even hour to hour; by the confusion of meeting so many new people so quickly; by the intrusiveness of yet another needle stick, or examination, or check of this or that; by the sheer numbers of new, unusual experiences that happen "all at once."

Now the primary doctor comes to see his patient who was hospitalized hours earlier. The doctor, too, enters his or her own trance, shifting his or her awareness upon entering the hospital. Even with the careful attention that children's hospitals and children's units in general hospitals pay to ambience and décor, there is no mistaking the different feel of a hospital. Tension is often in the air. Awareness of the disconcerting trance of hospitalization allows physicians to behave verbally and nonverbally in ways that can help to undo the alienating aspects of the patient's/family's spontaneous hypnotic experience.

Reframing language and suggestions can facilitate the therapeutic shift of those trance experiences from negative to positive. These approaches can begin as initial greetings that at once honor the reality of the patient's condition and situation, while providing hope and allowing the trance to begin to change:

> "I'm sorry to know that you aren't feeling well, and really glad to see that you are here so that you are already starting to improve. It was really smart of you and Mom and Dad to come to the Emergency Department when you did, because now you can start getting better."

While reviewing the history and examining the child, the doctor can often find some positive things to say about the examination in order to not limit or perpetuate the focus on those parts that are abnormal.

> "Well, your tummy is still pretty noisy from all that diarrhea. Your heart and lungs are just fine...that's really good and it probably means you'll be getting better faster than you thought.
>
> How was that IV when they put it in? I don't know if you'll need a different one or not, but in case you do, next time you could just pretend you're not even here, maybe already back at home, when they do it...they'll be so surprised when it hardly bothers you! Of course after your tummy is done resting it will pretty soon feel hungry and then the more you drink and eat, the stronger you'll feel and the sooner you'll be ready to go home."

The recognition that these statements represent not only kind and correct things to say, but also amount to powerful hypnotic suggestions, allows the clinician to think carefully and strategically about what to say when, and how.

The Trance of Life-Changing Diagnoses

Serious, life-altering diseases often present first in the acute care setting. Indeed, the aforementioned sense of heightened expectancy and uncertainty on the part of both parent and child that characterizes visits to the doctor often arise from the fear of getting "bad news." The possibility or certainty of a disease that will change a child's life (diabetes, cancer, and autoimmune disease) intensifies and alters both the child's and parent's states of mind. The evidence of this trance is supported by the nearly universal selective memory or amnesia that parents and children report later when they reflect on first hearing "bad news." Attending the family's vulnerable trance, the clinician's attention to minimal cues, pacing, leading, and careful choice of therapeutic suggestions is rendered even more powerful.

Clinicians dread being the bearers of this information and therefore often bring their own anxieties and guilt to the encounter. This has resulted in several efforts to study the challenge and phenomenology of "giving bad news" (Myers, 1983; Garwick, Patterson, Bennett, & Blum, 1995). None have noted, however, the opportunities clinicians have available to them to allow hypnotic strategies to help in those situations. For example the clinician's use of self-hypnosis can allow him or her to maximize his or her own comfort and, thereby, effectiveness, competence, confidence, and compassion (*see* Hypnosis for the Caregiver, below).

Significant diseases, for example the possibility of inflammatory bowel disease in a child with abdominal pain, bloody diarrhea and weight loss, are commonly first included in the differential diagnosis that is shared with the family after an interview and physical examination. It is a usual practice to defer considering psychological therapies for coping and psychophysiological control until a diagnostic evaluation is complete and contributing psychological causes have been ruled in or out. This practice follows the usual Cartesian duality separating mind and body. But once the specter of life-changing disease is raised, there is both a necessity to and a rich opportunity for investing in the child's capacity for self-comfort and self-regulation.

Teaching a child to use his ability to change physical sensation in anticipation of blood tests and intravenous lines or learning relaxation and mental imagery in order to cope with endoscopy and radiographic procedures provides the child with a focus for self-control in the midst of being investigated diagnostically. More fundamentally, as part of the initial interview and physical examination, the child can be helped to use those same abilities to begin to relieve the abdominal pain, cramps, and anxiety associated with uncertainty. In this case, hypnosis is not intended to be the primary therapy. Nor is it to be relegated to a minor role for symptom relief. Rather the clinician can consider hypnosis as co-therapy, deriving from the patient's own subconscious resources, balancing the allopathic interventions of medication, procedures, diet, and surgery.

Given our acculturation towards allopathic medicine, it is common for parents and adolescents to question the clinician's intentions when, early in the course of the evaluation, hypnotic methods are introduced. An adolescent might ask, "Are you telling me that you think this is all in my head?" The clinician can respond, "No. But I do believe that there is a lot of ability in your head and mind to help your body get better, in addition to whatever else you may need to do." Alternatively, as a method to evoke exploration, the clinician can respond with a question, such as, "I didn't say that…. is that what you think?" Then, let the journey continue.

When the child and family are struck at an acute visit with the sudden certainty of threatening disease—a malignant bone tumor or kidney failure—the trauma of such diagnoses threatens one's relationship to oneself. It is disorienting. In this fragile trance of alienation and incomprehension, the clinician's rapport, pacing, and leading are rendered more potent. While attempting to answer the child's, adolescent's and parent's many questions, the practitioner can also make reference to the child's innate strengths. Again, breathing and focusing and comfort can be suggested, interspersed between answers to questions. Sometimes after all the information that can be given is given in the trance of that encounter, the most graceful gift of the clinician is his or her presence and silence, enhancing and entraining the trance.

The Newborn

Having a baby is a hypnotic experience. Many childbirth preparation classes involve teaching pregnant women and their partners exercises in breathing, focusing, and dissociation that derive from hypnosis with proven benefit (Crasilneck & Hall, 1975; Chiasson, 1990; Rodger, 1990; Erickson, 1990; Kroger; 1990). Therefore, many young parents have been practicing hypnotic skills (without the label "hypnosis") in order to cope with birthing. This investment in internal resources can be carried forward to help with the life adjustment of caring for a newborn. Myla and John Kabat-Zinn (1998) have explored the use of meditative techniques in parenting.

The pediatrician's initial newborn examination is a special privilege that can serve as a catalyst for this transition. After meeting and congratulating the parent(s), we learn as much from observation as from the answers to the usual questions about how the pregnancy, labor, and delivery have progressed. We always examine a newborn in the mother's presence because observation of interaction between mother and baby begins the examination. The natural development of (hypnotic) rapport continues by listening to how the mother talks about the continuing evolution of the relationship with her newborn, who is now outside of her rather than inside. We know that a mother has already become sensitized to and engaged in this careful attention in response to the signals from her fetus throughout her pregnancy. Enhancing and promoting this intimate communication and relationship begins with acknowledging this fact, as in (directed to both mother and baby), "Now you finally get to meet face-to-face this person who you have been communicating with for so long. How wonderful!" One of our [LS] mentors, pediatrician Helen Nash of St. Louis, used to slowly trace her finger along an imaginary line from the mother's eyes to the eyes of the baby in mother's arms and say, "Palpate this" (Helen Nash, M.D., personal communication, July 1979).

Next is the observation of the newborn. In looking and listening before touching, we aim not only to learn about the infant and how she moves and how she quiets herself after crying; but also to model, especially for the first-time parent, the importance of paying careful attention to subtle cues of communication and movement offered by the infant. Pointing out aspects of infant's responses as they occur allows parents to validate for themselves that it is not only "Okay" and "right" but even good and desirable to "Look and listen before you touch." Demonstrating and modeling gentle, correct, and effective holding and rhythmic rocking of the infant goes a long way toward teaching parents an essential and effective hypnotic part of their relationship with their baby. We might legitimately call such soothing behavior "kinesthetic hypnosis." Fortunately this behavior is intuitive (subconscious) in even uncomfortable parents and so it allows for affirming suggestion. As an awkward father calms his infant daughter with gentle rocking, saying, "I am not sure how to do this," we can observe, "Sure you do. She is showing you how."

During the physical examination of the newborn, we talk to the infant conversationally to demonstrate our respect for the fact that the baby is resilient, responsive, and capable of understanding the reassuring tone of language if not the content. This serves to tell the parents, indirectly, what you are noting, "Well, your heart sounds strong and completely normal...you like showing me how you can hold your head up, don't you?" It also implicitly demonstrates a new relationship: the pediatrician will be a knowledgeable partner for their child. Sometimes we end the newborn examination by whispering audibly to the infant, "Now you be patient in teaching your Mommy and Daddy all they need to know about you. Have them call me if they don't understand you completely."

Finally, during the trance of pregnancy, there lurks the fear, often unexpressed, that the baby will not be healthy. Often, this fear is realized in the premature or term birth of an ill newborn who is removed from the mother's arms to an intensive care nursery. All of those same negative aspects of the trance of the hospitalized patient, above, are here intensified by the anxiety of the parent(s) towards their new son or daughter. When we have the opportunity to be the conduit for information from the intensive care nursery to the parents, we make every effort to follow four guidelines. First, we anticipate and absorb the parents' anxiety. Sometimes the most helpful statement is, "This is really tough, isn't it?" Next, we provide accurate information including the most difficult to accept: "We just do not know, yet." Third, and most important, we frame every improvement, however small, as resilience, because it is. This is an effort to prevent parents from developing a view of their growing son or daughter as weak and vulnerable in the future: "The reason he is getting off the ventilator is because he is tough and determined." Finally, we make suggestions for self-care for parents, including teaching them self-hypnosis, reminding them that this is the beginning of a long adventure in parenting during which they must care for themselves to be most available to their child.

Hypnosis for the Caregiver

Our work is rewarding and also full of stresses: our schedules, unanticipated demands on our time, receiving and giving bad news, administrative details, our own worries about our patients and the adequacy of our care for them and overall, the tension of being fully present and receptive at each encounter, and more. In addition, the authenticity and sensitivity with which we teach our patients and families about their own hypnosis is informed by our personal experience. Therefore, at every professional workshop that we teach, we strongly suggest to students of hypnosis, "The way to get experienced and good at using hypnosis with patients is first to get good with yourself."

The practice of self-hypnosis once or twice a day for 15–20 minutes—initially and solely for the purpose of practicing and getting good at it and for feeling good—will go a long way toward solidifying an implicit and personal understanding of the phenomenology of trance and the potential of trance. There are an infinite number of ways of doing self-hypnosis (Rossi, 1991; Yapko, 2003; Alman, 2001), but it is clear, much as we tell our patients, that "The more you do it the better you get."

Intimate familiarity with the components of one's own "stressed-out state"(e.g., tension in neck, stomachache, headache, irritability, being short-tempered or impatient) allows us to design the goals of our own trance as well as to cultivate its quick arrival as needed. It could be a simple and powerful as taking a deep breath in (through the nose to the count of 3) and exhaling slowly (through the mouth to the count of 6) (Weil, 1995) and noticing the relaxation that comes with that. It can be as simple, and as important, as mindfully noticing a few such breaths as we leave one examination room, giving ourselves the direction to let go of the previous moment and become present for the next patient.

Finally, there is the smile in the eyes of a young person to whom you have just given the gift of learning self-hypnosis, when you say, "You know, I do this, too."

> It's the humdrum, day-in, day-out, everyday work that is the real satisfaction of the practice of medicine; the million-and-a-half patients a man has seen on his daily visits over a 40-year period of weekdays and Sundays that make up his life. I have never had a money practice; it would have been impossible for me. But the actual calling on people, at all times and under all conditions, the coming to grips with the intimate conditions of their lives, when they were being born, when they were dying, watching them die, watching them get well when they were ill, has always absorbed me.
>
> I lost myself in the very properties of their minds: for the moment at least I actually became them, whoever they should be, so that when I detached myself from them at the end of a half-hour of intense concentration over some illness which was affecting them, it was as though I was re-awakening from a sleep. For the moment I myself did not exist, nothing of myself affected me. As a consequence I came back to myself, as from any other sleep, rested. (Williams, 1951)

References

Alman, B. (2001). Self-care: Approaches from self-hypnosis for utilizing your unconscious (inner) potentials. In B. Geary & J. Zeig (Eds.), *The handbook of Ericksonian psychotherapy* (pp. 522-40). Phoenix, AZ: The Milton H. Erickson Foundation Press.

Barnes, A. J., & Kohen, D. P. (2006). Clinical hypnosis as an effective adjunct in the care of pediatric inpatients. *Journal of Pediatrics*, 149, 563–565.

Brunnquell, D., & Kohen, D.P. (1991). Emotions in emergencies: What we know, what we can do. *Children's Health Care (Journal of the Association for the Care of Children's Health)*, 20(4), 240–247.

Chiasson, S. (1990). Group hypnosis training in obstetrics. In D. C. Hammond (Ed.), *Handbook of hypnotic suggestions and metaphors* (pp. 271–273). New York: W.W. Norton.

Crasilneck, H. B., & Hall, J. A. (1985). *Clinical hypnosis: Principles and applications* (2nd ed.). New York: Grune & Stratton.

Erickson, M. H. (1958). Pediatric hypnotherapy. *American Journal of Clinical Hypnosis*, 1, 25–29.

Erickson, M. H. (1990). Erickson's childbirth suggestions. In D. C. Hammond (Ed.), *Handbook of hypnotic suggestions and metaphors* (p. 281). New York: W.W. Norton.

French, G. M., Painter, E. C., & Coury, D. L. (1994). Blowing away shot pain: A technique for pain management during immunization. *Pediatrics*, 93(3), 384–390.

Garwick, A. W., Patterson, J., Bennett, F. C., & Blum, R. W. (1995). Breaking the news: How families first learn about their child's chronic condition. *Archives of Pediatrics and Adolescent Medicine*, 149, 991–997.

Hewson-Bower, B., & Drummond, P. D. (1996). Secretory immunoglobulin A increases during relaxation in children with and without recurrent upper respiratory tract infections. *Journal of Developmental and Behavioral Pediatrics*, 17(5), 311–316.

Jacknow, D. S., Tschann, J. M., Link, M. P., & Boyce, W. T. (1994). Hypnosis in the prevention of chemotherapy-related nausea and vomiting in children: A prospective study. *Journal of Developmental and Behavioral Pediatrics*, 15, 258–264.

Kabat-Zinn, M., & Kabat-Zinn, J. (1998). *Everyday blessings: The inner work of mindful parenting.* New York: Hyperion.

Kohen, D. P. (1980). Relaxation mental imagery (self-hypnosis) and pelvic examinations in adolescents. *Journal of Developmental and Behavioral Pediatrics*, 1, 4.

Kohen, D. P. (1986). Applications of relaxation/mental imagery (self-hypnosis) to pediatric emergencies. *International Journal of Clinical and Experimental Hypnosis*, 344, 283–294.

Kohen, D. P. (1995). Applications of relaxation/mental imagery (self-hypnosis) to the management of childhood asthma: Behavioral outcomes of a controlled study. *HYPNOS —The Journal of the European Society of Hypnosis in Psychotherapy and Psychosomatic Medicine*, 22(3), 132–144.

Kohen, D. P. (1997). Teaching children with asthma to help themselves with relaxation/mental imagery (self-hypnosis). In W. J. Matthews & J. H. Edgette (Eds.), *Current thinking and research in brief therapy: Solutions, strategies, narratives*—Annual publication of the Milton H. Erickson Foundation (pp. 169–191). New York: Brunner/Mazel.

Kohen, D. P. (2000). Hypnosis in the treatment of asthma. *The Integrative Medicine Consult*, 2(6), 61-62.

Kroger, W. (1990). Preparation for obstetrical labor. In D. C. Hammond (Ed.), *Handbook of hypnotic suggestions and metaphors* (pp. 293-296). New York: W.W. Norton.

Kuttner, L. (Director, Co-producer). (1986). *No fears, no tears: Children with cancer coping with pain.* Vancouver, B.C.: Canadian Cancer Society. [Videotape]. (Available from Fanlight Productions, www.fanlight.com, 1-800-937-4113.)

Kuttner, L. (Producer). (1998). *No fears, no tears—13 years later.* [Videotape]. (Available from C & W Bookstore, Children's & Women's Health Centre of BC, 4480 Oak Street, Rm. K2-126, Ambulatory Care Building, Vancouver, B.C. V6H 3V4, 1-800-331-1533, ext. 3, or http://bookstore.cw.bc.ca; also available from Fanlight Productions, www.fanlight.com, 1-800-937-4113.)

Lambert, S. A. (1996). The effects of hypnosis/guided imagery on the postoperative course of children. *Journal of Developmental and Behavioral Pediatrics*, 17(5), 307–310.

Myers, B. A. (1983). The informing interview: Enabling parents to 'hear' and cope with bad news. *American Journal of Diseases of Childhood*, 137, 572–577.

Olness, K., & Kohen, D. P. (1996). *Hypnosis and hypnotherapy with children* (3rd ed.). New York: Guilford Press.

Olness, K., McDonald, J. T., & Uden, D. L. (1987). Comparison of self-hypnosis and propranolol in the treatment of juvenile classic migraine. *Pediatrics*, 79(4), 593–597.

Reaney, J. B., Sugarman, L. I., & Olness, K. (1998). Taking biofeedback to where kids are. *Biofeedback*, 26, 30–32.

Rodger, B. P. (1990). Outline of hypnotic suggestions in obstetrics. In D. C. Hammond (Ed.), *Handbook of hypnotic suggestions and metaphors* (pp. 273–275). New York: W.W. Norton.

Rossi, E. L. (1991). *The 20 minute break—Using the new science of ultradian rhythms*. Los Angeles, CA: Jeremy P. Tarcher.

Sugarman, L. I. (1996a). Hypnosis: Teaching children self-regulation. *Pediatrics in Review*, 17, 5–10.

Sugarman, L. I. (1996b). Hypnosis in a primary care practice: Developing skills for the new morbidities. *Journal of Developmental and Behavioral Pediatrics*, 17, 300–305.

Sugarman, L. I. (2006). *Hypnosis in pediatric practice: Imaginative medicine in action* [DVD and learning guide]. Carmarthen, Wales, U.K.: Crown House.

Weil, A. (1995). *Spontaneous healing*. New York: Fawcett Columbine.

Williams, W. C. (1951). The Practice. In W. C. Williams, *The Autobiography of William Carlos Williams*. New York: New Directions.

Yapko, M. D. (2003). *Trancework: An introduction to the practice of clinical hypnosis* (3rd ed.). New York: Brunner-Routledge.

Chapter Fifteen

Perioperative Hypnosis

Thom E. Lobe, MD, NMD, ABMH

Previous books on pediatric hypnosis fail to discuss its use in the perioperative setting in sufficient detail to be of great practical use. Olness and Kohen's (1996a) classic work includes a chapter on hypnosis for Pediatric Surgery and Emergencies that briefly discusses pre-operative visits with children from the perspective of non-surgeons, including a section on pre-operative visits. Barber (1996), similarly discusses the use of hypnosis and suggestion for painful medical procedures. While thorough, it is written more from the perspective of an adult anesthesiologist than from a pediatric surgeon preparing a patient for surgery. And, while Barber's comments are mostly geared toward the adult patient, he comments that many of his suggestions also can be useful for children and adolescents. There are also some brief discussions about hypnosis and surgery in works by Brown and Fromm (1987), Crasilneck and Hall (1989), and more recently by Weitzenhoffer (2000). In general, there was little written at all before 1970 about pediatric pain in the hospital setting. Whether this was by choice (due to a dearth of written material), or because no one seemed to have enough experience to write the chapter, is difficult to say.

Surgical analgesia and anesthesia was one of the earliest applications of hypnosis. In the 1840s, James Esdaile (1846), a Scottish surgeon, performed more than 3000 minor and 300 major operations using hypnosis as the sole anesthetic. In recent years, hypnoanesthesia has been shown to be effective in many surgical procedures, including heart and lung surgery (Marmer, 1959), and a variety of pediatric procedures (Collision, 1972; Lewenstein, Iwamoto, & Schwartz, 1981; Nagle, 1961; Zeltzer & LeBaron, 1982).

Hypnosis as a substitute or adjunct in pediatric anesthesia is not new. Antitch (1967) reported using hypnosis for anesthesia in 3030 pediatric cases, out of which hypnosis was deemed successful 2907 times. In his experience, failures were due to the children's anxiety in emergency situations and to the therapist's failure to establish rapport. Others found hypno-induction in children's anesthesia equally effective (Betcher, 1958), and note that there is a statistically significant decrease in pre- and post-operative anxiety levels in children when hypnosis is used as an adjunct compared to when it is not (Olness, 1981).

Hypnosis has been shown to decrease anxiety and shorten the hospital stay in children undergoing surgery (Lambert, 1996), and in a recent review of the literature on procedure-related pain and distress in pediatric cancer patients, hypnosis appears to be a clinically valuable intervention (Richardson, 2006 ; Lobe, 2006).

It is interesting to note that some practitioners give intra-operative suggestions while the patient is under a general anesthesia. The suggestions can be given orally, but more often are in the form of a pre-recorded, therapeutic recording. Patients who listened to such recordings had fewer problems with post-operative nausea and vomiting, headaches, and muscular aches than did patients who listened to a neutral, non-therapeutic recording by the same voice (Lebovitz, Twersky, & McEwan, 1999). Further, pre-operative suggestion of rapid return of intestinal function after surgery has been shown to result in earlier return to function, a decreased hospitalization, and a significant hospital savings (Disbrow, Bennett, & Owings, 1993).

Minor surgical procedures can certainly be done in the office setting using hypnosis (Andolsek & Novik, 1980). The family members can be enlisted to help the child read a book, change disks in their ViewMaster, or whatever else helps keep the child's mind occupied while the procedure is being completed.

The First Encounter

To better explain how hypnosis can help children, imagine some apprehensive parents who just learned that their child needs surgery. Ever since the pediatrician told them the news, they have been on edge. Perhaps they have searched the Internet to learn more about their child's problem. Regardless, the questions and the fears mount: Will it be dangerous? Will it be safe? Will my baby be alright? Normal? Will there be a lot of PAIN?

And so, the family makes the trip to see the surgeon. Their pediatrician referred them. The parents are anxious—this isn't lost on the child. The child knows that something is up, something serious.

Enter the feared surgeon. He or she might as well be wielding a scalpel in hand. The child tries to hide, although that isn't really practical in the small exam room.

The surgeon smiles and greets them warmly. What the surgeon wears isn't as important as the fact that the surgeon isn't the imposing figure they all imagined. For the child and perhaps the parents too, the trance begins...

The surgeon skilled in the use of hypnosis will take advantage of this opportunity. Some children's surgeons practice hypnotic techniques unknowingly. In fact, that's probably true for many pediatric specialists. To a large extent, it's a matter of attitude, honesty, and the language that we choose to use.

It's common for pediatric specialists, including surgeons, to use humor and talk playfully with their patients. Once, for a hospital benefit, we did a video segment of one of my patients who had undergone 54 operations and was back for another. When I approached the 12-year-old girl in the pre-op area, she smiled and I probably said something silly to make her laugh. She was perfectly at ease. The reporters asked her how she felt. She answered by telling them that when I walked in and smiled, she knew that everything would be alright. They asked her why she had such confidence. She told them that, while she knew somewhere deep inside that the surgery was serious and that she might have a malignancy, when I made her laugh all her worries melted away. She knew that everything would be fine.

So...is that hypnosis? How did we get from the apprehensive patient and family about to undergo potentially life-threatening surgery, to such a relationship of trust?

Rapport is the key to all successful physician-patient-family relationships. When the patient and their family become comfortable with their doctor and give the doctor their trust, everything else seems to fall into place.

It is no accident that most pediatric surgeons are not like the stereotypical surgical personality: gruff, abrupt, seemingly disinterested, and unengaged with their patients. The pediatric surgeon is more likely to be closer in temperament and personality to a pediatrician, insofar as interacting with patients is concerned.

Most physicians who chose to care for children do so because they enjoy it. They like to talk and interact with the children, joke, play games, and, most importantly, listen to their patients. We all learn little "tricks" to distract the kids while we examine them. It's a matter of communicating effectively, and the kids are paying very close attention indeed. They pay attention to the words we use and to our body language. They are very adept at this.

We are taught by Laurence Sugarman and Daniel Kohen in Chapter Fourteen to find the hypnosis in the encounter—even if it's not our intention to induce a formal trance with the patient seemingly relaxed and with his or her eyes closed. It's all in the words we choose to use. The choice of words is important because the children are listening with anxious anticipation.

Sometimes it's as simple as answering a child's question. For example, Aaron, a 10-year-old boy, was in the pre-operative holding area, waiting apprehensively for his appendectomy. He asked me if it (the operation), was going to hurt. I placed my hand on Aaron's arm (a bit of non-verbal comfort), and answered by telling him with a smile that I didn't know how it was going to feel for

HIM. I didn't know if it was going to feel like an ache, or an itch, or a sore muscle (helping him begin to wonder, since none of those sounded too bad). I continued by telling him that he should expect to feel so much better after the surgery was over, that I wouldn't be surprised if he wasn't uncomfortable at all after the surgery was done!

It is a good idea to avoid the use of the "P" word. Don't talk about pain. Talk about comfort. Beware though: this approach backfired with one adolescent who was very concrete and literal and insisted that he wasn't "*uncomfortable*," he "*hurt...a lot*," and couldn't understand why I wasn't listening to him. Most patients know, however, (at least at a subconscious level), that we intend to help.

My pre-op conversation with Aaron was the first encounter one of my surgical residents had ever had with the power of suggestion. He was present with Aaron before the surgery and remarked to me later how he was amazed that Aaron was so comfortable after the appendectomy and, essentially, was ready for discharge home as soon as he left the post-anesthesia care unit (some still call this the recovery room).

I was speaking with the highly intelligent adolescent son of a physician about the boy's upcoming reconstructive surgery. The surgery is notorious as one of the most painful procedures we perform. Most surgeons who perform this surgery routinely use an epidural catheter post-operatively to make the patients more comfortable.

Jeffrey (the son) asked me what would happen if the catheter didn't work. I told him that we would use hypnosis. He looked at his father for reassurance and asked if that was possible. As though on cue, the physician-father confirmed that not only was it possible, but that he'd been hypnotized successfully in the past himself.

Jeffery asked me how the hypnosis worked. Being 12 years old, I figured that he was probably computer savvy. He confirmed this. I asked him to picture the cursor on the monitor and to note how it could be moved from one position to another and in so doing focused on another word or program. I suggested to him that the mind worked much like his computer. While the cursor can blink on one particular task, that doesn't mean the rest of the computer isn't still working on several other functions at the same time.

I further suggested to him that he could shift his mind, just like moving the computer mouse to change the cursor's position. As an example, I told him, I guessed that he hadn't given the first thought as to how his feet felt in his shoes, until my mention of it. Then, his attention shifted to his feet. He thanked me for the explanation and told me that he understood.

As always seems to happen to physician's family members, Jeffrey's epidural catheter was kinked and had to be removed before he went to the post-anesthesia care unit. The next morning I visited Jeffrey in his hospital room. He asked if he could go home. This was highly unusual because most of the children who have undergone similar extensive reconstructive surgery remain hospitalized for nearly a week for analgesia. He confirmed that he was comfortable. When I asked why he thought that was so, he reminded me that several weeks before, in my office, I had explained to him that he could remain comfortable, just by refocusing his attention on something other than the surgery.

There had been no formal induction, nor could one observe any of the phenomena usually noted when a patient goes deeper into a trance. Nonetheless, Jeffrey got the message and used it to remain comfortable. He was discharged home using only acetaminophen for discomfort and continued his smooth recovery.

Most patients seem to do better with coaching. For these children, a more formal session of hypnosis with suggestions for post-operative analgesia and return of bowel and bladder function may be the best option.

Patient Factors

Patients of any age who are about to undergo surgery suffer from a number of perceptions that serve to increase anxiety. Barber (1996) has described this in some detail for adult patients.

First, patients of any age feel rather helpless and dependent when they are about to undergo a medical procedure. It doesn't really matter how "nice" or "friendly" the staff are, when children leave their only source of safety and security, their fear dominates them. Remember, the patient will be removed from his or her parents to a strange place, someone is going to put a foul-smelling mask over the child's face (giving rise to fears of suffocation), and then stick cold monitoring pads or, worse yet, a needle somewhere into or onto him or her. A blood pressure cuff will squeeze the child's arm and in the midst of this, a stranger will hold the child secure while muttering something about not being frightened. Most children would be frightened by this time and have little sense of comfort.

With all this manipulation, most people will no longer feel in control. Often, despite many inadequate attempts to provide comfort, most young people wonder why they are being tortured so. Something got lost in the translation. The child feels like a victim who is passively assaulted by strangers claiming to want to help. How much more confusing for the child can it get?

Perhaps worse yet, the child is privy to the doctor or nurse reviewing the surgical "informed consent" with the parents. This is the document that lists the procedure and potential complications and which the parent's sign, acknowledging that they understand the risks. Therapist Reverend James Warnke, commenting on such documents, adds, "Accurate language is not necessarily therapeutic language."

For some strange reason (probably at the advice of its legal counsel), the hospital seems compelled to mention the worst of possibilities. Accordingly, the family and often the patient (whom everyone assumes is playing in the corner and not paying the least bit of attention), hears and assumes the worst.

The two rules for perioperative care in all young people are:

1. The child is *always* listening.
2. Choose your words carefully.

Most adults believe that the children are sufficiently preoccupied so as to not be listening to the adult side of the discussions; the serious stuff. Don't believe this for a minute! If the child is within earshot, he or she will catch every little detail.

Goals of Perioperative Preparation

The goals of preparing the child for surgery or a major procedure are simple if we only remember the basic goals for all hypnotherapy. The child must understand that he or she is the BOSS of his or her body and mind. Allowing the child to realize that he or she is in control can be critical to a successful and happy perioperative experience. At every step of the way, we want to foster the child's sense of self-mastery and allow the child to retain his or her dignity. We want the patient to be in total control of the experience. And, while we speak primarily about preparing the child for surgery, this discussion is equally true and relevant to any procedure including endoscopy, minor surgery, suture and drain removal, and dressing changes.

There are a number of observations of the human experience that are pertinent to our discussions of the perioperative management of children. Barber (1996, p. 213)) has outlined these nicely for us:

- Under stress and anxiety, patients become exquisitely susceptible to suggestion
- This heightened suggestibility extends from the time the intervention is contemplated until complete recovery
- Statements made during seemingly ordinary states of consciousness are as powerful as those given in an hypnotic circumstance
- In this state, patients seem to follow certain hypnotic principles: ("dominant effect" or "persons of superior authority") and tend to exhibit some signs of being hypnotized (focused attention, conscious amnesia, literal thinking, suspending critical judgment)
- Statements made by persons of authority directly involved in the patients care are particularly powerful, while statements made by others may have little or no effect.

- There appears to be a hierarchy to the patient's perception of authority (e.g., the person carrying out the procedure has the highest authority).

With these observations in mind, the key elements to preparing a child for surgery are:

- Information
- Instruction
- Suggestion

Information

The child should understand the experience that he or she is about to undergo in sufficient detail, described in age-appropriate language, so that there will be no surprises. Children like the familiar. They like to read and hear the same stories over and over again. If we tell them what they are about to encounter, as though it's the narrative of a story, they will begin to search for the familiar in the experience and will forget to be afraid.

They must be told every detail. I start with getting up the morning of the surgery and ask the kids to help me understand how the story begins. What will they wear? Who will help them dress? What color is their toothbrush? Then I remind them to not swallow the water or drink anything before the surgery when that is appropriate.

Ask them who will bring them to the hospital where the procedure is to be done. These are all details they can help provide. Sometimes they enlist the aide of their parents. That is helpful because it allows them to demonstrate that they are in control of their resources and support.

We talk about the trip to the hospital. Who will come with them? Some suggestions here are appropriate to encourage them to notice the details of the trip, the buildings they pass, the people they see, what other vehicles are on the road. There used to be a game for kids to play on road trips called "I Spy." There were all kinds of "I Spy" books for different types of vehicles, road signs, clothes people were wearing, animals, and so on. The kids would be so focused on filling up the book and finding all the different variations pictured that they'd forget about the fact that they'd been on the road for a long time. They were so focused on the task of finding all the possibilities that they usually arrived at the final destination before they knew it. On the way to the hospital for surgery they can play "I Spy" in their heads and keep count of all their "finds."

We talk about arriving at the hospital, where they will go first, and who they will meet and talk with. There are all sorts of age-appropriate, fun things to do after the patient arrives and is settled into a bed or pre-operative holding area. We talk about the fact that there will be lots of questions. Usually, there will be the same questions over and over again, by different people, at every stop along the way.

Eventually, the child will arrive at the pre-operative holding area, sometime shortly before the operation is scheduled. Here, the child will meet many new people: nurses, doctors, and others. There is usually a lot of activity because everyone is busy getting patients ready for surgery. The child will meet some of the nurses who will assist with the operation. The anesthesiologist will meet the patient. He or she may ask which scent the child favors so that the physician can choose the properly scented mask for anesthesia. Again, the patient is in charge and gets to choose.

When it is time to go to the operating room, some facilities will allow the family to stay with the child until they drift off to sleep. The child should be able to choose whether he or she wants this option if it's available. Usually the surgeon and anesthesiologist will talk about this beforehand so there are no surprises. And, so long as there aren't any significant medical issues, most pediatric-oriented facilities are accustomed to this.

The suggestion for the child to notice and think about all the new things that he or she will see on the way down the hall to the operating room can help the child to relax. Asking him or her to count the number of colored tiles on the walls or ceilings as he or she is rolled to the operating room on the gurney in anticipation of being quizzed for the answer is a good strategy to help keep the child thinking about something besides the anticipated procedure.

The patient should be told that the room may be a different temperature than the hall. Ask the patient to notice whether the operating room is warmer or cooler than the hallway.

After the child arrives in the operating room, a nurse usually puts some cool, sticky pads (monitor pads), on the chest, arms, or legs and will also place a special red-glowing clip or band aide-like device on a finger or toe. These are the various monitors for heart rate. The child should take notice when the beeping sound begins…is it fast or slow? The child should also notice how long it takes between beeps. He or she can often increase or decrease the interval between beeps, just by thinking about it. The child might want to try it and see how good he or she is at that. If the child can see the heart rate monitor, he or she can do the same with the peaks and valleys—they look like the outlines of mountains. The child can make the mountains wider, simply by thinking about them, again exercising self-regulation.

A nurse will often put a blood pressure cuff on an arm. This will inflate and deflate automatically. The child should know about this ahead of time.

Some operating rooms for kids have videos they can watch while they are going to sleep. We can ask them what movie they want to watch while they are in the holding area in order to set it up before the child arrives in the operating room. While in the office for the pre-operative visit ask the patient to bring in his or her favorite video or music—anything familiar helps the patient relax.

Small children like to hear stories they know or that they made up. I often ask about their favorite story in the holding area, record it, and then tell it back to the child as he or she is going to sleep. If the child doesn't have a story of his or her own, I make one up. Perhaps the child would like to go on a magic carpet ride to some far off land. Sometimes the kids prefer to go to a favorite or safe place. We use all this in our pre-operative preparation.

When the patients have learned self-hypnosis beforehand, they may prefer to use this to drift off into trance on their own, usually before the anesthesiologist places the mask over their face, administers any drugs, or starts any IVs. It is helpful for the child to know in advance what the mask or intravenous injection will be like. The mask they choose may have a scent they prefer, but the gases can smell bad. I tell the children that the mask is just like a jet pilot wears and the gas smells something like jet fuel. If they choose to get an injection of medicine in their intravenous line, they should be warned in advance that they will notice the medicine with a comment like, "I wonder what the medicine will feel like to YOU as it goes in your vein? It may feel sore, or like an itch, or you may not notice anything at all." This statement reinforces implicitly the fact that they control their own perceptions, and so they can change them for their own comfort.

I let the patients know what to expect when they wake up. Sometimes they regain consciousness in the operating room, other times it is in the post-anesthesia care unit. I let them know that the people around them when they awaken will all be familiar with hypnosis and ready to help with anything they need after the surgery. This ranges from simple reassurance that everything is alright, to reminding the patient how to "close their eyes, relax, and go to some special place."

I remind patients that they may be surprised to note how comfortable they feel after the surgery, how hungry they will be, and how well all their bodily functions will work, particularly the bladder and bowel. I let them know that they will be more and more comfortable every day and that, before long, they will be all healed and perfectly well.

Pre-Operative Instructions

This set of instructions is simple and usually given when the patient is in an effective trance.

Since much of post-operative discomfort is due to muscle spasm, I help the child pay attention to how he or she relaxes his or her muscles, particularly those of the body part on which the surgery took place. When the patient relaxes the muscles surrounding an incision, this goes a long way toward maintaining comfort. The greater the relaxation, the more comfortable the patient will be. Children can be told, accurately, that the sensations they may feel around the incision come from the body healing itself.

Knowing how to breathe deeply and slowly after surgery is calming and comforting. The patient should practice this before the surgery occurs so that there is a kinesthetic memory of proper breathing.

Just because we have taught the patient how to be comfortable after the surgery, doesn't mean that the body will respond any differently than it normally does to pain unless we suggest otherwise. Pain after some surgery is notorious for being accompanied by bladder and bowel dysfunction. After several patients developed urinary retention or intestinal ileus (paralysis) after surgery, despite their claims of no discomfort whatsoever, I began suggesting that their bladder and bowel would function normally after their surgery. This solved the problem. Metaphors work well for this. I suggest that the child may think in terms of faucets or valves, hoses or pipes, rivers, or whatever else comes to mind that may ring true in the child's imagination to represent the bladder and bowel.

I encourage young people to drink plenty of fluids and develop an appetite after their surgery. This tends to minimize the post-operative nausea and vomiting that often occurs as a result of the analgesics they may take. When the patients learn to be comfortable without medications for analgesia, post-operative nausea and vomiting are less of a problem.

Suggestion

Simple suggestions suffice. While in trance, after the suggestions for comfort, we offer suggestions to remind the rest of the body to function normally, "just as it always does." We specifically mention the bowel, bladder, and lungs. We want the patient comfortable and hungry so that they will maintain proper nutrition, so we talk about how the blood stream carries the food and vitamins to the area of the surgery to make it heal faster. Since we want the patient to void regularly so that they don't have to be catheterized, we give them suggestions about ease of voiding post-operatively. We also make suggestions regarding deep, comfortable breaths so that children will fill their lungs every time they breathe and avoid the complications of atelectasis and pneumonia.

Depending on the nature of the surgery, we may want the patient to protect a particular body part (Scott, 1976). For example, after a skin grafting procedure, we suggest that the most comfortable body position is the one that protects the integrity of the graft. If the graft is on the back, the patient may be instructed that he or she will feel most comfortable lying prone, and that any other position will be less comfortable. This type of suggestion is usually accompanied by a time limit, such as, "until you have healed the graft."

Several factors should be kept in mind when considering suggestions. First, they must be age appropriate. It doesn't help if a child does not understand our message. For example, learn the terms the child uses for urination, defecation, and other body functions, and then translate your language into the child's.

It is best if the suggestions are indirect, open ended, and permissive, thereby supporting the child's sense of independence and self-efficacy. Suggestions work better if they include all the senses, especially sound. This is particularly true when using hypnosis to help with induction of anesthesia because the perception of sound persists under most anesthesias. When the patient is invited to focus on the sound of the heart rate monitor, he or she can notice the interval between the beats: How long is it between beats? Does the length of the interval vary from beat to beat? Does the child notice how he or she can change the interval simply by willing it so? In so doing does the child notice how every time the interval changes the degree of relaxation becomes greater and greater?

It is effective to make suggestions self-perpetuating by linking them to recurring cues. There are plenty of such cues in the perioperative setting. The patient can be reminded that with every deep breath he or she will relax and be comfortable. Suggestions can be offered that every time the blood-pressure cuff inflates, or every time someone enters the room, it can be a reminder to take a deep breath and relax on exhalation.

Suggestions for comfort on awakening from anesthesia can make the process go more smoothly. These can be given with the patient in or out of trance. If the surgery is for abdominal pain, for example, a simple suggestion such as, "Imagine about how surprised you'll be when the surgery is all done and you notice how much better you're going to feel." Similar suggestions are useful for the post-operative patient who asks when he or she is going to feel better: "You'll feel better and better each day until, in a few days, it wouldn't surprise me if you don't have any discomfort whatsoever" Or "…will find your bowels moving regularly, just like they used to before you got sick."

Putting it All Together

The plan is to explain what to expect, teach self-hypnosis with the appropriate suggestions for surgery, have the children practice at home, and return to reinforce their skills before the day of surgery. They may then choose to use the hypnosis at the time of induction, after they awaken from anesthesia, and during the post-operative period until they no longer feel the need for it. They should expect to wake up comfortable and begin to use the hypnosis immediately in the post-anesthesia care unit and continue to use self-hypnosis in their hospital room and at home after their discharge from the hospital.

The use of hypnosis usually enters into the conversation as a natural part of the discussion of the proposed procedure, the expectation of any associated discomfort, and the options for controlling this possible discomfort.

While hypnosis can be used effectively as sole anesthesia to perform minor surgical procedures in children over 2 or 3 years of age, we will focus our discussions on the patient who is scheduled to undergo an operation under general anesthesia. Hypnosis can be discussed as an option along with other choices for pain control such as epidural catheters, patient-controlled analgesia (PCA) pumps, or parenteral and oral analgesic administration. Patients should be told what to expect insofar as possible discomfort, and appreciate our thoughts on the effectiveness and side effects of each modality. My experience is that children who choose hypnosis are sufficiently comfortable after surgery that they spend less time in the hospital and tend to require fewer post-operative analgesics (Lobe, 2006).

It is vital to explain hypnosis to families and answer any questions they have. I let them know that the goal is for their son or daughter to learn self-hypnosis, which is not only fun but also can become a valuable and lifelong skill. I explain that it can help improve performance in school, sports, and other extracurricular activities. After young people learn to use self-hypnosis, I explain that they often continue to use it into adulthood for situations that would otherwise be painful or stressful. When the family and child fully understand and agree, I ask them to sign an informed consent form for hypnosis to document their understanding.

To be most effective in teaching a child hypnosis, it is helpful first to learn the child's likes and dislikes, any special fears or concerns, something about family and friends, as well as where the child goes to school, lives, and plays. It is useful to include such information as favorite colors, sound, music, and familiar scenes in the language used for inducing and deepening the trance. Remember, children enjoy hearing stories and stretching their imaginations, especially when the images are theirs.

The child should be allowed to ask any questions he or she may have before learning how to go into a trance. This should be an enjoyable experience for them. Most children find the experience fun.

Induction

The induction should be tailored to the child. Any one of a variety of standard, age-appropriate induction techniques can be used.

My favorites, and those of the children are the Fingers Together, Balloon and Sand Pail, and the Arm Catalepsy techniques, although any induction will work (Olness & Kohen, 1996b).

I use going to a "Favorite Place" as a "deepening technique" and we spend most of our time there to ensure that the child has a clear image of where that place is, including all of its details and what he or she is doing there. We equate the child's choice with being safe. It's a place where the child is so very comfortable then everything else drifts away, and nothing can bother him or her.

While I do not need to know where that "favorite place" is, young people will usually tell me if asked. They will describe what they are doing, whether there is anyone else around, what they are wearing, what they are looking at or listening to, whether they are hungry and, if so, what they are eating. Each of these observations and be affirmed and reinforced by such comments as, "Great," "Wonderful," and "Isn't it comforting to know that you can do this so well?"

Some children go to a favorite park or playground. Some go on vacation with their parents, with friends, or alone, or to the beach or mountains. Some visit a friend's house and watch TV or play video games. And some simply crash in their bedrooms, flop on the bed, and listen to their favorite music. There is no end to the variation of Favorite Places they invent. A 9-year-old boy whom I prepared for a major procedure while writing this chapter told me that he was a seagull flying through the clouds, playing a game of hide-and-seek with his friends. Then he visited the Statue of Liberty in New York and flew across the country to see the Golden Gate Bridge. He liked to watch all the people and notice how small they seemed. After his operation, the nurses asked him to rate his pain on a scale of 1 to 10 (with 10 being the worst). He never rated it higher than a 2.

I suggest that they focus on their breathing and use the rhythm to relax. As they continue to relax and focus on remaining in their sanctuary, they are asked to notice how comfortable they are. With increased relaxation, I suggest that they begin to notice that nothing else bothers them as they assume control of their bodies and their minds. I remind them that the mind is like a computer. There are many functions going on simultaneously, mostly behind the scenes, and that the computer operator (or the brain) decides where to focus the attention. Other similar metaphors can work just as well, depending on the child's interest. Perhaps, instead of the brain, the child can identify with the sound and light technician, directing a rock concert and focusing everyone's attention on the action at center stage.

Suggestions can be given for time distortion: the duration of comfort can be expanded and discomfort contracted in time. And important safeguards can be added. The patient should understand that while comfortable in his or her special place, if a member of the healthcare team needs his or her attention to monitor or take care of anything important related to the patient's well being, then the patient should become sufficiently alert so as to be able to respond appropriately.

If the patient goes into a deep trance and the blood pressure begins to drop due to hemorrhage, or any other similar physiologic event occurs, it is important for the patient to pay attention to the caregivers, even if he or she chooses to remain in trance.

In order to include the unexpected, it is a good strategy to add a generic suggestion such as, "…and you might already be curious to discover what else you will encounter after the surgery that we haven't talked about and how pleased you will be after the procedure to learn how easily and naturally the procedure has gone for you." Or "…and anything else that you discover you need after your surgery that we haven't already talked about, your mind will provide just the right solution needed to keep you calm, safe, and as comfortable as you need to be for as long as you feel this is necessary."

The patient is always made aware of his or her choices. He or she can choose to focus on the Favorite Place rather than the site of the surgery, on being comfortable, or not. It is critical to acknowledge explicitly that the sensory experience is under the patient's control and, therefore, he or she can change it.

Post-operative suggestions are given to reinforce the experience. Some cue, such as a touch on the left or right shoulder, is suggested to remind the patient to take several deep breaths, close his or her eyes, and to transport him or herself to the Favorite Place, and to be as comfortable as need be for as long as necessary. This cue can be given by the patient's parents or a member of the healthcare team and will be used whenever someone perceives that the patient is uncomfortable. Or the patient can simply close his or her eyes, take a few deep breaths and transport himself or herself to his or her Favorite Place.

After the patient alerts from the initial trance, the post-hypnotic suggestion can be reinforced and the patient praised for doing so well. When the patient has been alerted, I answer any questions he or she may have. Then it is time to verify that the patient knows how to self-induce a trance so that he or she knows how to do self-hypnosis, reproduce the trance, and transport to the Favorite Place by the time he or she leaves my office. I assign the child the homework of practicing going into trance every day, adding that "The more you practice, the better you get."

While this discussion may seem like a lot, the trance and all the training averages about 15 to 20 minutes in length (although the patient usually has little perception of time during the experience).

I like to have the patients return to show me how well they are doing. This is an opportunity to answer any questions that child may have and to reinforce everything, especially the post-hypnotic suggestions. I schedule this within a week of the surgery, but it can be just as effective when done immediately before the patient goes to the operating room.

Implementation

In the operating room, I ask the patient whether he or she would like to use his or her self-hypnosis to go to his or her Favorite Place while the nurses and anesthesiologists do their jobs. Thus far, everything in the child's experience has usually been exactly as described, as though everyone was following a script. This is very reassuring for the child and goes a long way to diminishing or eliminating any residual anxiety.

Because the child already knows what to expect, he or she doesn't usually have any apprehension about going into trance to make the experience more enjoyable. Thus, most of the kids enjoy using their new skill and quickly go off to sleep before the anesthesiologist so much as administers the first of the anesthetic agents. Their facility with the induction serves as positive reinforcement and empowers the children with even greater confidence in their ability to control their comfort level after the procedure.

The children begin to emerge from their anesthesia in the operating room or in the post-anesthesia care unit, depending on the procedure and the anesthesiologist. I plan to be present as the child emerges and as soon as the child is sufficiently alert and is able to follow commands, I encourage him or her to go to his or her Favorite Place and remain as comfortable as he or she needs to be for as long as necessary. I reinforce all the suggestions that the child has been given and take the time to teach any nurses who are unfamiliar with the procedure how to touch the child's shoulder and remind the child to go to his or her Favorite Place if the child appears to be in any distress.

On the inpatient unit, the parents, nurses, aides, and others all are instructed in how to remind the patient to go to his or her Favorite Place for comfort. I also remind the patient to do this himself or herself whenever there seems to be more discomfort than the patient desires.

Some patients like to listen to a recording of their experience as a guide. I provide this for them and often prescribe listening to the recording every 4 to 6 hours (instead of taking analgesics). This gives them some extra security. Some patients use the recording and others do not. Every patient is different and so are the recordings. This is not a generic recording, but one of the training sessions cut to a CD, tape, or MP3 player, depending on the patient's desire.

The patients get the normal post-operative care for their procedure and, unless there are some specific concerns related to the surgery that keep the patient in the hospital, are told that they may go home as soon as they are comfortable enough, or as comfortable as they need to be. This often is on the day after surgery or the day after that. In either case, the children and adolescents dictate their care based on their level of comfort. My instructions on discharge are to continue to use the self-hypnosis for as long as needed.

During the entire stay in the hospital, we allow the children to take any additional analgesics they desire to assist them in remaining comfortable. Most simply take acetaminophen. While narcotic analgesics are offered, they usually do not need them.

Conclusion

The use of perioperative hypnosis can be extremely helpful to reduce hospitalization, the need for narcotic analgesics in children about to undergo major surgery (Lobe, 2006), and discomfort for diagnostic procedures in children (Butler, Symons, Henderson, Shortliffe, & Spiegel, 2005). As the preceding literature review has shown, little is really known about specific techniques and strategies or the psychophysiology of suggestion with children who need surgery. It is time to move forward from anecdote to evidence. There is a wealth of unanswered questions to be researched in order to understand how best to use hypnosis to help children find more comfort, be less afraid, and feel empowered when they undergo major surgical procedures.

References

Andolsek, K., & Novik, B. (1980). Use of hypnosis with children. *Journal of Family Practice*, 10(3), 503–507.

Antitch, J. L. (1967). The use of hypnosis in pediatric anesthesia. *Journal of the American Society of Psychosomatic Dentistry and Medicine*, 14(3), 70–75.

Barber, J. (1996). *Hypnosis and suggestion in the treatment of pain*. New York: W.W. Norton.

Betcher, A. M. (1958). Hypno-induction techniques in pediatric anesthesia. *Anesthesiology*, 19(2), 279-281.

Brown, D., & Fromm, E. (1987). *Hypnosis and behavioral medicine*. Mahwah, NJ: Lawrence Erlbaum.

Butler, L. D., Symons, B. K., Henderson, S. L., Shortliffe, L. D., & Spiegel, D. (2005). Hypnosis reduces distress and duration of an invasive medical procedure for children. *Pediatrics*, 115(1), e77–85.

Collision, D. R. (1972). Medial hypnotherapy. *Medical Journal of Australia*, 1, 643–649.

Crasilneck, H. B., & Hall, J. A. (1989). *Clinical hypnosis: Principles and applications* (2nd ed.). Boston: Allyn & Bacon.

Disbrow, E. A., Bennett, H. L., & Owings, J. T. (1993). Effect of preoperative suggestion on postoperative gastrointestinal motility. *Western Journal of Medicine*, 158, 488–492.

Esdaile, J. (1846). *Mesmerism in India*. London: London, Longman, Brown, Green & Longman.

Lambert, S. A. (1996). The effects of hypnosis/guided imagery on the postoperative course of children. *Journal of Developmental and Behavioral Pediatrics*, 17(5), 307–310.

Lebovitz, A. H., Twersky, R., & McEwan, B. (1999). Intraoperative therapeutic suggestions in day-case surgery: Are there benefits for postoperative outcome? *British Journal of Anaesthesia*, 82(6), 861–866.

Lewenstein, L. N., Iwamoto, K., & Schwartz, H. (1981). Hypnosis in high risk ophthalmic surgery. *Opthalmic Surgery*, 12(1), 39–41.

Lobe, T. E. (2006, in press). Perioperative hypnosis reduces hospitalization for patients undergoing the Nuss procedure for pectus excavatum. *Journal of Laparoendoscopic & Advanced Surgical Techniques*.

Marmer, M. J. (1959). *Hypnosis in anesthesia*. Springfield, IL: Charles C. Thomas.

Nagle, D. R. (1961). The use of hypnosis in pediatric anesthesia. *Journal of the Kentucky Medical Association*, 59, 140–142.

Olness, K. (1981). Hypnosis in pediatric practice. *Current Problems in Pediatrics*, 12(2), 1–47.

Olness, K., & Kohen, D. (1996a). *Hypnosis and hypnotherapy with children* (3rd ed.). New York: Guilford Press.

Olness, K., & Kohen, D. (1996b). Hypnotic induction for children: Techniques, strategies, and approaches. In K. Olness & D. Kohen (Eds.), *Hypnosis and hypnotherapy with children* (3rd ed., pp. 55–68). New York: Guilford Press.

Richardson, J., Smith, J. E., McCall, G., & Pilkington, K. (2006). Hypnosis for procedure-related pain and distress in pediatric cancer patients: A systematic review of effectiveness and methodology related to hypnosis interventions. *Journal of Pain and Symptom Management*, 31(1), 70–84.

Scott, D. L. (1976). Hypnosis in pedicle graft surgery. *British Journal of Plastic Surgery*, 29, 8–13.

Weitzenhoffer, A. M. (2000). *The practice of hypnotism*. New York: John Wiley & Sons.

Zeltzer, L., & LeBaron, S. (1982). Hypnosis and nonhypnotic techniques for reduction of pain and anxiety during painful procedures in children and adolescents with cancer. *Journal of Pediatrics*, 101(6), 1032–1035.

Chapter Sixteen

Hypnosis for Children with Chronic Disease

Ran D. Anbar, MD, FAPP

Hypnosis can be very beneficial to children coping with chronic disease. For example, it can be helpful in dealing with anxiety related to having a serious illness, and in ameliorating short and long-term discomforts associated with the disease or its therapy. For these reasons, it is my hope that most children diagnosed with chronic illness will be offered the opportunity to learn how to use hypnosis.

Chronic illness affects 10–30% of children (Pless, 1984; Newacheck, 1989; Newacheck, MacManus, & Fox, 1991). Examples of chronic illness include asthma, congenital heart disease, cystic fibrosis, diabetes, epilepsy, hemophilia, immunodeficiency, inflammatory bowel disease, juvenile rheumatoid arthritis, malignancies, and sickle cell anemia. Of these, 10% have severe disease by physiologic criteria (Perrin & MacLean, 1988). More than 80% of children with chronic illness survive into adulthood (Gortmaker, 1985).

In this chapter, we will review some uses of hypnosis by children with chronic disease. We will discuss further why hypnosis should be integral in the care of these children. A transcript of a hypnosis session is provided as an example, and specific hypnosis strategies valuable for children with chronic illness are highlighted.

Clinical Vignettes

Asthma

Beth— Improvement

Beth was a 9-year-old with asthma, documented by pulmonary function testing. Beth reported that often she became short of breath when she was anxious about her school tests, playing the piano at a music recital, or during soccer competitions. She was taught to use the hypnosis method of imagining herself listening to music, and relaxing with each beat. She also chose the image of opening her airways, which allowed her to "relax" her lungs when they were "tight." At follow-up visits, Beth reported that she had used hypnosis on a regular basis to control her shortness of breath. She stated that when she became very short of breath with exercise, hypnosis provided more relief than using inhaled bronchodilators.

Larry—No improvement

Larry was a 15-year-old with asthma and shortness of breath with exercise that only occasionally responded to bronchodilator therapy. There was concern that he did not use his medications. Larry was offered hypnosis and demonstrated a good ability to rapidly relax his breathing with the use of hypnotic imagery. Larry returned three months later stating that he was still short of breath as a result of exercise. He said he did not use hypnosis because he, "Didn't feel like it."

Comment

Indicators that patients with asthma may respond to the use of hypnosis include inadequate response to medical therapy, report of shortness of breath despite normal lung function (Anbar, 2001b), symptoms and signs suggestive of upper airway involvement (Anbar & Geisler, 2005), or reports that strong emotions or anxiety trigger some of their respiratory symptoms (Anbar, 2003). The improvement in asthma symptoms may be attributable to physiological as well as psychological factors (Hackman, Stern, & Gershwin, 2000).

Many children with asthma develop associated anxiety because they learn through experience that development of asthma symptoms, such as cough, may herald a severe asthma flare-up (ten Thoren & Petermann, 2000). Beth's improvement demonstrates that treatment of anxiety must be considered in a child with asthma.

Larry's case demonstrates that hypnosis can be ineffective if it is not applied by the patient, as is the case with many other therapies. Larry may have chosen to use hypnosis and ultimately benefited had the reasons "he didn't feel like" doing it been explored. For example, did he have fears or misconceptions about hypnosis that hadn't been addressed adequately? Was there a secondary gain to his shortness of breath? For instance, did he not wish to participate in athletic activities and his shortness of breath represented a face-saving way of avoiding sports? Behavior that is misconstrued as "non-adherent" or "resistant" to therapy often is self-protective.

Functional Abdominal Pain

Ian

Ian was a 16-year-old who had experienced recurrent abdominal pain since he was 3-years-old (Anbar, 2001c; Anbar, 2002b). He had undergone multiple diagnostic tests including radiological studies of his upper and lower bowels, an evaluation for acid reflux, a brain wave study, and blood work. These failed to uncover a physiological reason for his pain. Dietary modifications did not change his symptoms. When he awoke in the morning, he often was incapacitated with abdominal pain and developed diarrhea. During a typical month, Ian was relatively pain-free for an average of three days. He was unable to travel well due to his recurrent abdominal pain.

As a result of his medical problems, Ian was in a modified school program. This allowed him to begin school at 10:30 in the morning. In addition, he was an athlete who was unable to participate in as many sports as he would have liked, because he had to make up schoolwork in the afternoon. Ian enjoyed playing the acoustic guitar, and composing poetry and music. He stated that he did not have as many friends as he would have liked because of the time consumed by his recurrent abdominal pain.

Ian hypnotized himself by imagining an elevator in a hotel. He would descend 10 floors. The further down he went, the more relaxed he became. He then imagined going to a concert by singer and guitarist Dave Matthews. Ian was instructed, "Imagine a bright light above your head… I am not sure what color this light is, it may be white, yellow, or red, or any other color you might imagine. This is a healing light. As it passes through your body, this light will heal every nerve, every fiber, every muscle, and every cell in your body." When he completed this hypnosis experience, Ian reported that the light felt warm and pleasant. He said he was very relaxed, and that the experience seemed very real to him.

Over the subsequent week, Ian had five pain-free days as he regularly employed hypnosis. He was congratulated on the great improvement of his symptoms. Ian was very interested in learning other uses for hypnosis, such as how hypnosis could be used as a tool to improve his creativity as a musician. His physician agreed to explore this with Ian. Allowing a patient to extend his utilization of hypnosis can serve to strengthen his belief in its effectiveness, thereby making hypnosis an even better medical therapeutic tool. One of the skills Ian was taught was how to allow his subconscious to type using "Automatic Word Processing" (Anbar, 2001a). Ian took this opportunity to write a poem about what it felt like to be hypnotized, which was first published in *Clinical Pediatrics* (Anbar, 2002b):

All these senses I feel deep inside
Deafening silence to my ears
A cold breeze on my skin
Give me goosebumps as I stare into space

The feel of the cloud is warm and soft

like a comforter by a warm fire
My mouth is filled with the taste of something
So hard to describe, sweet, sour, salty, an equal amount of each

All this I feel in a moment's time
Every second may differ in various ways
but I try to remember the good feelings
of being safe and calm and relaxed...

Ian then wrote a poem about what it felt like to have had abdominal pain for 13 years (Anbar, 2002b):

This feeling I get sometimes
Like an internal blast
Ready to explode
How long will it last

Waiting, feeling, not knowing what to expect
When will the suffering end
No medicine to heal me
How far will I bend?

Intense at times
I struggle to see
What's always lurking
Inside of me

That's all I can remember...it used to be longer

Ian's subconscious reported having written this poem several months prior to typing it. However, when Ian finished hypnosis, he denied that he recognized either poem.

Five months later, Ian reported minimal abdominal complaints. He was attending school on a regular schedule: He arrived at 7:30 am along with all the other students, and completed his school day in the early afternoon. This allowed him to compete in his school's soccer league on a daily basis. Ian shared the following poem, which he had composed consciously, regarding the dramatic improvement in his health:

Amazing this relief I feel
Like a burden lifting off of my shoulders
Not a worry in the world
As life seems so much more fulfilling

I'm waiting to fall on my face
But now I know I will rise back up
I have never known a life like this
Where happiness has no limit

Now I will try to live life to its fullest
Almost as if I have another chance
As I step out into the world

With a whole new perspective on life

Ian did not experience any significant recurrence of abdominal symptoms during 6 years of follow-up.

Comment

As demonstrated by this case, chronic symptoms of long-term duration can resolve within a few weeks of application of self-hypnosis. Automatic Word Processing, as used by Ian, can help patients understand or resolve psychological issues that are associated with their symptoms (Anbar & Savedoff, 2005/6). Ian's use of poetry to describe the experience of hypnosis, as well as his characterization of his abdominal status before and after use of hypnosis, provides an unusual window through which to appreciate its potential impact on patients with chronic disease. Prior to the typing, he may have chosen not to be aware of the poetic description of his abdominal pain because such awareness might have provoked uncomfortable feelings. He may have decided to reveal the poem to himself because his pain had improved. Further examples of the utility of hypnosis in resolving somatic symptoms are described in Chapter Eleven.

Ventilator-Dependent Patient

Daniel

Daniel was a 21-year-old college student with profound weakness resulting from Spinal Muscular Atrophy, type II. He was completely dependent on a ventilator to breathe for him. He developed a serious pneumonia, for which he required three weeks of antibiotic therapy, as well as aggressive chest physiotherapy and inhalation therapy. Daniel also learned hypnosis in order to relieve his anxiety during this acute illness. He used imagery of going down a staircase to a beautiful park. Notably, when Daniel imagined himself on the third step of the staircase the pressure required to ventilate his lungs decreased by nearly half. After 15 minutes of hypnosis, Daniel's blood oxygen level rose by 30%. Following each hypnosis session his ventilator pressure and oxygen level remained at their improved levels for 3 to 6 hours. Daniel reported that he felt much better after using hypnosis. Daniel again used hypnosis successfully when he next developed pneumonia.

Comment

As Daniel was monitored by "technology," his case demonstrates some physiological effects of hypnosis. The enhancement of Daniel's lung function may have been the result of hypnosis-induced relaxation that led his chest wall muscles to yield better to the ventilator administered breaths. Alternatively, hypnosis may have led to improvement of neuromuscular coordination that led to better function of his respiratory system. Research studies are required to help understand the hypnotic mechanism of action in this setting.

Vocal Cord Dysfunction

Tom

Tom was a 15-year-old who presented with a 5-year history of shortness of breath and chest pain during exercise that persisted despite therapy with multiple asthma medications including albuterol, salmeterol, cromolyn, and flunisolide. When Tom experienced respiratory distress he found it difficult to inhale, and developed associated mid-sternal chest pain. His mother had witnessed these episodes and described him as having a "panicked look" when they occurred. Often, he developed a loud noise upon inspiration (stridor). On occasion, Tom lost consciousness following an episode. The episodes prevented him from trying out for the varsity basketball team. An exercise stress test showed that when Tom developed chest tightness he had no associated lung function abnormality, nor cardiac arrhythmia. An echocardiogram was normal.

Tom was interested in learning hypnosis. He employed the image of his throat turning black when he was having trouble breathing. By imagining his throat turning a contrasting red, Tom felt he could normalize his breathing. He was also given the suggestion—during his only hypnosis session with the pulmonologist—that sometimes his subconscious would take care of the breathing problem before he would become consciously aware of it. Tom reported that within a day of the hypnosis his shortness of breath had nearly resolved. Three months later Tom reported using hypnosis on a weekly basis, and explained that once he realized the control he was able to achieve with hypnosis he no longer worried about his breathing.

Comment

Tom's case illustrates a patient who may have developed anxiety or panic due to recurrent episodes of apparent asthma associated shortness of breath. (Anbar, 2001b; Baron & Marcotte, 1994). Such anxiety could have caused further shortness of breath and vocal cord dysfunction, which can cause stridor (Anbar & Hehir, 2000;

Fritz, Fritsch, & Hagino, 1997). Tom may have responded well because anxiety is very amenable to treatment with hypnosis.

Adherence

Sean—Improvement

Sean was a 14-year-old with cystic fibrosis, who had difficulties in adhering to his therapies. As is routine practice at his Cystic Fibrosis Center, he had been offered the opportunity to learn how to use hypnosis given its potential helpfulness in coping with a chronic disease (Anbar, 2000b). He reported he enjoyed hypnosis and had used it to control anxiety, ease pain when undergoing medical procedures, and to improve his athletic performance. A suggestion was given to Sean to employ the imagery of an invisible door in front of his mouth that would block entry of food—unless he unlocked the door with his pancreatic enzymes. Once Sean began employing this image, he no longer neglected to take his enzymes.

Six months later, Sean returned for routine follow-up at the Center. He reported using hypnosis on a daily basis to help with relaxation and his athletic performance. However, he had stopped taking all medications except for his enzymes. It was then suggested that the door in front of his mouth had multiple locks, all of which needed to be opened with use of each of his prescribed medications before he could eat. Sean then became entirely adherent to his prescribed therapies.

Sally—No improvement

Sally was a 17-year-old with diabetes mellitus who was non-adherent with her insulin and diet. She agreed to use hypnosis to increase her level of adherence, but stated she could not enter a hypnotic state. She denied the ability to visualize, and also declined to acknowledge her eyelids becoming tired when she fixated on a spot on the wall.

Comment

Use of hypnosis can improve adherence to medical therapy by allowing a patient to develop new mental strategies to reach a desired goal (Anbar, 2000b). However, as the case of Sally illustrates, the patient is in control when it comes to hypnosis. Despite her verbal agreement to do hypnosis, an important clue that she was not allowing herself to be interested was her denial of eyelid fatigue, as all people can feel this phenomenon, if they are willing to feel it. Once again, as in Larry's example, "resistance" indicates that important information likely has not been addressed with the patient.

Pain during Blood Drawing

Melinda—Improvement

Melinda was a 9-year-old with acute lymphocytic leukemia who was very fearful of blood drawing (phlebotomy). She would typically scream, cry, and require restraint for routine blood work. She was very good at hypnosis, and was taught how to induce "glove anesthesia" by imagining that her hand was coated by a numbing medicine, and encased in two thick gloves. Subsequently, Melinda was able to transfer the numbness from her hand to the antecubital fossa. Then, she reported no pain when she underwent phlebotomy. She was so excited by her new skill that she eagerly anticipated her next opportunity to undergo a blood test. Again, to her delight, she experienced no pain. Thereafter, Melinda chose to use hypnosis whenever she underwent phlebotomy. She stated that it made her feel more in control of the situation, as opposed to using a topical anesthetic cream.

Luke—No improvement

Luke was a 15-year-old who learned to use hypnosis to control his asthma associated shortness of breath. As an aside, he asked to be taught how to induce glove anesthesia. He denied being able to achieve numbness with the imagery utilized for Melinda.

Comment

Instruction in glove anesthesia (Hammond, 1990) may be taught to all interested patients with chronic illnesses who require any painful procedures. As many pediatric patients are successful in inducing numbness, it is possible that Luke would also have been successful, had the right imagery and sufficient time been taken with him. In addition, as opposed to Luke, Melinda had a large incentive for hypnosis to work; it is under such circumstances that hypnosis is most likely to be successful (Udolf, 1987).

Literature Review

The impact of chronic illness includes disruption of the normal process of child development encompassing physical, personal-social, cognitive, and moral dimensions (Cerreto & Travis, 1984). As described in Chapter Seven, these disruptions can become traumatic experiences.

Symptoms in patients with chronic disease result from acute, chronic, and recurrent discomforts. These arise from the disease, are caused by therapies, or develop as a result of psychosocial factors. Patients' experience of their symptoms is dependent not only on the physical nature of the discomfort, but also on the patients' emotional, psychological, and spiritual states. Social factors usually contribute to the impact of symptoms in patients' lives. Assessment of symptoms, in part, is based on patients' subjective impressions, which are affected by their general attitudes and beliefs that arise as a result of their personal histories. (Anbar & Hummell, 2004; Tsao & Zeltzer, 2005).

Evaluation of symptoms involves review of physical and psychological factors. Patients should be asked to describe the onset, duration, and frequency of their symptoms. The nature of a symptom can be described by its location and distribution, quality, and intensity. Psychological factors that impact the perception of symptoms include anxiety, depression, substance abuse, and certain behaviors (e.g., non-adherence to therapy, physical activities that trigger pain, and reinforcement by family members attending to the patient when he or she reports the symptom). In order to gain insight into how patients think about their symptom, they should be asked about its meaning, when it is most bothersome, what will change when their symptom improves, and about their expectations of therapy for the symptom (Anbar & Hummell, 2004).

Children with chronic illness are twice as likely to develop mental health problems, such as attention deficit hyperactivity disorder, misconduct, and school and adjustment problems, as compared to healthy peers (Cadman, Boyle, Szatmari, & Offord, 1987; Lavigne & Faier-Routman, 1993). However, only 25% of these children with a significant mental health problem receive mental health services (Cadman et al., 1987).

Chronic illness can affect children's mental status through intrinsic factors including the age of the child at the onset of the illness, the course of the illness (e.g., progressive, stable, or with exacerbations), prognosis (e.g., expected improvement, persistent, fatal), its impact on the child's mobility and cognitive abilities, predictability of the associated symptoms, and visibility of the illness. Extrinsic factors include the family's economic status, accessibility of treatment, and the effectiveness of parenting of the child (Pless, 1984; Perrin & MacLean, 1988).

Interventions aimed at decreasing the impact of chronic illness on a child include providing the child and his or her family with education about the disease, helping to strengthen the family unit, teaching parents to reinforce their child's self-help activities, providing external support to assist families with handicapped children, and engaging the support of the child's teachers, school administrators, and peers (Perrin & MacLean, 1988; Bauman, Drotar, Leventhal, Perrin, & Pless, 1997).

In order to prevent mental health problems, children with chronic illness should be encouraged to attend school on a regular basis, perform household chores to the best of their abilities, and spend time with friends (Perrin & MacLean, 1988).

Stress management training for the affected child also can be of great benefit. Such training may include contingency coping exercises, relaxation skill training, and social skill training (Alexander, Cropp, & Chai, 1979; Perrin & MacLean, 1988). Each of these stress management skills can be achieved with hypnosis. For example, ego-strengthening (see below) can help improve self-esteem, which in turn enables the child to cope more capably with stressors associated with chronic illness. Anxiety reduction (see below) helps patients relax, which helps place them in a better position to assess and react to their symptoms appropriately (Anbar, 2000b; Anbar, 2002a). Anxiety reduction also helps patients interact better socially, which allows them to receive enhanced support from their peers.

Hypnosis also can be useful in the treatment of chronic disease because it can affect patients' perception of their disease. Hypnosis has been shown to reduce acute pain, chronic pain, depression, anxiety, and dependence on pain medications. Further, it is more effective in controlling pain than placebo, relaxation, distraction, or alpha-feedback (Udolf, 1987; Olness & Kohen, 1996).

There are many published examples of the successful use of hypnosis in the treatment of chronic disease. Hypnosis has been used successfully to control discomfort and pain associated with cancer, fibromyalgia, HIV, juvenile rheumatoid arthritis, and sickle cell disease (Dinges et al., 1997; Haanen et al, 1991; Walco, Varni, & Ilowite, 1992; Langenfeld, Cipani, & Borckardt, 2002; Rucklidge & Saunders, 2002; Wild & Espie, 2004). Hypnotherapy has been shown to improve adherence to prescribed therapies of adolescents with diabetes, with an associated improvement of their blood sugar control (Ratner, Gross, Casas, & Castells, 1990). In one study, hypnosis appeared to reduce the need for transfusions in patients with hemophilia (LeBaw, 1992). In controlled studies, hypnosis has been shown to greatly improve irritable bowel syndrome (Whorwell, Prior, & Faragher, 1984; Whorwell, Prior, & Colgan, 1987).

Clinical Strategies

The goals of clinical hypnosis for patients with chronic disease include reducing anxiety from acute and chronic symptoms, reducing discomfort from the disease and medical procedures (*see* Chapters Fourteen and Eighteen), helping control reactions that result from stress, providing a coping skill, and increasing the patient's self-esteem. Achievement of any of these goals helps patients become more confident in their abilities to help themselves, which allows them to achieve further goals more easily.

Not only does hypnosis empower the patient with chronic disease, but providing hypnosis instruction to patients empowers the healthcare provider by allowing him or her to help chronically ill patients even when medications have been insufficient to control their symptoms (Anbar, 2000a; *see also* Chapter Nineteen).

A generic case example of the verbatim instructions that might be used by a healthcare provider helps illustrate how hypnosis may be taught for treatment of a patient with chronic disease.

Generic Case Example

"Before we get started, you need to understand that all hypnosis is self-hypnosis. Contrary to what you might see in cartoons, hypnosis is not sleep. When you are doing hypnosis you know what's going on and you can stop at anytime you want to. Do you know why?"

"That's right. It's because you are in control. You already do hypnosis, you just don't realize it. For example, have you ever been bored in school?"

"What did you do when you were bored?

"What did you do if there was nothing to doodle on?"

"That's right. When you daydream (or zone out), that's hypnosis. Can you imagine what your room might look like, or what a favorite song might sound like?"

"Those are examples of hypnosis. So you see, you already know how to do hypnosis. What I can teach you, if you like, is how to use hypnosis to help you feel better. Would you like to know how to do that?"

"Good. One way that hypnosis works is through images in the mind. An image in the mind can affect the way your mind and body work. For example, have you ever played with magnets?"

"What do they do?"

"That's right. When the positive pole faces the negative pole the magnets attract. That's where the saying comes from: 'Opposites attract.' Now, hold your hands about 4 inches apart, and imagine, with your eyes open or closed, whichever is more comfortable, that your hands are giant magnets that can attract themselves all by themselves."

"That's right. Notice how the hands are coming together. Some people say that their hands tingle or feel warm as they come together, and others feel something else."

"That's right. Now that your hands are stuck together let me show you something else. Leave the magnets there. Don't let those hands separate. When I count to three, your job will be to leave the magnets there and try to separate the hands. I think you may be surprised by how that will feel. One… Two… Don't take the magnets away… Three!"

"How did that feel? How did it work? Was it magic? Was it something I did? Or did you do something? What did you do?"

"Now you begin to understand how an image in the mind can affect the body. Would you like another example?"

"Put both hands up in front of you. Now, imagine that in one hand you are holding a bucketful of wet sand, like you might have played with on the beach when you were younger. And in the other hand, imagine holding strings that are attached to many helium balloons of different colors. Now, notice how the hand holding the bucket can become heavier and heavier, while the hand holding the balloons can become lighter and lighter—all by itself."

"How did you do that?"

"Very good. Now, do you like relaxing?"

"Good. Then let me show you how you can relax with hypnosis. First I will tell you what you can do. Then you can do it. Afterwards we'll talk about the experience. In a few moments you can imagine going to a safe, relaxing place of your choice. It can be a place you've been to, a place you'd like to go to, or even an imaginary place. Now, once you are there, you can imagine what you might see, hear, smell, touch, and taste. Do you know why you want to imagine with all your senses?"

"The more you use your different senses the more real the experience can become, and the more relaxed you can be. Brain studies have shown that when you imagine a sense, you actually activate the same part of the brain that becomes active when you are literally experiencing that sense. Does that make sense to you?"

"In your relaxing place is there a place to sit or lay down comfortably?"

"Good. Then once you arrive in your relaxing place I will ask you to find a place to sit or lay down comfortably. Then, I will talk to you about relaxing from your head to your neck, to your arms, to your legs, down to your toes. How do you think you will feel then?"

"That's right. Now, here is an important part. You get to pick your own personal relaxation sign. This is a sign that you can use anytime you want to relax without using hypnosis. I suggest you pick a one-handed sign. Some people choose to touch their index finger to their thumb, while others cross their fingers, or make a fist. What would you like your sign to be?"

"Very good. Once you make your sign in hypnosis, you can stay in your relaxing place for as long as you like. You can imagine being there for a minute, an hour, a year, or even forever. In hypnosis, time can mean whatever you want, so this will only take a few moments in real time. Once you are ready to return you can raise your hand and I will give you a few more instructions."

Once the patient indicates that he or she is ready to begin, the therapist provides instructions similar to those described above. Note that no further mention is made of eye closure, which is only necessary if the patient feels it would be helpful. Once the patient raises his or her hand during hypnosis the instructions continue as follows:

"Very good. Now, before you come back you can tell yourself four things: First, congratulate yourself for your excellent use of your imagination. Second, remind yourself to practice your hypnosis every day for at least two weeks so that you can become very good with it. Hypnosis is a mind/body skill, so the more you use it, the better it becomes. Third, remind yourself that whenever you want to relax without the use of hypnosis all you need to do is to make your relaxation sign. Finally, now your mind is open to suggestions. You can offer good suggestions to yourself. The more you tell yourself these things the more they can come true. For example, you might tell yourself that you like how you feel right now and that you want to feel this way for the rest of the day. Or, you could tell yourself that you will become better and better at controlling discomforts that you may encounter. You might even imagine how good it will feel when you are better. After you have told yourself all of the good things you need to hear—when the time is right, and you will know exactly when that time is—then come back."

Once the patient indicates he or she is back to usual awareness, the therapist asks:

"Very good. How do you feel?"

"What has changed?"

"How did you do that?"

"What did you like about the experience?

"Is there anything you didn't like, or wish was different?"

"Would you like to feel something neat?"

"Make your relaxation sign."

"What just happened?"

"Now you realize that you can control how you feel. The more you do hypnosis the more in control of yourself you can become. Isn't that great to know?"

"Good job."

Specific Hypnosis Techniques

Patients vary in their abilities to use various hypnosis techniques. In order to decide which techniques might work best for an individual patient, the therapist should consider the patient's medical condition, motivation for change, interests, and developmental age (Sugarman, 1996). Patients should be offered the opportunity to use different techniques, so that they can help identify those that are most helpful for them.

The following techniques typically are beneficial for use with children who developmentally are 7 years of age or older. For children younger than 7 years, hypnosis almost invariably needs to be modified, as described in Chapter Two.

Ego-strengthening

Ego-strengthening is a central component of clinical hypnosis for both establishment of rapport and a feeling of self-efficacy. The patient who believes in his or her abilities is more capable of achieving improvement. Ego-strengthening suggestions should be given before, during, and after hypnosis. Also, patients can be advised to give themselves ego-strengthening suggestions at home. Examples of ego-strengthening suggestions include:

Before Hypnosis
"You already know how to do hypnosis."

"Each person has an ability to help themselves."

"It's impressive how you have insight into the way your symptoms change in response to stress in your life."

During Hypnosis
"That's right... You are doing well."

"You appear to be very relaxed."

"Congratulate yourself for your excellent use of your imagination."

After Hypnosis
"What changed [*as a result of your hypnosis experience*]? How did *you* do that?"

"You did very well."

"Now you realize that you can control how you feel."

Suggestions Patients may give themselves at Home
"I will become better and better at controlling discomforts that I may encounter."

"Every day, I come closer and closer to achieving my goals."

"Each time I do hypnosis it will become easier and easier."

Anchoring Gesture

While in hypnosis, an anchoring gesture is established as a post-hypnotic suggestion (e.g., a "relaxation sign"). This allows patients to pick a signal that will trigger the feelings achieved within hypnosis. For preschool and some elementary school-age children, a tangible anchor is useful, such as a smooth stone, or seashell. I keep a supply of both in my office. For older children and many adolescents, a physical anchor, such as touching their fingers together, often is useful. For older adolescents and adults, anchors can be an image, or a word (for example, a mantra.)

Patients can be encouraged to use their anchoring gesture multiple times a day as an ego-strengthening exercise, and to broaden its utility.

Anxiety Reduction

Many patients with chronic disease develop anxiety as a result of associating symptoms with unpleasant experiences such as physical discomfort or medical intervention. Such anxiety can lead to intensification of their symptoms, such as increased shortness of breath in a patient with asthma (Anbar, 2003), or increased pain associated with cancer (Kuttner, Bowman, & Teasdale, 1988). When anxiety is not recognized as a comorbid condition, affected patients may be treated unnecessarily with medications targeted at their medical condition (Anbar, 2003). Not only are these medications often ineffective in such instances, but sometimes they have significant side effects that cause further deterioration of a patient's health. For example, a patient with asthma might be treated with chronic steroids by mouth for anxiety-induced shortness of breath, which leads to the development obesity and brittle bones without relief of his or her symptoms. Instead, hypnosis could have been used to relieve the patient's shortness of breath (Anbar, 2003).

There are many ways that hypnosis might be used as a tool to reduce anxiety. Some of these techniques include imagery, progressive relaxation, breathing, self-suggestions, and rehearsal. Other techniques are described in Chapters Five and Ten.

Imagery
"Imagine going to a safe relaxing place of your choice. Pay close attention to what might be perceived there with each of your senses."

Allowing patients to choose their own imagery often is more effective than use of imagery proposed by the therapist. Patient chosen imagery is likely to be more meaningful to the patient, and will not include disturbing thoughts that might be introduced inadvertently by the therapist. For example, the therapist might propose imagining a beach to a patient who has had a near-drowning experience, with a resultant negative response from the patient. Additionally, when patients are asked to create their own imagery it is implied that they hold the key for resolution of their issues, which is ego-strengthening.

Progressive Relaxation
Each phrase in the following sequence may be paced with the patient's breathing.

> "When you are ready, relax your forehead... Now, let that wonderful feeling of relaxation spread to the muscles around your eyes... down to your cheeks... your jaw... down your neck.... That's right... Down to your shoulders... arms... and hands... Very good...Now, take a deep breath and let it out slowly. Notice how your chest can relax... as you do that... Now, take a deep breath and let it out slowly. Notice how your belly can relax... as you do that... and let the relaxation spread to your legs... and your feet... That's right."

Breathing
> "Find the spot in the middle of your body that is relaxed. Nod your head when you have located this spot... With each inhalation, bring in a feeling of calm...That's right...And with each exhalation you can spread the relaxation outwards...Toward your upper chest...And your abdomen...That's right... down your legs, and down your arms...Very good... And into your neck and toes and face and forehead...Good job."

Self-suggestion
> "Remind yourself that whenever you want to relax with the use of hypnosis, all you need to do is to make your relaxation sign."

Using Automatic Word Processing (Anbar, 2001a), a patient can be taught how to express himself or herself through typing, while in hypnosis. This process allows the patient to discuss, and sometimes begin to resolve emotionally, meaningful material in a state of relatively low anxiety. The method enables patients to give themselves suggestions (Anbar & Savedoff, 2005/6). For example, a patient might choose to tell himself or herself to focus on good feelings from the present time rather than anxiety-provoking future possibilities (Anbar, 2001a). Additionally, patients can choose to forget what they have typed, and thus not deal with some psychologically intense issues on a conscious level, until they are ready.

Rehearsal

"Whenever you feel uncomfortable you can use hypnosis, or your relaxation sign, to help yourself feel better. Would you like to test this?" If the patient responds affirmatively, the therapist continues, "When you are ready, remember how it felt to be uncomfortable. Imagine this feeling with all of your senses. Allow this feeling to grow as intense as you wish. When you want it to stop, make your relaxation sign. Notice how you immediately become comfortable again, even though the cause of the discomfort might remain."

Time Distortion

Time distortion can be utilized to shorten the apparent length of uncomfortable medical therapies, thus making them more tolerable. Conversely, time distortion may be used to gain increased benefit from pleasurable or beneficial hypnotic experiences. For example, the patient might be told, "You can stay in your relaxing place for as long as you like. You can imagine being there for a minute, an hour, a year, or even forever. In hypnosis, time can mean whatever you want, so this will only take a few moments in real time."

Positive Visualization

By imagining a future better than the present, patients can help direct themselves towards improvement or recovery. Hypnotic techniques to accomplish this goal include imagining a future in which the patients feel better, is improving continually, is capable of coping well with their illness, or has recovered entirely.

Role of the Parent

Parents are often very involved in the care of a child with a chronic illness. Young children (under 8 years of age) frequently want their parents to help with hypnosis. For example, the young child may enjoy having his or her parent tell a calming story. Older children generally prefer to do hypnosis on their own. Application of self-hypnosis fits well into the important childhood task of achieving self-mastery (Olness & Kohen, 1996). Thus, parental involvement with hypnosis for the older child may be counter-productive. At times, parents must be counseled explicitly to avoid discussing their child's use of hypnosis.

A good indicator whether a child's use of hypnosis should be monitored or guided by a parent, is to ask the child about his or her preference. This query might be framed as, "Are there certain situations in which you would want your parent to help with doing hypnosis?" For example, children might want parental involvement during times of exacerbation of their disease (e.g., a sickle cell disease crisis.) At such times children often regress in their abilities to help themselves, and even older ones may desire parental involvement.

Sometimes, it is helpful to offer parents the opportunity to learn self-hypnosis so that they can better appreciate its applications with their children. Further, because chronic childhood diseases can have profound effects on family function (Varni, Katz, Colegrove, & Dolgin, 1996; Mastroyannopoulou, Stallard, Lewis, & Lenton, 1997), self-hypnosis utilized by the parents or siblings can benefit the entire family (*see* Chapter Thirteen).

Caveats

All healthcare providers who practice clinical hypnosis should have professional training in the care of patients with the health issues for which they utilize hypnosis. In this way, the healthcare provider will be capable of assessing whether patients' symptoms should be treated appropriately with hypnosis, and whether medical therapy also is indicated. For example, if a patient's symptoms are a side effect of a medication, the best therapy may be to switch or discontinue the medication rather than use of hypnosis for the symptoms.

Patients with chronic disease should consult with their healthcare provider before employing hypnosis in order to ameliorate their chronic or new-onset symptoms. Otherwise, there is a potential that the patients will not receive proper medical attention for their symptom. Patients and their families should be counseled that there are limits to the usefulness of hypnosis, and they should not expect a "miracle."

Symptoms of patients with chronic illness can arise as a result of physical or psychological issues. Therefore, the practitioner using hypnosis should formulate a treatment plan based on the assessment of the primary cause of the patients' symptoms. For instance, if the primary cause of a symptom is a psychological coping reaction (e.g., a conversion disorder), symptom removal without attention to the patient's psychological issues might cause the patient significant distress. Further, in formulating hypnotic suggestions, the therapist should keep in mind the cultural norms that might be related to the patients' symptoms.

Instruction of hypnosis to uninterested patients is unlikely to be of benefit since the efficacy of hypnosis is based upon the patients' desires. In order to assess whether a patient is a good candidate for hypnosis, the patient should be asked if he or she wants their symptom to improve. Patients who answer tentatively (e.g., "Um, yes," or, "I'm not sure"), should be offered the opportunity for further exploration into whether they want to use hypnosis to help themselves. A good strategy in this setting may be to tell patients to consider whether they want to learn how to use hypnosis during the interval between successive appointments.

Patients should not be urged to use hypnosis if they are uninterested. Not only will the hypnosis be less likely to be helpful in this setting, but the patients would be less likely to feel ownership of the experience. Thus, the sense of self-mastery achievable with hypnosis will be negated, and deprive the child from gaining an important tool for dealing with his or her chronic disease on a long-term basis.

Finally, hypnotizability scales do not correlate well with clinical outcome of hypnosis in children (*see* Chapter Four). One reason for this may be that children are often unmotivated to cooperate with administration of such scales. For this reason, a low level of response to hypnotizability testing should not preclude use of hypnosis for clinical reasons in children, and typically hypnotizability scales are not used in clinical practice with children (Olness & Kohen, 1996).

Conclusion

Five months after learning how to use hypnosis, just after sharing the poem he had written consciously about his healing, Ian wanted to know if his subconscious had written any new poems. His subconscious replied (Anbar 2002b):

The smell of happiness
fills me with joy
as every day
better than the next one

A breeze of wind
feels different
as do all other feelings
in this new state of health

I never thought I could feel so incredible
so strong, so healthy, so happy
not even looking back at the problems before me
instead I look ahead to what lies in the future

Filled with joy my life is so much better
as every breath that I take I am more thankful
to everyone who has helped me
and to everyone who will continue to

Ian's subconscious beautifully illustrates the potential incredible outcome of hypnosis work. Surely, everyone with a chronic illness deserves a similar opportunity to use hypnosis in order to gain more control over his or her life.

References

Alexander, A. B., Cropp, G. J. A., & Chai, H. (1979). Effects of relaxation training on pulmonary mechanics in children with asthma. *Journal of Applied Behavior Analysis, 12,* 27–35.

Anbar, R. D. (2000a). Of mind, body, and modern technology. *Clinical Pediatrics,* 39:433–436.

Anbar, R. D. (2000b). Self-hypnosis for patients with cystic fibrosis. *Pediatric Pulmonology,* 40, 461–465.

Anbar, R. D. (2001a). Automatic word processing: A new forum for hypnotic expression. *The American Journal of Clinical Hypnosis,* 44, 27–36.

Anbar, R, D. (2001b). Self-hypnosis for management of chronic dyspnea in pediatric patients. *Pediatrics,* 107, e21. Available at: http://www.pediatrics.org/cgi/content/full/107/2/e21

Anbar, R. D. (2001c). Self-hypnosis for treatment of functional abdominal pain in childhood. *Clinical Pediatrics,* 40, 447–451.

Anbar, R. D. (2002a). Hypnosis in pediatrics: applications at a pediatric pulmonary center. *BMC Pediatrics,* 2:11. Available at: http://www.biomedcentral.com/content/pdf/1471-2431-2-11.pdf

Anbar, R. D. (2002b). Self-expression through poetry in hypnosis. *Clinical Pediatrics,* 41, 195–196.

Anbar, R. D. (2003). Self-hypnosis for anxiety associated with severe asthma: A case report. *BMC Pediatrics,* 3:7. Available at: http://www.biomedcentral.com/1471-2431/3/7

Anbar, R. D., & Geisler, S. C. (2005). Identification of children who may benefit from self-hypnosis at a pediatric pulmonary center. *BMC Pediatrics,* 5:6. Available at: http://www.biomedcentral.com/1471-2431/5/6

Anbar, R. D., & Hehir, D. A. (2000). Hypnosis as a diagnostic modality for vocal cord dysfunction. *Pediatrics,* 2000. 106, e81. Available at: http://www.pediatrics.org/cgi/content/full/106/6/e81

Anbar, R. D., & Hummell, K. E. (2004). Self-hypnosis for pain management in patients with cystic fibrosis. *Pediatric Pulmonology*, Suppl 27, 148–149.

Anbar, R. D., & Savedoff, A. D. (2005/6). Treatment of binge eating with automatic word processing and self-hypnosis: a case report. *The American Journal of Clinical Hypnosis*, 48, 191–198.

Baron, C., & Marcotte, J. E. (1994). Role of panic attacks in the intractability of asthma in children. *Pediatrics*, 94, 108–110.

Bauman, L. J., Drotar, D., Leventhal, J. M., Perrin, E. C, & Pless, I. B. (1997). A review of psychosocial interventions for children with chronic health conditions. *Pediatrics*, 100, 244–251.

Cadman, D., Boyle, M., Szatmari, P., & Offord, D. R. (1987). Chronic illness, disability, and mental and social well-being: findings of the Ontario Child Health Study. *Pediatrics*, 79, 805–813.

Ceretto, M. C., & Travis, L. B. (1984). Implications of psychological and family factors in the treatment of diabetes. *Pediatric Clinics of North America*, 31, 689–710.

Dinges, D. F., Whitehouse, W. G., Orne, E. C., Bloom, P. B., Carlin, M. M., Bauer, N. K., Gillen, K. A., Shapiro, B. S., Ohene-Frempong, K., Dampier, C., & Orne, M. T. (1997). Self-hypnosis training as an adjunctive treatment in the management of pain associated with sickle cell disease. *The International Journal of Clinical and Experimental Hypnosis*, 45, 417–432.

Fritz, G. K., Fritsch, S., & Hagino, O. (1997). Somatoform disorders in children and adolescents: A review of the past 10 years. *Journal of the American Academy of Child & Adolescent Psychiatry*, 36, 1329–1338.

Gortmaker, S. L. (1985). Demography of chronic childhood diseases. In: N. Hobbs & J. M Perrin, (eds.) *Issues in the Care of Children with Chronic Illness*. San Francisco: Jossey-Bass.

Haanen, H. C., Hoenderdos, H. T., van Romunde, L. K., Hop, W. C., Mallee, C., Terwiel, J. P., & Hekster, G. B. (1991). Controlled trial of hypnotherapy in the treatment of refractory fibromyalgia. *Journal of Rheumatology*, 18, 72–75.

Hackman, R. M., Stern, J. S., & Gershwin, M. E. (2000). Hypnosis and asthma: A critical review. *Journal of Asthma, 37*, 1–15.

Hammond, D. C., ed. (1990). *Handbook of Hypnotic Suggestions and Metaphors.* New York: W.W. Norton.

Kuttner, L., Bowman, M., & Teasdale, M. (1988). Psychological treatment of distress, pain, and anxiety for young children with cancer. *Journal of Developmental and Behavioral Pediatrics, 9*, 374–381.

Langenfeld, M. C., Cipani, E., & Borckardt, J. J. (2002). Hypnosis for the control of HIV/AIDS-related pain. *The International Journal of Clinical and Experimental Hypnosis, 50*, 170–188.

Lavigne, J. W., & Faier-Routman, J. (1993). Correlates of psychosocial adjustment to pediatric physical disorders: A meta-analytic review and comparison with existing models. *Journal of Developmental and Behavioral Pediatrics, 14*, 117–123.

LeBaw, W. (1992). The use of hypnosis in hemophilia. *Psychiatric Medicine, 10*, 89–98.

Mastroyannopoulou, K., Stallard, P., Lewis, M., & Lenton, S. (1997). The impact of childhood non-malignant life threatening illness on parents: Gender differences and prediction of parental adjustment. *Journal of Child Psychology and Psychiatry, and Allied Disciplines, 38*, 823–829.

Newacheck, P. W. (1989). Adolescents with special health needs: Prevalence, severity, and access to health services. *Pediatrics, 84*, 872–881.

Newacheck, P. W., MacManus, M. A., & Fox, H. B. (1991). Prevalence and impact of chronic illness among adolescents. *American Journal of Diseases of Children, 145*, 1367–1373.

Olness, K., & Kohen, D. P. (1996). *Hypnosis and Hypnotherapy With Children.* 3rd ed. New York: Guilford.

Perrin, J. M., & MacLean, W. E. (1988). Children with chronic illness: The prevention of dysfunction. *Pediatric Clinics of North America, 35*, 1325–1337.

Pless, I. B. (1984). Clinical assessment: Physical and psychological functioning. *Pediatric Clinics of North America, 31*, 33–45.

Ratner, H., Gross, L., Casas, J., & Castells, S. (1990). A hypnotherapeutic approach to the improvement of compliance in adolescent diabetics. *The American Journal of Clinical Hypnosis, 32*, 154–159.

Rucklidge, J. J., & Saunders, D. (2002). The efficacy of hypnosis in the treatment of pruritis in people with HIV/AIDS: A time-series analysis. *The International Journal of Clinical and Experimental Hypnosis, 50*, 149–169.

Sugarman, L. I. (1996). Hypnosis: Teaching children self-regulation. *Pediatrics in Review, 17*, 5–11.

ten Thoren, C., & Petermann, E. (2000). Reviewing asthma and anxiety. *Respiratory Medicine, 94*, 409–415.

Tsao, J. C., & Zeltzer, L. K. (2005). Complementary and alternative medicine approaches for pediatric pain: A review of the sate of the science. *Evidence-based Complementary and Alternative Medicine, 2*, 149–159.

Udolf, R. (1987). *Handbook of Hypnosis for Professionals*. Northvale, NJ: Jason Aronson.

Varni, J. W., Katz, E. R., Colegrove, R. C. Jr., & Dolgin, M. (1996). Family functioning predictors of adjustment in children with newly diagnosed cancer. *Journal of Child Psychology and Psychiatry, and Allied Disciplines, 37*, 321–328.

Walco, G. A., Varni, J. W., & Ilowite, N. T. (1992). Cognitive-behavioral pain management in children with juvenile rheumatoid arthritis. *Pediatrics, 89*, 1075–1079.

Whorwell, P. J., Prior, A., & Faragher, E. B. (1984). Controlled trial of hypnotherapy in the treatment of severe refractory irritable bowel syndrome. *Lancet, 2*, 1232–1234.

Whorwell, P. J., Prior, A., & Colgan, S. M. (1987). Hypnotherapy in severe irritable bowel syndrome. *Gut. 28*, 423–425.

Wild, M. R., & Espie, C. A. (2004). The efficacy of hypnosis in the reduction of procedural pain and distress in pediatric oncology: A systematic review. *Journal of Developmental and Behavioral Pediatrics. 25*, 207–213.

Chapter Seventeen

Hypnosis for Children with Elimination Disorders

Linda Thomson, PhD, MSN, CPNP

A hypnotherapeutic approach can be extraordinarily beneficial for children with elimination disorders. The lives of children with these embarrassing problems are shrouded with shame and secrecy. The social and emotional consequences for the child and family are substantial. After establishing a therapeutic alliance, anxiety reduction, relaxation, increasing self-awareness, self-control, and ego-strengthening are integral parts of hypnosis with children. Each of these treatment goals are elements that help children with dysfunctional elimination to resolve their problem themselves by learning in hypnosis to control what they never knew they could. The resulting increase in self-efficacy and self-esteem is magical. While physical pathology is rarely the cause of enuresis or encopresis, the skills in self-regulation afforded with hypnotherapy are powerful adjuncts even when rare organic causes require allopathic treatment.

Enuresis

To Pee or Not to Pee

Tia, Chris, Amy, and Mark

Tia was a 12-year-old girl who went to Girl Scout camp wearing diapers at night because she had nightly enuresis. She hid the wet diapers in the bottom of her sleeping bag and lived in fear that the other campers would find out. This year she wanted to go to camp without the shame of being a "sleepwetter" (Tia's term for nocturnal enuresis) and be able to sleep over at her friends' homes without diapers. In the past, Tia had unsuccessfully used imipramine and read a children's book about bedwetting. She had also tried a vibrating enuresis alarm but found it annoying. When it went off she was already wet. She also reported that with the alarm, she worried all night and then didn't feel well rested in the morning. Tia also had a very noticeable facial tic. That, however, did not bother her. She wanted to stop wetting the bed.

Chris' family recently moved about 1,000 miles so that his parents could assume new positions as house parents at a boarding school. Ten-year-old Chris was not happy about the move and leaving all his friends. He became depressed and was prescribed a selective serotonin reuptake inhibitor (SSRI). Over the years Chris had occasionally wet the bed, but now it was a nightly occurrence.

At age 11 Amy had been on desmopressin acetate (DDAVP) for two years and still continued to wet two nights per week. She wanted to be able to stop wearing diapers and stop taking pills.

It was after Mark's 9-year-old check-up that he returned to the office to learn to control his enuresis that occurred four or five times per week. Mark said if he could stop wetting his life would be better because he would "be like normal." He wanted to be able to sleep over at a friend's house without diapers. Mark also wanted to have more time in the mornings to watch cartoons instead of showering and changing the sheets.

Evaluation and Medical Management

One of the most common behavioral and urological problems presented to pediatric clinicians is nighttime bedwetting. *Primary nocturnal enuresis* is urinary incontinence during sleep in a child who is over 6 years of age and has never been consistently dry for more than six months. Five to seven million American children are affected (National Kidney Foundation home page, 2003). The condition is three times more likely to occur in boys. Twenty percent of 5 year olds wet the bed. The annual spontaneous resolution rate is 15%. By the age of 10 the prevalence of bedwetting is about 5%. At age 18, one percent of teens have not achieved nocturnal continence (Mosier, 1998).

Many possible causes and explanations for enuresis have been proposed. Nocturnal enuresis rarely signals a kidney or bladder problem. Five percent of children with enuresis will have an organic cause for their condition (Lawless & McElderry, 2001). Doubtful, but previously postulated, etiologies have included small bladder size, poor bladder muscle control, and sleep disorders. Others have attributed nocturnal enuresis to personality disorders, neuroses, and difficulty with arousal from sleep. Constipation may contribute to the frequency of nocturnal enuresis. A stool filled rectum may restrict bladder expansion. The frequent rubbing on the bladder from a full rectum may alter the brain's interpretation of the sensations of a full bladder. Some studies suggest a deficiency of nocturnal production of the anti-diuretic hormone (ADH). This deficiency in the endogenous regulator of urine output results in over-production of nighttime urine.

Heredity plays a significant role in enuresis. Three out of four children with enuresis will have a positive family history in one or both parents. This may relate to an inherited deficiency or maturational delay in ADH production. When a child has had a prolonged period of nocturnal continence and then begins to urinate during sleep, this is called *secondary enuresis*. Physical causes such as a urinary tract infection must be ruled out. Secondary enuresis often has psychological causes. Stress from any source, but commonly a parental divorce, may result in bedwetting. The possibility of sexual or other abuse should also be explored in a child who begins with enuresis after a long period of continence.

Although enuresis itself does not pose a serious physical health risk, it can have potentially damaging effects on the child's emotional well-being and self-esteem. The condition may be a source of shame and embarrassment and have profound effects on the social, emotional, and behavioral health and everyday life of the child and his entire family. A study by Chang et al. (2002) suggests that compared to age and gender matched controls, children with enuresis have lower social competence and school performance. The research by Hagglof et al. (1997) indicates that self-esteem is significantly impaired for patients with enuresis when compared to controls. Decreased self-esteem may result in more behavioral problems and antisocial behavior. Children with enuresis frequently avoid social contacts and age-appropriate peer activities such as sleeping at relatives' or friends' homes and summer camp.

Even though nocturnal enuresis is a common condition, it can seem like a huge and over-whelming problem to the child and family. Children with enuresis viewed bedwetting as the third most stressful situation in their life, surpassed only by parental divorce and arguments. Sixty-one percent of parents feel that bedwetting is a significant problem, although only 33% have consulted their child's healthcare provider concerning the condition. Sixty-eight percent of parents of 3- to 14-year-olds report that their child's problem of bedwetting was never raised by the health provider during routine examinations (Mosier, 1998). It is believed that as many as 90% of children with enuresis are undiagnosed and untreated. Parental misunderstandings about bedwetting may lead to inappropriate parental behavior such as belittling, shaming, punishments, and withdrawing privileges. These negative and punitive techniques often make the problem more difficult to manage and further decrease the child's self-esteem.

There are a variety of approaches and treatments for enuresis. Perhaps the most widely studied behavioral intervention for nocturnal enuresis is conditioning therapy using moisture sensitive alarms. Urination triggers an auditory or vibratory alarm designed to wake up the child. The alarms have a high drop out rate as it may take as long as 6 months to obtain adequate control (Mosier, 1998). Sixty-five percent of individuals did not wake to void and slept through the buzzer and the wetting (Blum, 2004). The success rate for conditioning therapy is extremely variable but may be as high as 70% with a 30% relapse rate (Mosier, 1998). The alarms are not without their problems. Often they fail to wake the child but arouse other family members. The child may find the noise frightening or very annoying because by the time the alarm wakes them they may already be quite wet. Some children take the alarms off in sleep, subconsciously avoiding the intrusion.

Studies of the bladder stretching approach have produced contra-dictory results (Blum, 2004). The theory is that retention control training will increase functional bladder capacity. The child is asked to hold his or her urine during the day for progressively longer periods of time. This requires a strong patient commitment and, at best, is 30% effective.

Although fluid restriction before bedtime seems logical, it has never been demonstrated to be effective (VonHoecke, Baeyens, Walle, & Hoebeke (2003)). It has often been suggested that the parent should arouse the child several hours after sleep onset and take him or her to the toilet. This strategy is problematic for two reasons. First, several hours after bedtime the child is in a deep stage of sleep and not really awake even though he or she may walk to the bathroom with the parent. Therefore, this practice encourages the child to empty the bladder while sleeping, not to associate a full bladder with awakening (Butler, 1998). Second, it guarantees failure of the child's autonomous search for control. If the bed is dry, the child did not do it on his or her own. If the bed is wet, the child has failed both himself or herself and his or her parents.

Pharmacologic management is based on various pathophysiologic explanations for enuresis: uninhibited detrussor spasm, relative nocturnal polyuria and decreased sleep arousal. Since the 1960s imipramine has been used for bedwetting. Banerjee et al (1993) divided 50 children with nocturnal enuresis into two groups. Half were treated with imipramine and half with hypnosis. After three months, 76% of the imipramine group and 72% of the hypnosis group were dry. After treatment was discontinued, all 72% of the hypnosis group remained dry, while only 24% of the imipramine group was continent at night. Imipramine can be toxic at excessive doses or with patients who have cardiac conduction defects.

In 1990 the antidiuretic hormone analogue DDAVP was approved for the treatment of nocturnal enuresis. DDAVP is expensive and the relapse rates after discontinuation are high. DDAVP has also been combined with oxybutinine, a smooth muscle relaxant, in certain select populations.

Hypnotherapeutic Approach

It is not surprising that relapse rates are high for pharmacologic management and alarms because they externalize the locus of control. The reason for success is attributed to the pill or the buzzer. Hypnotherapy empowers the child with an internal locus of control, has no medication or equipment costs and no negative side effects.

In an early study by Olness (1975), 40 children with enuresis were taught self-hypnosis. Thirty-one resolved their bedwetting, most within the first month after just one or two visits. Six others improved. Of the three who did not improve, one was experiencing significant secondary gain and had no desire to be dry, one was not invested in practicing self-hypnosis, and the third had a urological abnormality.

In a large study of 257 children who used hypnosis to resolve enuresis, Kohen, Colwell, Heimel, & Olness (1984) found 44% achieved 30 consecutive dry nights and continued to be dry at a 12-month follow-up. Another 31% showed significant improvement. Over-involvement by parents and lack of motivation were the factors most related to failures in achieving nocturnal continence. Most of the 257 children had already tried two or three other treatment modalities. Separate studies by Kohen et al. (1984) and Stanton (1979) concluded that improvement in enuresis with hypnosis will be seen within the first one to four sessions. If the child has not improved within the time frame, it is unlikely that they will improve with this therapeutic modality (Gottsegen, 2003).

In the hypnotic approach to enuresis, the first step in the evaluation is a thorough history while building rapport with the child. The clinician gets to know the child apart from his or her problem. Five percent of children with enuresis have an organic cause for the nocturnal incontinence (Lawless, 2001). An appropriate medical evaluation must attempt to rule out physiologic causes such as urinary tract infection, constipation, diabetes insipidis and mellitus, hyperthyroidism and spinal dysraphism. For the child who is motivated to resolve his or her nighttime problem, learning that the clinician is joining together with him or her as a partner with the confidence that the clinician can help the child help himself or herself can be a monumental relief. While acknowledging that the child's bedwetting is nobody's fault and empathizing that it is annoying, the clinician determines the child's thoughts and worries about his or her nocturnal incontinence.

The history should include the process of toilet training, when diurnal continence was achieved, developmental delays, and whether the child has ever been dry at night and for how long. Prior to the first visit a nocturnal enuresis questionnaire can be completed by the child and parents and then reviewed as part of the history process (*see* Appendix at the end of this chapter). It is important for the clinician to ascertain how the problem has been dealt with in the past. Does the child awaken at night after urinating or does he or she sleep through until morning? Does the child wear a diaper at night? Who strips the bed and takes the sheets to the laundry area? Is the child responsible for his or her personal hygiene in the morning? What other enuresis treatments have been tried in the past? What are the parental attitudes about the child's condition? Most importantly, why does the child want to be dry? How will his or her life be better? What would the child like to be able to do that he or she feels he or she cannot do now? In the context of rapport building and history taking, the clinician begins to reframe the problem from "wet" to dry: beds are referred to as completely dry, mostly dry, or somewhat dry.

With the child's self-esteem at stake, the problem continues to be reframed. The clinician reminds the child that for 1,439 minutes each day, the child's brain and bladder work together perfectly. There is just one minute at nighttime that needs to be worked on. Appropriate to the developmental level of the child, the physiology of the brain-bladder-kidney connection is explained. The clinician may suggest having a telephone conversation between the brain and bladder. The bladder tells the brain it is full and needs to be emptied and the brain responds either to keep the sphincter muscle tight or the brain wakes the child up so that he or she can go the toilet. The child may be given the suggestion that he or she has a tool belt that contains all the tools needed to repair any faulty wiring between the brain and the bladder.

The clinician may suggest that the brain is like a computer that can be programmed for success. After determining whether the child would prefer to hold his or her pee through the night until morning or wake during the night to use the toilet, the clinician suggests that the preferred solution becomes the default setting on the brain's computer. However, the alternative solution is programmed in by the child as a backup. It is important for the child in trance to rehearse both scenarios in his or her imagination. The mental rehearsal is continued through waking up in the morning feeling dry and proud. The child may be given the suggestion to thank the parts of his body that worked so well and especially himself as the computer programmer who knew just the right way to program his or her brain's computer for success.

Other techniques include visualizing the bladder as a balloon blown up and tied with a very strong, safe, tight knot. The knot stays tied until the morning when the child arrives in the bathroom and unties it. Sports metaphors can be useful. If the child enjoys playing offense, the suggestion can be given that he or she is very good at waiting for just the right moment and then putting the ball exactly where it needs to go. If the child's interest is in defense, the metaphor changes slightly to noticing how nothing gets past him or her on the field unless he or she wants it to. Being the captain and telling all the players how to work together perfectly as a team can also be helpful.

Utilizing the child's reasons for wanting to be dry, the clinician may suggest the child visualize that time in the future fully experiencing the feelings of pride, happiness and excitement as he or she sleeps over at a friend's, attends summer camp, or goes on a vacation. Imagining a walk in the forest noticing how the birds fly from their nests, the chipmunks leave their burrow, and a deer wakes and moves from its sleeping place, and then all return to their warm, dry, sweet-smelling nests, is another metaphorical approach. The clinician may also read the child the story of Sugar Man, a meerkat who wets the bed from *Harry the Hypno-potamus: Metaphorical Tales for the Treatment of Children* (Thomson, 2005).

Keeping a calendar of success is important. This helps children visualize their progress and encourages future success. In trance, the child may imagine the calendar filled with happy, smiley faces or stickers and then a time this month or next when the calendar is no longer needed. Fundamentally, self-monitoring aids in dissociation, reframing and control of the problem by putting it down on paper.

It is important that the child own the problem. The child must be responsible for voiding before bed, stripping the sheets if wet and delivering them to the laundry, and personal morning hygiene. The child is encouraged to practice self-hypnosis nightly, checking in on the brain-bladder communication, visualizing success and perhaps reciting the mantra "Tight, tight, tight through the night, night, night." The parent is reminded not to remind the child about anything that pertains to the child's ownership of the problem. The parent, however, may offer praise for success. Ego-strengthening and the language of possibilities is a vital part of the hypnotic approach to enuresis: "I wonder what you will decide is the best part of being the boss of your body when you have been dry for two weeks?"

Tia

Tia was seen three times over a 5-week period. She conquered having dry beds after the second session. Tia practiced her self-hypnosis nightly and kept a calendar of her success. She was motivated and had a very specific goal in mind. In a follow-up conversation 5 months later, Tia's mother reported that not only had the hypnosis been helpful for Tia's enuresis, but her facial tic had also dramatically decreased. Three years later, when Tia entered high school, her tic increased. Tia knew that she had benefited from hypnotherapy in the past in controlling her "sleepwetting." Now she wanted to use it to eliminate her facial tic.

Chris

After multiple hypnosis sessions with Chris, there had been no change in his nightly enuresis. The possibility that Chris' nocturnal incontinence was the result of his SSRI was considered. In collaboration with Chris' therapist, he was weaned off the medication. His enuresis stopped, but the depression returned. Chris did not like the way he felt when he was not using the medication. He made the decision that he would rather feel well and wet the bed, than be dry and be depressed. The SSRI was re-instituted and the nightly enuresis recurred.

Amy

Amy practiced her self-hypnosis nightly including the mantra "Tight, tight, tight through the night, night, night." Using developmentally appropriate language, specific suggestions about increasing her own production of anti-diuretic hormone were given as she continued to decrease her dose of DDAVP. Along with the suggestions about making less urine during the night came a new mantra: "Make less for more success." At a follow-up visit 5 months after beginning hypnosis, Amy was dry every night and had stopped taking her DDAVP.

Mark

One month after Mark's first hypnosis session he returned with his calendar of success. His enuresis had decreased to one or two nights per week. His wet nights were reframed as mistakes, not failures, and mistakes can be corrected. Following the second session, Mark remained dry usually by awaking to go to the bathroom. He was also very happy to report at follow-up that he'd had a very successful sleepover.

Summary

Hypnosis may be the primary treatment for enuresis. It may also be used in conjunction with an alarm or medication. The clinician may suggest, "I wonder how wonderful it will be for you when you beat the buzzer." The child may also be encouraged to imagine that part of the brain (the posterior pituitary) that produces the anti-diuretic hormone, sending it a message to increase production so that the kidneys can make less urine during the night. When children are successful with their dry beds with hypnosis their self-esteem soars because they know they did it themselves. Their success was intrinsic, not dependent on a pill or a buzzer.

Encopresis

To Poop or Not to Poop

Drew, Benny, and Zach

Drew is a 10-year-old, fourth grade student with primary retentive encopresis. He was having explosive, large bowel movements once every 7 to 10 days. Occasionally he would make it to the toilet, but usually not. He had daily fecal soiling. According to his parents, he has never been motivated to do anything about the fecal soiling. Now, however, he would like to sleep over at a friend's house and go to overnight camp in the summer. Drew was now motivated and asked his parents to make an appointment to see me.

Drew achieved diurnal urinary continence just before entering kindergarten. Having bowel movements on the toilet had always been a problem. At 6½ his fecal soiling had been going on for about one year. Initially his parents were patient with the problem because Drew had started kindergarten and his parents were going through a divorce. They thought his problems were related to those issues and interpreted his fecal soiling as a willful decision not to go to the bathroom and interrupt his play. They tried all sorts of negative reinforcement and punishment without any change. Then they tried praise and positive reinforcements.

His physical exam was entirely normal other than the palpable dilated loops of bowel in his abdomen. Radiographic studies confirmed marked constipation with the presence of a large amount of stool in the colon.

Five-year-old Benny showed no interest in toilet training until well past 3 years old. By 4½, toilet training for stools was described as a "huge struggle." Benny refused to have a bowel movement anywhere but in his underwear. He had daily fecal soiling and bowel movements every 3 or 4 days. He was seen by a therapist who recommended negative reinforcement. Like many children with encopresis, Benny was misdiagnosed with oppositional defiant disorder. At age 5 he was evaluated by a gastroenterologist who suggested polyethylene glycol (Miralax), phenolphthalein (Ex-Lax), and making Benny responsible for helping his mother clean his underwear. When he returned to the gastroenterologist two months later, there had been no progress.

Zach was adopted from Guatemala at 4 months of age by an older professional couple. According to his mother, Zach was difficult to toilet train and never wanted to sit on the toilet seat so would withhold stool. Zach, now 7, was having a bowel movement every 3 to 5 days in his underwear with daily soiling. About every 3 weeks his stools were so large that they clogged the toilet.

Zach's problem had caused significant marital stress. His mother described Zach's father, a psychiatrist, as an angry person who dealt with other people's problems all day long and did not want to handle problems in his own home. The mother's and father's methods of coping with Zach's encopresis were quite different. The father was punitive and demeaning; the mother was sympathetic but ineffectual. She described Zach as a normal, well-adjusted, delightful 7-year-old in every other way but this.

Zach had a thorough evaluation with a pediatric gastroenterologist that revealed no organic cause for his retentive encopresis. He was also seen by a psychologist who misdiagnosed him with oppositional defiant disorder.

Evaluation and Medical Management

Encopresis is the term used when children beyond the developmental age for being toilet trained have stools in unacceptable places, usually their underwear. This may vary and fluctuate from fecal soiling to entire bowel movements outside of the toilet. Retentive encopresis is most often caused by or the result of the voluntary, self-perpetuating withholding of stool. Functional constipation results in overflow incontinence and most often has its beginnings with toilet training. Hypnotherapy, along with an initial catharsis and a consistent treatment plan, can have a significant positive effect on this difficult and frustrating problem.

During toilet training the child may decide that he or she does not like having a bowel movement on the toilet. Perhaps the child is more comfortable in a squatting position or hiding behind the couch. He or she may have fears about the toilet or the possibility of falling in, which at that age is not entirely unrealistic. Perhaps the child has not developed the patience to sit still long enough to complete the task of defecation. For these and other reasons the youngster may decide he or she just will not go at all rather than go in the toilet and the child withholds his or her stool. The child becomes very good at ignoring the urge and holding it in until he or she can no longer retain the stool. He or she then passes a large constipated stool that can be quite painful.

Developmentally, young children are literal, primary process thinkers. If it hurts to have a bowel movement, they are quite sure that they never want to do that again, so they continue to retain feces. This is not an abnormal response, but rather a basic attempt to avoid pain. The fear of having a painful bowel movement is reinforced each time they pass a hard, constipated stool. In turn, this establishes a self-perpetuating, cycle of stool-withholding. Animism, giving life and feelings to inanimate objects, is common in preschoolers. They may refer to their feces as "bad poops" for being the cause of their discomfort. The medical morbidities of this functional constipation include impaction, abdominal pain, anal fissures, hemorrhoids, rectal bleeding, urinary tract infections, and overflow diarrhea around the fecal mass.

The belief that the child with encopresis will "just grow out of it" has never been substantiated. VanGinkel, Reitsma, Buller, van Wijk, Taminiau, & Benninga (2003) did an 8-year follow-up on 8 children with encopresis. Constipation persisted in 4 out of the 8 children into young adulthood. Three out of the four who were successful with a regimen of enemas, laxatives, and a high fiber diet had frequent relapses. The researchers determined that the involuntary loss of feces had a major negative impact on the psychosocial functioning of the affected individual.

The psychological and social morbidities for both the child and the family can be devastating. These children commonly carry with them a fecal odor and may live in constant fear of being discovered, teased, and ridiculed. Children with encopresis and overflow soiling are commonly rejected by classmates, teachers, and even parents. This certainly can result in maladaptive social, developmental, and relational problems. The toll on self-esteem can be enormous. The child may suffer from anxiety, withdraw, and become depressed. At the time of diagnosis, many children with encopresis have behavioral problems including oppositionality, anxiety, depression, inattention, and hyperactivity. At times it can be difficult to determine which came first—the encopresis or the behavioral problems (Buttross, 1999). The child also becomes insensitive to the smell of his or her incontinence and tries desperately to appear indifferent to the problem. To save face and avoid shame, the child may hide the soiled underwear behind dressers, under beds, and in closets.

The first step in the clinical evaluation of the child with encopresis is to establish a therapeutic alliance with the child. This rapport and sense of trust is essential when working with a child with this emotionally charged condition. Another essential step in the evaluation is a thorough history including previous methods of management, the child's coping mechanisms, and his or her feelings about the problem and its effects on his or her life. The developmental, behavioral, and health history may elucidate pathophysiologic factors. A complete physical examination is needed to rule out any specific physical problems that may contribute to the constipation. Organic disorders such as hypothyroidism, spinal defects, abnormalities of calcium metabolism, and aganglionic megacolon need to be established or excluded. The presence of a physical condition does not preclude the use of hypnosis. The family and psychosocial history are also important and, of course, critical to understand.

Management of the child with encopresis with overflow soiling starts with demystifying the condition. The child lives in fear of exposure and most likely is the only child he or she knows with this problem. The child may be quite sure that he or she is the only one in the world who soils his or her pants, other than babies. Sometimes the child may be relieved just to know this problem has a name because then he or she is not the only one with the problem. Both the child and the parent need to understand that encopresis is not voluntary or intentional and is not the child's fault, but it is the child's responsibility. A developmentally appropriate explanation of the pathophysiology of encopresis should be given to both the child and the parents. The clinician joins with the child as a team to help him or her effectively restore bowel function and self-esteem. As with enuresis and all clinical problems, the clinician must know the child separate from the problem, thereby establishing a therapeutic alliance.

For any behavioral management to be effective, a thorough but gentle colonic clean-out must be accomplished with the understanding and involvement of the child. Given the control issues and autonomy needs inherent in encopresis, the use of enemas, suppositories or other intrusive techniques (such as digital disimpaction) should be avoided unless necessary to ensure a successful clean-out. If they are needed, they must be done with as much cooperation and control on the part of the child as possible. Abdominal roentgenograms can be done before and after the catharsis and shown, with explanation, to the child to help his or her imagery and understanding of the problem.

When the large intestine is empty, then the biobehavioral maintenance program can be implemented. The family and significant others such as babysitters, teachers, or school nurses need to be informed about and involved in implementing the management plan. It is important that they be educated about encopresis so that their words and actions do not undermine success and the youngster's self-esteem.

As part of the maintenance plan the child is asked to sit on the toilet after breakfast and after supper each day. An appropriate amount of time might be one minute for each year of age up to a maximum of 10 minutes. It is also helpful when the child can place his or her feet on a small stool that allows the knees to be higher than the hips as the child sits on the toilet. It is suggested that he or she keep a favorite book or video game in the bathroom for use during this time. The child is praised for sitting even if no bowel movement resulted. Of course, extra praise is given when the child defecates before the timer goes off and beats the buzzer. A diet rich in fiber with plentiful amounts of water is encouraged. Initially the child with retentive encopresis may need a daily dose of a laxative, stool softener, mineral oil, or polyethylene glycol to keep the stools soft. A goal, however, is that by making dietary adjustments these products will no longer be necessary.

It is necessary for the parents and the clinician to understand and appreciate the fact that incontinence for the child with encopresis is unanticipated. The child with encopresis may not feel the urge to defecate in the same way as children without this problem. Because the child has absent or greatly diminished perceptual awareness of the need to have a bowel movement he or she should never be punished for fecal accidents. The vast majority of accidents in patients with retentive encopresis and overflow soiling are not willful acts of defiance, nor do they represent laziness or immaturity. Although the child should not be penalized for incontinence, he or she must be taught, expected, and helped to assume ownership of the problem and needs to be held accountable for sitting twice a day on the toilet for a specified period of time, caring appropriately for soiled underwear, and taking medications if prescribed. The parents are responsible for the initial clean-out, providing a diet rich in fiber along with any stool softeners or laxatives, and generous amounts of praise for their child's increasing responsibility.

Children benefit from keeping a calendar of success. As mentioned with self-monitoring of enuresis, calendars also potentiate dissociation and control. The calendar may include stickers or smiley faces for sitting on the toilet, having a bowel movement on the toilet, having clean underwear, and for taking medication. Success begets success. As the child sees the progress he or she is making, it encourages him or her to continue the maintenance program. The calendar may also reveal problem areas such as an afternoon accident happening after forgetting the morning toileting routine.

Hypnotherapeutic Approach

Hypnosis can augment and enhance the biobehavioral approach to encopresis. The addition of hypnotherapy to the management gives the child the responsibility for his or her own solution and the opportunity to be in control of his or her bodily functions. The child has a phobia about defecating predicated on pain. In the trance state, the child can be taught to imagine sitting on the toilet in comfort instead of in fear and anticipation of discomfort. The child can imagine having a bowel movement easily and comfortably and how good and how proud that makes him or her feel. Of course, the child gets to use self-hypnosis while sitting on the toilet, associating its effects with success.

The hypnotic trance state decreases a patient's anxiety and may be used to increase motivation and sense of control. The patient's motivation can be reflected back in trance. Perhaps the child will chose to imagine a sleepover, summer camp, or a family vacation. Hypnosis must be personalized to the developmental level and specialized interests of the child. Biofeedback has also been used to teach patient's with encopresis sphincter control and may be combined with hypnosis. However, some patients may feel that the use of a biofeedback anal sphincter probe is intrusive.

In a study by Olness (1977), 20 children with encopresis were divided into two groups. In addition to medical management, half were taught self-hypnosis and half received biofeedback training of the anorectal sphincters. Eight out of ten children in the self-hypnosis group were successful and nine out of ten in the biofeedback group. In another study, Olness (1976) concludes that success is chiefly the result of the children being responsible for their own solutions.

Metaphors can be very powerful and fun for children. Metaphors allow the child to gain a new perspective as he or she views the problem in a non-threatening, engaging, and memorable way. Metaphors can bypass natural resistance to change and offer a possible solution by generating new patterns of consciousness and expanding the boundaries of the subjective experience.

Putting things where they need to go at just the right time can be incorporated into a sports metaphor such as shooting a basket or making a soccer goal. If the child is interested in sports, mastery metaphors about being the captain of the team and telling all the players exactly what he or she would like them to do can be useful. The hypnotherapist may suggest noticing how all the child's muscles work together perfectly. The child may imagine a boat traveling down a winding river. Just before the river is ready to empty into the ocean, there is a drawbridge. It opens twice a day to let the boats go through. If a boat needs to pass through at any other time, the boat can toot its horn to signal the guard of the bridge to work the controls that open the bridge and allow the boat to easily pass through (Thomson, 2005).

Another metaphor suitable for children with encopresis concerns a gatehouse. A tractor trailer truck drives up to the gate house. The guard is asleep and doesn't open the gate. Motorcycles come up behind the big truck and decide to go around and sneak right under the gate. Then the big 18-wheeler decides to crash the gate. The guard's boss has a decision to make. He can either fire him for sleeping on the job or give him another chance. He decides to give him another chance. Then the boss discovers that the battery for the alarm inside the guard house that is supposed to signal the guard when a vehicle is coming needs to be replaced because it hasn't been used in a long time. The guard promises his boss not to fall asleep, the alarm is working again, the gate has been repaired, and traffic is moving along just right when the gate is opened by the guard at just the appropriate times (Thomson, 2008, publication pending).

The therapeutic alliance and rapport between the child and the clinician is vitally important to the success of the hypnotic intervention. Consistency and long term follow-up of children with encopresis is necessary. Many have been the victim of erratic management for years, fluctuating between punitive coercion and intentional avoidance and disregard.

Ego-strengthening is part of every hypnotic strategy. Hypnosis is structured to reinforce the child's confidence, sense of personal responsibility, and mastery. When a child has successfully conquered his or her problem with encopresis, the child and the family are forever grateful. A huge burden has been lifted allowing self-esteem to flourish. It is true that the clinician has given the child an incredible gift—a tool to tap into his or her own inner strengths and resources. However, it is the child who needs to be credited with the success.

For Drew, Benny, and Zach the pain–retention cycle was explained in a developmentally appropriate manner and the problem reframed. The three "nots" were discussed with each child: He was "not" the only child with this problem; it was "not" voluntary; and it was "not" his fault, but it was his responsibility. Each child's motivation to change was assessed and treatment goals established. An initial clean-out was instituted. Polyethylene glycol was added to a diet newly rich with fiber. Sitting on the toilet after breakfast and supper was agreed upon in order to help the child capture and increase his awareness of the gastrocolic reflex. He would assume all responsibility for his personal hygiene, the first rinse of any soiled underwear and putting them in the laundry. Each child would keep a calendar of success.

Drew
For Drew the goals of the hypnotherapy were realized in 5 sessions over a 2-month period. Using the trance state, Drew visualized letting stools pass comfortably and easily into the toilet while sitting comfortably relaxed. Drew imagined future success and a time without the problem. Ego-strengthening suggestions were given to enhance self-efficacy, and mastery metaphors were incorporated into each hypnotic session.

Drew was motivated to learn to resolve and control his humiliating problem. He had a specific goal in mind of attending summer camp and stuck to the plan. He assumed ownership of the problem and practiced his self-hypnosis regularly when sitting on the toilet and at bedtime. Within the first month, his encopresis had improved dramatically and by the end of the second month had virtually resolved. At one year follow-up he was continuing to do exceptionally well and had used his skills of self-regulation and self-hypnosis to help himself with another problem related to anxiety.

Benny

Benny was seen five times with tremendous improvement and success. Benny brought his Super Duper Pooper Chart with him to each visit. He got a sticker for just sitting on the toilet in the morning and another for sitting after supper, a sticker for having a bowel movement in the toilet, and another for a day with clean underwear. With Benny, no formal hypnotic induction was ever needed. Together we had read the story of "Lonnie the llama" who had encopresis from *Harry the Hypno-potamus: Metaphorical Tales for the Treatment of Children* (Thomson, 2005). Benny thrived on the positive reinforcement of the Super Duper Pooper chart. Parental support, consistency, and the therapeutic alliance that developed all contributed to his success. The careful use of language, esteem building, and ego-strengthening were also important.

Zach

For Zach success did not come easily. Six weeks after the initial visit his parents had still not done the initial clean-out because it had been inconvenient; there was never a good time. According to the mother, there wasn't time in the morning for him to sit on the toilet either. She didn't think Zach would like the Miralax so she hadn't gotten any yet. Despite our plans to the contrary, the father was still in charge of washing Zach's bottom.

Zach enjoyed hetero- hypnosis that was full of mastery metaphors, ego-strengthening, and imagining success, but he rarely practiced self-hypnosis. He began sitting on the toilet for the first time. However, he was literally up against a brick wall. His abdomen was still full of stool; no catharsis had ever been attempted. The Visiting Nurses Association was contacted to come to the home to do the enemas due to the family's inability to accomplish this task

Visits to my office were very sporadic. Seven months later, there were no consistent toileting practices, no Miralax being given, and the parents were still cleansing his bottom. Zach was having continuous fecal soiling, large amounts of stool in his underwear and none in the toilet. He routinely hid his soiled underwear. According to the mother, the father was verbally abusive to Zach and to her, and the marriage was deteriorating.

Two years after first beginning hypnosis, the parents were divorcing. Zach was refusing to rinse out his underwear and was hiding it all over the house. He would not sit on the toilet and was having daily bowel movements in his pants. The child's efforts need to be supported not thwarted. The not-so-subtle message that Zach received was that his problem was an annoying inconvenience to his parents, the cause for many an argument, and that supporting him in his quest to solve it was not all that important. Despite this troubling problem, at least it gave him a measure of control in his family. Dysfunctional family systems are a common saboteur of a child's motivation for self-regulation and development.

Summary

These cases represent the importance of having all family members in acceptance and agreement with the plan. Although the child needs to assume ownership of the problem, consistent, loving support is needed from the parents. The parents are responsible for the initial clean-out. The parents need to secure and provide the prescribed laxatives, suppositories or stool softeners, and bring the child in for regular follow-up appointments. If the morning or evening schedule does not allow for relaxed toileting time, then the schedule needs to be readjusted to make this a priority for the child.

Hypnosis is not *the* treatment for encopresis. It can be a highly successful adjunct to treatment. Medical management and parental support are critical pieces. Encopresis requires a positive, supportive team approach.

Conclusions

These clinical examples are representative of the success and failure of hypnotic work with children with elimination disorders. Tia, Amy, and Mark assumed ownership of their problem with enuresis; they were motivated to make changes and had specific goals in mind. Their parents, while being supportive, gave the children the space and the freedom to autonomously become the boss of their "pee." Although Chris was unsuccessful in having all dry beds, he learned valuable skills that he can use and adapt to meet other situations in his life. Someday he will decide to control his enuresis despite the SSRI. When that time comes, he knows that he has a caring, competent professional who will partner with him in his quest for self-mastery. In the case of Drew and Benny, hypnotic intervention for encopresis was combined with supportive parents who accomplished an initial catharsis and followed through with the maintenance program and regular visits. That combined with the youngsters' efforts to be the boss of their poops helped them overcome this devastating disorder. In Zach's case he was trying hard, but hard, hard stool and his parents' inability to see his needs over their own obstructed his success.

The therapeutic alliance between clinician and child that is an integral part of the hypnotic intervention is a vitally important factor in determining the success of hypnosis. Joining with the child as a partner supports and empowers the child to take charge of his or her body and his or her "pee" or "poop." Getting to know the child separate from the enuresis or encopresis and making it fun for him or her is fundamentally important. For children with an elimination disorder, "fun" has never been linked with their embarrassing condition. Incorporating therapeutic metaphors into the treatment helps the child view the problem from a different perspective: altering, re-interpreting, and re-framing. The best and most effective metaphors are the ones the children develop themselves. Their creativity and imaginative ability are boundless. The relaxation response and ego-strengthening that are integral to every hypnotic experience are also beneficial and reinforcing adjuncts to the medical management of an elimination disorder. Self-confidence flourishes when children learn to control what they never knew they could by tapping into their own inner strengths. This self-efficacy and self-mastery enhance self-esteem. The child has been given an incredible gift. He or she now owns these self-regulatory techniques and can use them throughout his or her life for his or her own benefit.

References

Banerjee, S., Srivastav, A., Palan, B. M. (1993). Hypnosis and self-hypnosis in the management of nocturnal enuresis: A comparative study with imipramine therapy. *American Journal of Clinical Hypnosis.* 36(2), 113–119.

Baumann, F. W., Hinman, F. (1974). Treatment of incontinent boys with non-obstructive disease. *Journal of Urology*, 111, 114–116.

Behrman, R. E., Kliegman, R. M. & Jenson, H. B. (2000). *Nelson textbook of pediatrics* (16th ed.) Philadelphia: WB Saunders.

Benninga, M. A., Voskuijl, W. P., Taminiau, J. A. (2004). Childhood constipation: Is there light at the end of the tunnel? *Journal of Pediatric Gastroenterology Nutrition.* 39(5), 448–464.

Bloom, D. A., Seeley, W. W., Ritchey, M. I., McGuire, E. J. (1993). Toilet habits and continence in children: An opportunity sampling in search of normal parameters. *Journal of Urology*, 149, 1087–1090.

Blum, N. J. (2004). Nocturnal enuresis: Behavioral treatment. *Urologic Clinics of North America,* 31(3), 499–507.

Browne, S. E. (1997). Brief hypnosis with passive children. *Contemporary Hypnosis.* 14(1) 59–62.

Butler, R. J. (1998). Annotation: Night wetting in children, psychological aspects. *Journal of Child Psychology and Psychiatry,* 39, 453–463.

Buttross, S. (1999). Encopresis in the child with a behavioral disorder: When the initial treatment does not work. *Pediatric Annals,* 28(5), 317–321.

Chang, S. S., Ng, C. F., & Wong, S. N. (2002). Hong Kong Childhood Enuresis Study Group. Behavioral problems in children and parenting stress associated with primary nocturnal enuresis in Hong Kong. *Acta Paediatrica,* 91, 475–479.

Claydon, G. S., & Lawson, J. (1976). Investigation and management of long-standing chronic constipation in childhood. *Archives of Diseases of Childhood*, 51, 918–923.

Collison, D. R. (1970). Hypnotherapy in the management of nocturnal enuresis. *Medical Journal of Australia*, 1, 52–54.

Culbert, T., Kajander, R., Reaney, J. (1996). Biofeedback with children and adolescence: Clinical observation and patient perspective. *Journal of Developmental and Behavioral Pediatrics*, 17(5), 342–350.

DeLorijn, F., vanWijk, M. P., Reitsma, J. B., vanGinkel, R., Taminiau, J. A., & Benninga, M. A. (2004). Prognosis of constipation: Clinical factors and colonic transit time. *Archives of Diseases of Childhood*, 89(8), 723–727.

DiLorenzo, C., & Benninga, M. A. (2004). Pathophysiology of pediatric fecal incontinence. *Gastroenterology*, 126(Suppli 1), S33–40.

Doleys, D. M. (1977). Behavioral treatments for nocturnal enuresis in children: A review of the literature. *Psychological Bulletin*, 84, 30–54.

Edward, S. D., & van der Spuy, H. I. (1985). Hypnotherapy as a treatment for enuresis. *Journal Child Psychology and Psychiatry*, 26, 161–170.

Fleisher, D. R. (1976). The diagnosis and treatment of disorders of defecation in children. *Pediatric Annals*, 5, 700–722.

Forsythe, W. I., & Butler, R. J. (1989). Fifty years of enuretic alarms. *Archives of Diseases of Childhood*, 64, 879–885.

Forsythe, W. I., & Redmond, A. (1974). Enuresis and spontaneous cure rate study of 1,129 enuretics. *Archives of Diseases of Childhood*, 49, 259–263.

Friman, P., & Jones, K. (1998). Elimination disorders in children. In T. Wartson & F. Gresham (Eds.) *Handbook of child behavior therapy*. New York: Plenum Press.

Glicklich, L. B. (1951). An historical account of enuresis. *Pediatrics*, 8, 859–876.

Gottsegen, D. (2003). Curing bedwetting on the spot: A review of one session cures. *Clinical Pediatrics*, 42(3), 273–275.

Hagglof, B., Andren, O., Bergstrom, E., Marklund, L., & Wendelius, M. (1997). Self-esteem before and after treatment in children with nocturnal enuresis and urinary incontinence. *Scandinavian Journal of Urology and Nephrology*, Supplement 183: 79–82.

Halpern, W. I. (1977). The treatment of encopretic children. *Journal of the American Academy of Child Psychiatry*, 16, 478–499.

Hobbie, C. (1989). Relaxation techniques for children and young people. *Journal of Pediatric Health Care*, 3(2), 83–87.

Jarvelin, M. R., Moilanen, I., Vikevainen-Tervonen, L., & Huttman, N. P. (1990). Life changes and protective capacities in enuretic and non-enuretic children. *Journal of Child Psychology and Psychiatry*, 31, 763–774.

Johnson, M. (1998). Nocturnal enuresis. *Urologic Nursing*, 18(4), 259–275.

Kohen, D. P., Colwell, S. O., Heimel, A., & Olness, K. N. (1984). The use of relaxation/mental imagery (self-hypnosis) in the management of 505 pediatric behavioral encounters. *Journal of Developmental and Behavioral Pediatrics*, 5(1), 2–25.

Kohen, D. P. (1990). A hypnotherapeutic approach to enuresis. In D. C. Hammond (Ed.), *Handbook of hypnotic suggestions and metaphors*. New York: W.W. Norton.

Kolvin, I. (1973). *Bladder control and enuresis*. Philadelphia: Lippincott.

Lawless, M. R., & McElderry, D. H. (2001). Nocturnal enuresis: Current concepts. *Pediatric Review*, 22, 399–406.

Levine, M. D. (1982). Encopresis its potentiation, evaluation and alleviation. *Pediatric Clinics of North America*, 29(2), 318.

Levine, M. D. (1981). The schoolchild with encopresis. *Pediatrics in Review*, 2(9), 285–290.

Levine, M. D. (1982). Encopresis. *Psychosocial Issues in Child Health Care*, 80, 696–699.

Loening-Baucke, V. (1990). Modulation of abnormal defecation dynamic by biofeedback treatment in chronically constipated children with encopresis. *Journal of Pediatrics*, 116, 214–222.

Mantle, F. (1999). Hypnosis in the treatment of enuresis. *Pediatric Nursing*, 11(6), 33–36.

Miller, K. & Atkin, B. (1992). New insights into the cause and treatment of bedwetting. *Family Practice Recertification*, 14(7), 129–142.

Milling, L. S., & Costantino, C. A. (2000). Clinical hypnosis with children: First steps toward empirical support. *International Journal of Clinical and Experimental Hypnosis*, 48(2), 113–137.

Moffatt, M. (1989). Nocturnal enuresis: Psychological implications of treatment and nontreatment. *Journal of Pediatrics*, 114, 697–704.

Mosier, W. A. (1998). Update on childhood enuresis. *The Clinical Advisor*, 32–34.

National Kidney Foundation. (2003). Available at: http://www.kidney.org

Olness, K. N. (1975). The use of self-hypnosis in the treatment of childhood nocturnal enuresis: A report on forty patients. *Clinical Hypnosis*, 14, 273–279.

Olness, K. N. (1976). Autohypnosis in functional megacolon in children. *American Journal of Clinical Hypnosis*, 19, 28–32.

Olness, K. N. (1977). *Comparison of hypnotherapy and biofeedback in management of fecal soiling in children.* Paper presented at the annual meeting of the Society for Clinical and Experimental Hypnosis, Los Angeles.

Olness, K. N. (1977). How to help the wet child and the frustrated parents. *Modern Medicine*, 45, 42–46.

Olness, K. N., McParland, F. A., & Piper, J. (1980). Biofeedback: A new modality in the management of children with fecal soiling. *Journal of Pediatrics*, 96, 505–509.

Olness, K. & Kohen, D. P. (1996). *Hypnosis and hypnotherapy with children,* (3rd ed.). New York: Guilford Press.

Owens-Stively, J., McCain, D., & Wynne, E. (1986). *Childhood constipation and soiling: A practical guide for parents and children.* Minneapolis: Behavioral Pediatrics Program, Minneapolis Children's Medical Center.

Parker, P. H. (1999). To do or not to do? That is the question. *Pediatric Annals*, 28(5), 283–290.

Rushton, H. G. (1989). Nocturnal enuresis: Epidemiology, evaluation and currently available treatment options. *Journal of Pediatrics*, 691–696.

Schmitt, B. D. (1990). Nocturnal enuresis: Finding the treatment that fits the child. *Contemporary Pediatrics*, 2, 70–97.

Stanton, H. E. (1979). Short-term treatment of enuresis. *American Journal of Clinical Hypnosis*, 22, 103–107.

Sussman, D., & Culbert, T. (1999). Pediatric self-regulation. In M. D. Levine, W. B. Carey, A. C. Crocker (Eds.). *Developmental-behavioral pediatrics* (3rd ed.). Philadelphia: W. B. Saunders.

Teets, J. M. (1992). Enuresis: Nursing diagnosis and treatment. *Journal of Community Health Nursing*, 9(2), 95–101.

Thomson, L. (2002). Hypnosis for habit disorders. *Advance for Nurse Practitioners*, 59–62

Thomson, L. (2005). *Harry the hypno-potamus: Metaphorical tales for the treatment of children*. Carmarthen, Wales, U.K.: Crown House.

Thomson, L. (2008, publication pending). *Harry the hypno-potamus: More metaphorical tales for the treatment of children*. Carmarthen, Wales, U.K.: Crown House.

Tilton, P. (1980) Hypnotic treatment of a child with thumbsucking, enuresis and encopresis. *American Journal of Clinical Hypnosis*, 22, 238–240.

VanGinkel, R., Reitsma, J. B., Buller, H.A., van Wijk, M.P., Taminiau, J.A., & Benninga, M.A. (2003). Childhood constipation: Longitudinal follow-up beyond puberty. *Gastroenterology*, 125(2), 357–363.

VonHoecke, E., Baeyens, D., Walle, J. V., & Hoebeke, P. (2003). Socioeconomic status as a common factor underlying the association between enuresis and psychopathology. *Journal of Developmental and Behavioral Pediatrics*, 24, 109–114.

Wicks, G. (2005). Bedwetting and toileting problems in children. *Medical Journal of Australia*, 596.

Appendix: Nocturnal Enuresis Questionnaire

Nocturnal enuresis means urinating, wetting, or "peeing" in the bed at night. Your answers to the following questions about this problem will help me to understand how best to help you with it. These questions are about you, the patient. Parents or guardians and children/adolescents can complete this form together. Circle, check, or write in the answer that best tells about you.

Young person's name _____

Preferred or nickname _____

Special pronunciation _____

Birth date _____   Today's date _____

Person helping to complete this form _____

1. How old were you when you started urinating in the toilet during the day? _____ years
2. How many nights each week do you usually stay dry?
   0   1   2   3   4   5   6
3. What is the longest you have ever been dry every night in a row?
   a. _____ Days   b. _____ Weeks   c. _____Months
4. Please check any and all of the following ways you have ever used to stay dry at night. Circle any of them you are using now.
   ____ Diaper or "Pull-up"   ____ Alarm Clock wakes at night
   ____ Drinking little or less after dinner
   ____ Accupuncture/Accupressure   ____ Hypnosis
   ____ Trying to remember to keep dry ____ Parent wakes at night
   ____ Keeping "Dry Night" calendar
   ____ Punishment for wet nights   ____ Rewards for dry nights
   ____ Enuresis Alarm (Device that makes noise/vibrates when wet)
   _____ (Brand Name of Device)
5. Have you ever used any of these medicines to treat enuresis?
   (Check all that apply)
   ____Imipramine (Tofranil) Dose:_____
   ____Desmopressin (DDAVP) Dose:_____
   ____Oxybutinin (Ditropan) Dose:_____
   ____Homeopathic medicine_____
   ____Herbal Substance: _____
   ____Other: _____

6. Do you sometimes drink caffeinated drinks (soda, tea, coffee) during or after dinner?   Yes   No
7. When you need to urinate during the day, do you have to go right away?   Yes   No
8. Do you sometimes urinate in your clothes by accident during the day?   Yes   No
   If "Yes" how many times each week? 1   2   3   4   5   6   7   7+
9. Do you sometimes have a bowel movement (BM, "poop") in your clothes by accident during the day? Yes   No
   If "Yes" how many times each week? 1   2   3   4   5   6   7   7+
10. Is it hard for you to have a bowel movement most days?   Yes   No
11. Do you take any medicine to help you have bowel movements most days?   Yes No
    If "Yes," what medicine(s)?_____
12. Do you have any other medical or health problems? Yes   No
    If "Yes," please check all that apply
    ____ Learning problems
    ____ Attention Deficit Disorder (ADD, ADHD)
    ____ Diabetes   ____ Constipation
    ____ Kidney/bladder problems   ____ Bladder infections
    ____ Sleep problems   ____ Seizures
    ____ Allergies: _____
    ____ Something else:_____
13. Do you take any other medicines?   Yes   No
    If "Yes," what medicine(s):_____
14. Did either of your parents, or any uncles, aunts or cousins have enuresis as a child?   Yes   No
    If "Yes," who:
    ____Mother   ____Father
    ____Sister   ____Brother
    ____Cousin   ____Aunt (Mother's Side)
    ____Uncle (Mother's Side)   ____Aunt (Father's Side)
    ____Uncle (Father's Side)
15. Is enuresis a problem for you? Yes   No
    If "Yes," check all reasons why it is a problem that fit for you, circle the most important one.
    ____Can't do sleepovers   ____Embarrassing on vacations
    ____Have to wash my sheets/pajamas a lot
    ____Getting teased   ____Parents are upset
    ____Don't like wearing diapers
    ____Don't feel good about myself
    ____Can't get a new bed   ____Something else:

    _____

Thank you for answering these questions. If there is more you want us to know, or if there are questions you want us to answer for you, or if you'd like to draw a picture, please use a clean piece of paper.

Chapter Eighteen

Hypnosis for Children and Adolescents with Recurrent Pain

Laurence I. Sugarman, MD, FAAP, ABMH

Although the world is full of suffering, it is full also of the overcoming of it.
Helen Keller, 1903,
U.S. blind and deaf educator (1880–1968)

In the American Desert there lives a species of lizard commonly called the ground skink (family *Scincidae*). At full-size, more than half of its body is comprised of its tail, which it counts on most predators to grab. As a mechanism of escape, it practices *autotomy*, or self-amputation (Aaron M. Bauer, 1993). When assaulted by an eagle for example, its tail detaches, leaving the rest of the skink free to run away and grow a new one. When its tail comes off, a signal is sent to the skink's brain. Because the skink has a primitive brain, that signal probably does not evoke deep emotion, meaning, poetry, or persecution. It is only a message to scurry away to some-place safe and grow a new tail.

Pain is just a signal, if you are a ground skink.

The use of hypnosis for pain is perhaps the longest studied and most dramatic of all forms of hypnotherapy. In part, this is because of the power pain holds in our lives. Pain is the ultimate metaphor. Many of the problems that bring young people to us for care—anx-iety, sleep disturbance, elimination disorders, depression, coping with chronic disease—can be experienced as "painful." If, as in the context proposed in Chapter One, hypnotherapy is a skill set that helps young people become more adaptive during formative years, then the ability to master life's pains early on is a powerful investment. It could be argued that the clinician who understands how to help the child or adolescent with chronic or recurring pain *can help* anyone; or, that the child who learns to manage pain and suffering with equanimity, *can do* anything.

This chapter is specifically *not* about acute pain experiences. Chapter Fourteen, "Integrating Hypnosis in Acute Care Settings," addresses acute pain, both procedural and spontaneous. Nor is this chapter about chronic persistent pain. Although some children and adolescents experience constant pain lasting greater than three months, recurring pain is more common. The realms of acute, chronic, and recurrent pain largely overlap. Each acute pain experience colors and informs subsequent discomfort both neurologically and psychologically. Indeed, sometimes it is difficult to know, in a given child's history, when acute episodes of pain become a more persistent experience. As we shall see, recurrent acute pain episodes can heighten pain sensitivity both peripherally (outside the brain and spinal cord) and within the central nervous system to play a role in the evolution of recurrent pain syndromes (Fitzgerald & Howard, 2003). Common recurrent pain syndromes in childhood and adolescents are listed in Table 18.1. For most, our understanding of the pathophysiology and treatment is insufficient, and allopathic therapies (medication and surgery) are inadequate. This is why there is great potential for research aimed at the role of hypnosis and, more broadly, self-regulation training, in preventing chronic and recurrent pain in children and adolescents.

What Is Pain?

The International Association for the Study of Pain defines pain as "An unpleasant sensory and emotional experience associated with actual or potential tissue damage" (International Association for the Study of Pain, 1979, pp. 249–252). This definition captures the essential dual nature of the pain experience: it intertwines both physiological and psychological variables. Nociception refers to

Table 18.1: Recurrent Pain Syndromes and Diseases that Commonly Cause Recurrent Pain in Children and Adolescents

- Abdominal Migraines
- Complex Regional Pain Syndrome (reflex sympathetic dystrophy)
- Discogenic back pain
- Dysmenorrheal
- Endometriosis
- Headaches
- Hemophilia
- Fibromylagia
- Hypermobility Syndromes
- Irritable Bowel Syndrome
- Migraine Headaches
- Pelvic Pain (as a sequel of pelvic inflammatory disease)
- Pain related to a variety of chronic diseases (Fabry Disease, Cystic Fibrosis, Neurofibromatosis, Juvenile Rheumatoid Arthritis)
- Recurrent Abdominal Pain
- Recurrent Postoperative Pain
- Sickle cell disease

the component of pain that is solely attributable to the amount of tissue damage without regard to the developmental, emotional, historical, and other psychological components. Interestingly, we do not have an equally simple term for these other components, even though the pain experience, especially recurrent pain, is rarely directly proportionate to its nociceptive portion. Clinicians have long recognized the lack of a one-to-one correlation between the extent of tissue damage and the degree of suffering. From an evolutionary perspective, it makes sense that as higher brain functions evolved, so would the complexity of interpretation of the pain signal. This higher level of complexity grows disproportionately to the nociceptive elements and more proportionately to the pain's meaning. With this complexity comes a higher capacity for suffering, and "also of the overcoming of it" (Keller, 1903). As Dabney Ewin put it, "The strain of the pain is mainly in the brain" (D. Ewin, personal communication, November 1, 1998).

There is a tendency, when physiological evidence is lacking, not to believe the child or adolescent (or adult) who says he or she is in pain. This leads to an under appreciation of suffering and alienation: the opposite of rapport. There has been a tendency for healthcare providers to view recurrent pain syndromes as exclusively organic or psychogenic, "real" or "fake." In fact, the majority of pediatric recurrent pain syndromes have real pain that results from the interplay of physical, psychological, temperamental, and environmental factors leading to what has been called "biopsychosocial dysfunctional pain" (Poole, Schmitt, & Mauro, 1995, pp. 47–77). For whatever reasons young people say they feel pain, whether it is a wholly conscious misrepresentation of conflict (malingering) or a deeply subconscious somatic discomfort, it represents some form of distress. It is still a signal that needs to be addressed. As Schechter, Berde and Yaster (2003) put it, "Pain is whatever the individual experiencing it says that it is and exists whenever he or she says that it does" (p.14).

Relevant Neurobiology of Pain

Our understanding of the neurobiology of pain can be divided into *peripheral* and *central* components even though these regions influence each other. The reader is referred to basic texts on the subject, and especially *Pain in Infants, Children, and Adolescents* (Schechter, Berde, & Yaster, 2003) for a thorough examination of the known psychophysiological mechanisms of the pain experience. There are three concepts that can be gleaned from this literature that are relevant to the role of hypnosis in the treatment of pain. The first is *transduction*, a term that generally refers to changing one form of energy into another. In the nervous system, transduction refers to the conversion of stimuli detected by receptors on cells to electrical impulses that are then transported to the nervous system, as in the conversion of sound waves to neural impulses in the ear. The next term is *plasticity*. This refers to the ability of the nervous system to alter its sensitivity in response to stimuli. This is accomplished through a variety of mechanisms, including altering cellular response thresholds, growing more receptors, making more synapses between cells, recruiting cells, and growing new cells or cell death. The third term refers more commonly to the psychological realm, but as we shall see, impacts the other two. It is *dissociation*, the treatment of something as distinct or unconnected.

It is the ability to dissociate, to separate oneself from a normally connected experience that can allow an individual to alter both the transduction and plasticity of pain.

In order to understand the influence of transduction and plasticity on the experience of children and adolescents, let us track pain pathways in a young nervous system. When a noxious stimulus, a needle for example, punctures the skin, that sensation is transduced by sensors (so-called nociceptors and others) that respond to mechanical, thermal, and chemical stimuli. Not only are these sensors fully present at birth, but also they are more sensitive (having lower thresholds) in infants than in adults. With recurrent stimulation, a variety of factors, including H^+, K^+, serotonin, histamine, prostaglandins, cytokines, and nerve growth factors, stimulate intracellular gene expression thereby allowing a lower intensity of stimulus to evoke pain (Woolf & Costigan, 1999). This constitutes plasticity in the cells that transduce stimuli in the periphery. In addition, repeated inputs, via nerves carrying this transduced stimulation, activate cells in the spinal cord such that they respond to normal inputs in an exaggerated and extended manner. These cells, in turn, send increased impulses to higher centers of the brain where they project, through the thalamus and limbic systems, to higher centers including the somatosensory cortex and the anterior cingulate cortex (Rainville, Duncan, Price, Carrier, & Bushnell, 1997). These higher centers enact associations of meaning, emotion, and sympathetic nervous system activation (the "fight or flight response") (Woolf & Manion, 1999, pp. 1959–1964). In addition, this increased input stimulates more brain plasticity, further augmenting sensitivity by a mechanism yet to be elucidated (Fitzgerald & Howard, 2003). Originating in higher centers of the brain, descending pathways modulate the output of nociceptive neurons in the periphery (Dubner & Ren, 1999). These descending inhibitory controls are immature at birth and still maturing in adolescence (Fitzgerald, 1991). The lack of descending inhibition in young children means that an important intrinsic analgesic system is lacking, and the effects of noxious stimuli on the central nervous system may therefore be more profound than in the adult (Fitzgerald & Howard, 2003).

The persistent nature of sensitization is exemplified in two studies. In the first, infants who were circumcised without anesthesia displayed a stronger pain response to subsequent routine vaccination at 4 and 6 months than uncircumcised infants. Anesthetic applied prior to circumcision attenuated the pain response to subsequent vaccination (Taddio, Katz, Ilersich, et al., 1997). A study of children aged 6 to 17 years with chronic juvenile arthritis shows that background recurrent pain alters acute pain thresholds. Both inflamed joints and noninflamed paraspinal areas show reduced pain thresholds that remain even when the primary inflammation has subsided, suggesting a central cause for sensitization (Fitzgerald & Howard, 2003). In summary, human beings generally respond to repeated injury with increased sensitivity in order to protect themselves. This tendency towards hypersensitivity is accentuated in early years and informs subsequent behavior.

How is Pain Detrimental?

Regardless of the relative contributions of nociceptive and psychosocial components of pain, ongoing pain hurts us. Repeated pain contributes to "rewiring" of neural pathways in the spinal cord and brain leading to increased and ongoing pain sensitivity in infants as young as 24 weeks (Fitzgerald, 1994; Porter, German, & Anand, 1999). Repeated acute pain triggers the release of a cascade of hormones and other chemical substances that further amplify pain responsiveness and activate the sympathetic nervous system. The stress hormones that are part of this autonomic response increase the metabolic rate and, when they persist, have significant injurious effects on the cardiovascular, gastrointestinal, immune, and hematological systems. In this way the physiological processes that heighten sensitivity and vulnerability to pain contribute to a vicious cycle of more pain, disability, and vulnerability (Schechter et al., 2003). Furthermore, these conditioned physiological responses can be triggered simply by the threat of pain, dissociated from actual nociception, such that chronic or recurrent pain becomes a learned, self-perpetuating behavior (Fordyce, 2001). However it is derived, for whatever original, protective reason, recurrent and chronic pain becomes a maladaptive psychophysiological reflex. The interruption of these neurohumoral cascades with timely, effective therapy prevents these detrimental effects. As compared to the ground skink, human beings, especially young human beings, require attachment, empathy, rapport, and support to limit the injury caused by pain itself (Kuttner, 1996).

Factors that Contribute to Recurrent Pain

All recurrent pain first starts with an isolated incident. Multiple factors then lead to subsequent recurrence and periodicity: organic cycles (dysmenorrhea), conditioned responses (the smell, sound, other sensory stimuli of the school bus or the classroom), lowering thresholds (heightened sensitivity to stimuli), social and behavioral reinforcement (friends or family expect me to have a headache), negative feedback of co-morbidities (sleep, diet, exercise, generalized disability), and self-protection (pain keeps me from . . .) (McGrath & Hillier, 2003). These reinforcers have various potencies and patterns that must be engaged and addressed as part of undoing these cycles. It is important that the clinician keep in mind that recurrent pain can involve increased sensitivity at all levels from receptors in the periphery to the cerebral cortex. Finally, after enough cycles, to some degree, the recurrent nature of pain can become a product of the negative expectancy of the patient: "It happens because I expect it to." A critical piece of any hypnotic strategy that hopes to change this negative expectancy is helping the young person have the courage to imagine it can be different.

What is Different about Pain in Young People?

There are three facets to this question's answer: (1) the attitudes of adult care providers; (2) the child's and adolescent's development; and (3) the interaction of the two. The first and second facets are discussed below. It is within the third realm, informed by the other two, that therapy does or does not occur. That domain is the subject for the latter half of this chapter, and indeed, all the chapters of this text.

Clinical Attitudes about Pain in Children

Before the 1970s, the medical literature is essentially devoid of any formal reviews or research specifically addressing the management of pain in children (Schechter et al., 2003, p. 3). A 1968 survey revealed that only 2 of 60 postoperative pediatric patients received any analgesia, and only 26 of 180 children admitted to an intensive care unit over a 4-month period received any opioid analgesics. The authors wrote, "Pediatric patients seldom need medication for relief of pain. They tolerate discomfort well. The child will say he does not feel well or that he is uncomfortable, that he wants parents and often he will not relate this unhappiness to pain" (Swafford & Allen, 1968, pp. 131–136). Twenty-five years later another postoperative survey reported that 75% of pediatric patients had insufficient analgesia and 40% complained of moderate to severe pain (Mather & Mackie, 1983).

We can speculate on the historical reasons for this neglect of pediatric pain treatment. Certainly, our relative ignorance of neurological and psychological development with regard to pain informed this attitude. In part, this mind-set was the result of the perpetuation of standards of practice: We do what we always do. Lack of information about pharmacology in infants and children, fear of over-medicating, and contributing to opiate addiction drove many to conclude that the young patient's ongoing discomfort was a lesser evil then pharmacotherapy. One cannot help but wonder if an antecedent of this blindness towards the pain experience of infants and children originates in the childhoods of the clinicians themselves as a form of "learned helplessness": "I put up with this pain as a child. You can, too" (Schechter et al., 2003, pp. 1–13). No matter how the past attitudes of professionals were justified, they were ripe for change.

Over the last two decades a revolution has taken place in the management of pain in infants, children, and adolescents in clinical settings. This dramatic change has been driven by our new appreciation of the profound conditioning effect of early pain experience. We have learned that children are not insensitive to pain but *hyper*sensitive in early life. The neurobiological and psychodevelopmental research that led to these new understandings broke down old myths and produced a blossoming of clinical efforts to recognize, assess, and holistically treat pain experiences in children and adolescents.

In this chapter, we will make use of this understanding to form an approach to the hypnotherapy of children and adolescents in pain. The reader is urged, however, to keep in mind that our knowledge of developmental biology and psychology still falls short of explaining the physiological mechanisms by which hypnosis helps children control pain. In essence, these descriptions of science and research constitute no more than our current, professional, authoritative, Western cultural metaphor for understanding pain. As Kay Thompson tells us:

> [T]hose people who work in surgical situations and who work with pain patients assume that pain relief, if it's utilizing hypnosis, must follow the [known] neurological pathways. That is not a valid assumption. [Y]ou have to be aware that hypnosis violates some of the physiological and neurological kinds of expectations. That's all right. That's what hypnosis is so good for. ... Once you ... set aside your assumption that you know how the world works, then it opens a great many things to you as a person, in order to believe in the things that other people can do. ... (Kane & Olness, 2004, p. 323)

In the consultation room or at a hospital bedside, interacting with one child, all of our well-researched understanding may carry no more weight than that child's own imagined metaphor.

Developmental Aspects of Pain in Children

With increasing age, pain perception is modified by accumulated experience and the responses of those around us. As a general trend, the attribution of meaning to pain and the appreciation of the ability to modify perception with psychological capacities increase with cognitive development. Infants will respond with reflexic crying and withdrawal; an 8-year-old may respond with anger and/or regression; and a mature adolescent may describe the experience in detail, explaining how she coped and what she learned about herself (McGrath & Hillier, 2003). However, while children's overt distress during medical procedures decreases with age, there is little evidence that there are age-related differences in pain perception or persistence. The primary determinants of pain perception and persistence seem to be one's cumulative pain experience more than age (McGrath & Hillier, 2003; Bennett-Branson & Craig, 1993; Palermo & Drotar, 1996; Gidron, McGrath, & Goodday, 1995).

Psychological Meanings of Recurrent Pain in Children and Adolescents

There are an infinite number of attributions of meaning that attach over time to our experiences, particularly our painful ones. When pain is associated with various memories and social experiences it can accumulate diverse psychological functions. Olness and Kohen (1996) have listed types of emotional significance, including (1) punishment, (2) gaining attention, (3) identification with a similarly affected loved one, (4) avoidance of feared or undesired situations, (5) remaining attached to a loved one (as in school phobia), (6) gaining status, (7) subconscious, unexpressed hostility, (8) controlling others, and (9) assuring prolongation of life in the case of a young person with life-threatening illness (pp. 192–193). While the reader ought not consider this list complete, it is a valuable framework from which to start. Most importantly, unless such motivating factors are uncovered and engaged, it is unlikely that the young person can let go of pain. As Kaye Thompson puts it, "When everything that can be done and should be done, has been done, there is no longer any reason to have the pain" (Kane & Olness, 2004, book front).

A 16-year-old young woman came in with a month-long headache "on top" of her head. So far, an extensive evaluation resulted in the conclusion that "Nothing is wrong." She told me, "It started when I bumped my head on the doorjamb getting out of a car." After a lengthy and careful description of the discomfort, her neurological evaluation, CAT and MRI scans, and the medications she had used unsuccessfully since she had "bumped" her head, I remembered to ask her the events preceding the injury:

"Exactly how did you bump your head?"

"I told you. I was getting out of a car."

"What car?"

"It doesn't matter."

"It doesn't?"

"Why does it matter?" [*Angrily.*]

"Why does it matter?" [*Softly.*]

"My boyfriend's car ... we had a fight. ..." [*She starts to cry.*]

"Does it matter?"

"And he got in an accident after that," [*now fully in tears.*]

"This must really be hurting you a lot."

What is Hypnoanalgesia?

There is no single sensory organ that is responsible for pain as the ear is for hearing or the eyes are for seeing. As we have seen, the neurobiological landscape of pain ranges from the somatic periphery to multiple brain centers. Therefore, as yet, there is no single site at which to study *hypnoanalgesia,* the psychophysiology of pain control apparently mediated by hypnosis. Significant research efforts have been made to dissect out and measure the components of pain that are affected by hypnosis. These efforts are fraught with problems. What measurable physiological correlates or proxies (blood pressure, heart rate, skin conductance) vary tightly with the pain experience? How do we control for the desire of patients to deny pain in order to please the doctor or researcher? How do we control for formal hypnosis versus "waking suggestion" or other social variables? How can we ethically perform laboratory research on hypnosis and pain in children to compare them with adults? Most of these problems remain unresolved.

We know that the ability to control pain hypnotically correlates better with the ability to dissociate and imagine than with the ability to relax (E. R. Hilgard & J. R. Hilgard, 1994; Appel & Bleiberg, 2006; Miller, A. Barabasz, & M Barabasz, 1991). We know that it does not really matter whether we call the interaction "hypnosis" or not for most patients in clinical settings (E. R. Hilgard & J. R. Hilgard, 1994). We know opioid antagonists do not block hypnoanalgesia so that hypnotic pain control does not seem to be mediated by endorphins, the endogenous neurotransmitters that block pain (Goldstein & Hilgard, 1975; Katz, Sharp, Kellerman, Marston, Hershman, & Siegel, 1982). We know that, on average, the subject's report of the degree of discomfort is its best measure. We also know that in laboratory settings, sympathetic nervous system correlates of pain (increased blood pressure and heart rate) may respond to painful stimuli even when a subject in hypnosis reports significantly less discomfort than controls (E. R. Hilgard & J. R. Hilgard, 1994). Hilgard's (1974) theory of alternative cognitive controls in which a portion of our awareness dissociates itself and neglects pain, or aspects of it, has served as the leading model for our understanding of hypnoanalgesia for thirty years (pp. 301–316).

There are exceptions to this model that hint at the diversity of hypnoanalgesic effects. Karen Olness (1996) reports that during her personal experience using hypnosis as the sole anesthesia during surgical procedures, "I felt no pain, nor did my autonomic measures suggest that some other part of me was perceiving pain" (pp. 197–198). Despite the controversy, we are beginning to anchor this psychological model in neurobiology. For example, we know that there are areas of changing metabolic activity in the brain on Positron Emission Tomography (PET) imaging depending on a subject's focus on pain in and out of hypnosis (Rainville, Carrier, Hofbauer, Bushnell, & Duncan, 1999). There are separate neuronal pathways for affective aspects of pain (perceived unpleasantness) distinct from nociception. Rainville has shown that hypnotic suggestion for dissociating unpleasantness from pain perception results in variations in PET images in the anterior cingulate cortex, but not the somatosensory cortex. These findings directly link hypnotic suggestion about pain affect with frontal lobe-limbic activity (Rainville et al., 1997). Raz has allied electroencephalographic mapping with functional magnetic resonance imaging as a multidimensional probe for brain activity in hypnosis (Raz, Fan, & Posner, 2005). This has yet to be applied to pain or young people, but it promises great insight. Finally, in pursuit of cellular markers for hypnotic control of pain, Rossi has proposed a model for studying the up-regulation (increasing sensitivity) that occurs in the central nervous system in response to tissue injury as a way of investigating "how hypnotic suggestion achieves its inflammatory and pain relieving effects" (Rossi, 2002, pp. 221–222). In sum, we are focusing with ever higher levels of resolution on the problem of understanding how and where we self-regulate pain and its attendant physiological effects.

There is no doubt that eventually we will be able to observe changes in markers of gene expression emanating from individual cells in brain centers that mediate consciousness of pain and correlate incontrovertibly with hypnotic interaction. There will be verification at a cellular level that hypnoanalgesia is a "real" phenomenon. There will always be doubters, and hypnoanalgesia will probably be less effective for them, be they clinicians or patients. In the meantime, the ultimate proof that hypnosis helps young people manage life's pain is their word.

Relevant Literature Review

There is a huge volume of literature documenting the effectiveness of hypnosis for pain control in the laboratory and in clinical settings for adults. There is a much smaller volume about hypnotherapy for children with recurrent pain. The majority of research has focused on children with headaches, the most pervasive of recurrent pain syndromes in children (Abu-Arafeh & Russell, 1994). In perhaps the most persuasive study of hypnosis for children with juvenile migraine, Olness and colleagues demonstrated in a prospective, partially placebo-controlled trial that hypnosis was superior to propranolol and placebo (Olness, McDonald, & Uden, 1987). Numerous other studies have shown that hypnotic techniques were effective in the management of headaches (Olness & Kohen, 1996; McGrath, 1999; Holden, Deichmann, & Levy, 1999; Kohen & Zajac, in press). In addition to headaches, hypnosis has been shown to be helpful as primary or adjunctive therapy in the treatment of recurrent pain related to chronic illnesses, recurrent abdominal pain, malignancies, sickle-cell disease, hemophilia, and juvenile rheumatoid arthritis (Olness & Kohen, 1996; Hilgard & LeBaron, 1984). While anecdotal reports and descriptive series abound, there is still a paucity of reports in the mainstream professional literature. More prospective, controlled trials are needed in order to support the legitimate role of hypnosis in helping children with recurrent pain.

Approaching the Child with Recurrent Pain

Guidelines for Hypnotherapy of Young People with Recurrent Pain

1. *All pain is a real sensation for the patient as he or she defines it.* It may not be somatically based pain or clearly definable by our present understanding of neuroscience. Similarly, whatever the patient says "helps," "does help," even if it makes little clinical sense to the clinician. This principle requires the clinician to become aware of his or her own pain prejudices that can subtly reflect a lack of confidence in the young patient.

2. *A careful evaluation ought to include not only potential physical causes but also the contributions of sleep, diet, exercise, and other environmental factors.* Medical and lifestyle interventions ought to deal with structural components that are in themselves disruptive and painful. Olness and Libby (1987) report an extensive evaluation and psychological treatment of a girl with recalcitrant headaches, who ultimately proved to be suffering primarily from carbon monoxide poisoning due to a faulty furnace. I have been asked to use hypnotherapy to help a

number of children with recurrent headaches or abdominal pains who have responded to changes in sleep schedules, diet, and exercise. One boy resolved his headaches completely when a careful dietary history revealed that his headaches were temporally related to an increased intake of peanut butter. Incidentally, he successfully went on to use hypnosis so that peanut butter no longer induced a headache because, as he said, "I don't like having headaches but I do like eating peanut butter."

3. *Clarify the role of recurrent pain in the family's ecology.* How do the parents understand their child's pain experience? What are their beliefs and fears regarding the pain's etiology? Their faith that the child can improve is at least as important as the clinician's. Often it is easier for a child to have a problem than anybody else in the family. If a child will not be seen alone— either the parents insist on coming in the room during the therapy or the child insists that they accompany him—this constitutes evidence that the family is part of the pain's perpetuation. As much as parents can be part of the problem they can also be part of the solution. Boyce (1992) has noted that the self-efficacy that arises from hypnotherapy can help loosen enmeshed parent-child relationships in which the child is seen as vulnerable.

4. *Always use the young person's own language and imagery, once elicited, to describe his or her experiences.* This powerful, simple principle reinforces rapport: The young person hears his or her own words, and their acceptance, from the mouth of the authoritative healthcare provider. The reinforcement of this language engages those resources, both conscious and subconscious, that relate to the young person's pain. This also means that it is best to avoid prescribing imagery. Finally, as this symptom, and so its descriptors, change with the therapeutic process, the clinician is an archivist of the young person's experience, monitoring his or her learning.

5. *Consider "resistance," lack of cooperation, and difficulty developing rapport self-protective: something is being left out.* For example, a young girl with unexplained recurrent headaches engages in

self-monitoring, but does not practice self-hypnosis and shows little interest during visits. Then, at a home visit, during a particularly severe headache, she whispers tearfully to the clinician, "If I make it better who will believe that it's real?" *See* the clinical vignette "Lisa" in Chapter Four [rape case].

Framing Hypnotherapy for Recurrent Pain: Applied Dissociation

The concept of *dissociation* can be a useful and unifying theme when considering how to help a young person with recurrent pain. Here, "dissociation" is not used in the traditional sense that is attributed to Janet and Hilgard (Pierre, 1925; Hilgard, 1974). The reader is asked to consider the term in a broader, simpler context: dissociation as disconnecting, as in the skink from its tail. For the clinician, this means developing rapport and understanding the young person apart from his or her pain. For the family, this may mean understanding their son's or daughter's recurrent pain as an entity within the family separate from the child. For the young person, this may mean learning to understand pain as the elemental signal that it is, dissociating from the emotions and resulting disability, and then learning to change that signal and use it differently. This may start with separating the "head" and "stomach" from the "ache," removing possessive terms so that "my pain" becomes "that pain," then reframing the headaches as a group of shifting multisensory images or changing number on a scale.

This notion of dissociation, as deconstruction and reconnection, is powerful for two fundamental reasons. First, it utilizes a natural subconscious ability (*see* Chapter Four) that arises spontaneously in the trance of pain. Second, the ability to dissociate enables us to examine and experience in a creative way. Rossi (2002) effectively argues that novel experiences in and out of hypnosis facilitate brain plasticity, rewiring, gene expression, and ultimately the changing of maladaptive subconscious reflexes. So the hypnotic ability to dissociate provides a psychophysiological link to the neurocellular processes that alter our responsivity to pain.

Helping Young People Dissociate from Pain

Self-Monitoring

Brown and Fromm (1987) note that *self-monitoring* is the first step in all behavioral change. When we become mindful of conditioned subconscious responses (breathing for example) we change that experience, at least for that moment. Self-monitoring can be used as a way to repeatedly exercise that mindfulness, extend rapport, change the role of the symptom in the family, embed posthypnotic suggestion, and suggest positive change. By reframing the recurrent pain as number or some other varying image to observe, self-monitoring can be a powerful tool that aids dissociation. In addition, the introduction of a self-monitoring scale creates the cognitive room for a range of experience. There is not only "Pain" or "No Pain." There can also be a little pain, a bit more, enough to be in the way, and more. If there are gradations of discomfort, then there are also degrees of coping. The introduction of self-monitoring, exemplifying these elements, is illustrated in the following vignette.

Peter

At our first visit, while describing his headaches, 14-year-old Peter is asked,

L. Sugarman [LS]: Have you ever kept track of these?

Peter: Not really.

LS: Well, it would be interesting if I could follow you around every day by shrinking myself down and sitting on your shoulder or making myself invisible to everybody but you. Then I could check in and see how you're doing and keep you company.

[Peter responds with evident interest—eye contact, open posture, a smile—so this constitutes the building of rapport, a partnership.]

LS: Of course I can't do that in reality. So it would help me help you if you could keep track on paper of how your head is feeling every day so that you can tell me about it when we next meet and you won't have to remember. OK? [*Here, self-monitoring is introduced as a way to extend rapport. Peter is to keep track for me, not himself. This framing can undo some potential opposition that may arise from a sense of inefficacy: "This may not work for me but I'll do it for him." Note also that he is not going to keep track of "headaches" but how his "head feels," an implicit reframing suggestion.*]

LS: Let's do that by making up a number scale with zero being normal. What does it to go up to? What number would represent the worst possible headache? [*Having Peter choose the range of the scale is an effort to involve him in ownership, further ensuring coop-eration. In my experience most patients have the scale go to 10, but 7 or 23 is fine, too. Peter chooses 10.*]

LS: Thank you. So let's get this straight. Zero is normal, right? Now 10 is the worst possible headache you can imagine. That would be like your head is actually exploding or something! I don't even want to think about that. You can't really have a 10. If I gave you a really hard intelligence test and you got every question right then I would know two things: You are really smart, and I need a better test. [*This series of statements serves two purposes. First, it makes the scale inclusive. Because Peter's head is not really going to explode he can't have a headache that rates a 10. Second, the metaphor of the intelli-gence test is intended to be ego-strengthening.*]

LS: Now that we know that the scale goes from normal to impossi-ble, what number would you give your head at this very moment?"

[*Peter looks up and to the right for a moment then says,*]

Peter: I don't know. Maybe a 2 or 3?

LS: You don't know. It is maybe a 2 or 3, right? Good. But which one is it: a 2 or a 3? You'll need to decide so you will only need to write one number down when you keep track. [*More attempts get owner-ship, commitment, and embed suggestions for self-monitoring.*]

[*Peter chooses 3.*]

LS: OK. It's a 3. It seems to me that you do very well coping with a 3. [*Labeling lower numbers as more effective better coping.*] At what number do you need to stop what you are doing because you have to concentrate on coping with the head ache?

[*Peter pauses, looks away, and then says,*]

Peter: It depends on what I'm doing. [*he labels higher numbers as less coping.*]

LS: Right. As you keep track, notice how it can be helpful to you. Now do this experiment: Do whatever you need to do to make it a 2. I'll be quiet.

[*Peter closes his eyes, furrows his forehead in concentration, takes a couple of breaths, then opens his eyes and says,*]

Peter: It's a 2.

LS: Great. It'll be interesting to figure out how you do that so that you can do it even better. From now on, whenever you pay attention to the number for how your head feels, also notice how you turn it down. [*Two embedded suggestions: Peter already knows how to help his head feel better (and has displayed the physical cues that correlate with that act) and paying attention to a number for how his head feels has now been linked to the suggestion to make it feel better.*] So, now you can carry a number with you on the screen in your mind, just like some television channels do, for how your head is feeling at that moment. And you can learn how you change it when you concentrate on it. If you carry that around with you in the back of your mind all day, then at the end of the day when it's time to write down how your head has felt, it will be easy to know the average number, the highest it went, and the low number for the most comfortable you made it feel. Those are the numbers to write down, so that you can bring them to me on the calendar when we get back together. OK? [*With these words the dissociation of the headache as a range of numbers on a screen that can be varied with concentration (or "mindfulness") for the purpose of informing the clinician is complete.*] Now keeping track of this is just between you and me. This is not for your parents or anybody else. Will you need your parents to remind you to do this?

[*Peter shakes his head, "No."*]

LS: But your mother is going to be really curious about whether you're keeping track as I asked you to and what numbers you're putting down. What should she do about that?

[*Peter shrugs.*]

LS: How about this: If she really can't help it, she could ask, "So, how's that calendar coming along?" or she could simply ask, "What number are you giving your head today?" If your mother begins to bother you about this, let me know. [*Turning to the mother*] You know none of us want to do something when we are nagged about it. [*Here we dissociate the mother from the son's care of his head, giving the mother of a task of not nagging*.] But what should you do when you've been feeling fine and you forget to write down numbers on the calendar?

[*Like most performance-driven people, Peter says that he should fill in the blanks that he forgot after the fact.*]

LS: No. I suggest that you give yourself a break and leave a blank space. You're a human being. You don't have to be perfect. You can forget your headaches if you need to. [*More rapport, acceptance, and an embedded suggestion to forget headaches.*] So you understand all of this?

[*Peter repeats back the exercise of self-monitoring.*]

LS: Great. Now we can get started on seeing how to help your head to feel better. By the way, is your head still a 2, or have you changed it again …?

"Taking a History": Using Evocative Descriptors, Creating New Potentials

With experience, all clinicians learn that the initial interview is more than the collection of data. It is an opportunity to build rapport, introduce new frames of understanding, and promote positive expectancy. In the case of a child or adolescent whose life has been ruled by recurrent pain, the initial interview is also an opening for the clinician to know the child distinct from the pain that seems to have him or her and, in that interaction, engage those aspects of his or her identity and self that are distinct from the pain. A questionnaire, such as the "Rainbow Babies and Children's Hospital General Academic Pediatrics Imagery Discomfort Questionnaire," allows the clinician to collect a wide variety of information, including likes, dislikes, enjoyable activities, and imaginative capacities (Olness & Kohen, 1996). When this is reviewed with the child as the visit begins, it can introduce new ways of understanding, or reframe, the young person's discomfort. Preprinted questionnaires, rating scales, and forms are useful only if they are reviewed actively with the young person, as the catalyst for engagement. Paper forms cannot replace therapeutic communication.

Traditionally, physicians are taught the mnemonic: Onset, Palliative/precipitating factors, Quality, Radiation, Severity, and Timing to describe a patient's pain. In this setting, the list can continue to include more imaginative descriptors including the color, shape, texture, malleability, smell, temperature, and affect. This augmented, multisensory description allows further characterization of pain as a separate entity and opens potential for how the characteristics vary as the young person "makes it better." There is value and reliability in children's headache drawings, and their utilization by the clinician tells the child: "Your imagination is an important part of how you get better" (Stafstrom, Goldenholz, & Dulli, 2005, pp. 809–813).

Allison

Ten-year-old Allison is seeking relief from her migraine headaches. She brings in her Imagery Discomfort Questionnaire for review. Not only has she completed the form but she has drawn a picture of her headache on the back. After some discussion, what used to be Allison's migraine headaches have become "that yellow-green-smelly-squishy-wet-throbbing-blob-behind-my-eyes." This allows the clinician to ask, based upon the previous reframing of the headache as Allison's creation,

> **LS**: So how does it change when you make it better? Would you like to do an experiment? First, find out whether you can relax in that chair and concentrate better on that yellow-green-smelly-squishy-wet-throbbing-blob-behind-the-eyes with your eyes open or by letting them close … I will wait and watch. Whichever your eyes find most comfortable, let them stay that way, then let your head nod when you know.

> [*Allison closes her eyes slowly, opens them, then closes them again, with immediate eye-movements beneath the lids, then relaxes her facial muscles as she leans back in her chair and subtly nods.*]

> **LS**: Good. The next part of the experiment is to find out what part of the yellow-green-smelly-squishy-wet-throbbing-blob-behind-the-eyes you will change first and how that will feel. Either let your head nod again or let your voice come out of hypnosis to talk … whichever is most comfortable for you … when you are ready. …

This hypnotic interaction can continue in this way as Allison learns to practice changing the richly detailed multisensory imagery of what used to be simply a "headache." This is, in fact, dissociative, and we can wonder what is happening with those old neuronal connections that used to encode "headache" as she performs her novel experiments.

In a related example, 8-year-old Bethany sent me a drawing after she had successfully stopped having migraines with hypnosis as the sole therapy. The picture was unsolicited, a gift. A large pink, furrowed brain fills the page. The frontal region is occupied by a large rectangular space over which the word "Migraines" is crossed out and "New Stuff" is written in. In the space are icons representing buying clothes, playing with friends, playing videogames, and "other stuff." Next to the space is a door and hanging by the door is a large key. The key is labeled, "My Hypnosis."

Not Allowing the Pain to "Go Away"

A young person's description of the resolution of his or her discomfort creates an opening for reframing and focusing on internal resources. Brian has been frustrated by irritable bowel syndrome and has stated, "None of that medicine really works on me." Note that the clinician's language implicitly suggests changes in the patient's discomfort. The clinician separates the "stomach" from the "ache," only refers to the symptom in the past tense, and uses his authority to express faith in this early adolescent's ability to help himself. He also abruptly shifts Brian's attention and stimulates his curiosity by acting out a metaphor and using confusion.

Brian

Twelve-year-old Brian says: I have stomachaches.

LS: You have stomach [*pause*] aches? All different kinds?

Brian: No, it's the same stomachache. It just comes and goes.

LS: Oh, I see. It's that same stomach ... ache that you've learned to have and get rid of over and over.

Brian: I guess so [*confused.*] I mean I get a stomach ... ache and then after while it goes away.

LS: Well, actually it can't go away on its own. ... I can stand up and walk out of this room all by myself without anybody asking me. I can

---

439

do this because I'm a person who can think by myself and control my own body. Watch. This is me going away [*Clinician stands and walks out the door, closes it behind him, knocks, comes back in and sits down.*] You got that?

[*Brian nods, looking incredulous.*]

LS: Good. Now, on the other hand, if you suddenly ordered me out of the room that would be *you* getting rid of *me*. That uncomfortable feeling in the stomach that you had isn't some alien being that controls itself, though I bet it has felt that way. It Is something that happens in your body in some way that you don't know yet. When it seems to go away it's because you really do something that you don't yet know that you *do* know how to do to make yourself feel better. How do you feel about what I just said?"

Brian [*listening intensely replies*]: I don't know … kind of good and bad. I mean I never thought of it that way … so it's good that I can do this and bad that I don't know how.

LS: Right. [*the clinician affirms*] So what would you like to learn first?

Without any formal hypnosis, much of the therapeutic work has already been done. Brian now has a frame in which he expects he can learn to feel better.

Doing What the Pain Says to Do

A tenet of hypnotherapy is that the patient already has the subconscious resources sufficient to solve their problem. The therapist's role is to provide the rapport that evokes those capacities. Every young person with recurrent pain presents us with the opportunity to access those inner agencies because sometimes it feels better. Patients are often mindful of how they feel when they are uncomfortable and can answer our persistent questions about "the pain." But the answer often lies in how they feel better. Essentially, a path towards changing pain recurrence begins with doing what the pain asks us to do before we have it. This approach is exemplified in the following vignette.

Billy

Billy is 8 years old. He says the belly pain starts when "I don't know what's going to happen or when it's noisy on the school bus and when my big sister is bossy. Mom says it's stress or something."

    LS: [*Rather than focusing initially on the triggers or the discomfort, the clinician asks*]: So what do you do about that?

    Billy: What do you mean?

    LS: When your belly wants attention by being uncomfortable, how do you help it? [*Note the implicit reframing in this question.*]

    Billy: I don't know.

    LS: Sure you do.

    Billy: [*Pause.*] Um, sometimes I go up to my room and have wars with my Guys.

    LS: Your Guys?

    Billy: My Transformers [*plastic action figures with weapons and fighting abilities that can change from creatures into machines*].

    LS: Wow. Yeah. Your Guys are Transformers. Right! … So I wonder how your guys help your belly get what it needs. [*This is exactly when the therapist resists the strong temptation to start prescribing imagery and strategies in favor of the child's own creativity!*]

Over the next thirty minutes, the clinician and Billy play with pretend Transformers and Billy demonstrates how the Transformers solve problems and make him feel better. The Transformers are imagined in part because the clinician has none and also because real ones are not as effective or creative.

> [*Finally, the clinician asks*] **LS**: So, Billy, I am wondering if you could take our special Transformers with you and play with them whenever and however you want, even just in your mind, to give your belly attention before it asks by bothering you.
>
> The session closes with Billy practicing using his special Transformers for a self-hypnotic exercise to keep his belly feeling better.

Utilizing Ideomotor/Ideosensory Capacities: How Our Brains Change Our Pain

Ideomotor and ideosensory phenomena form a powerful piece of hypnotic engagement for young people living with recurrent pain. Because children and adolescents experience an undeniable link between suggestion and somatic feeling/action with ideodynamic phenomena, the seeds of creating a new relationship between mental and somatic processes are deeply sown. Moreover, there is a neurobiological basis for enlisting ideodynamic capacities. Rossi (2002) indicates that, in hypnosis, ideomotor activity, particularly involving the hands and arms, activates large areas of neuronal activity for genomic involvement and brain plasticity.

Out of respect for what we do not know about the young person's pain and its emotionally charged attribution, I generally approach ideodynamics by avoiding initially the pain itself, even when the child or adolescent is in pain at the time. I use what they bring— his or her hands together in his or her lap, a bouncing leg and foot, one hand on the arm of the chair and one in the lap—as a starting point to help evoke awareness of how to positively change sensation and motor activity in that body part. Then I suggest that he or she wonder, and thereby entrain subconscious processes, how this new understanding will help him or her, in time, to approach the pain. Finally, I ask him or her to consider the ideosensory component as both a post-hypnotic suggestion and an "anchoring signal" for the purpose of remembering his or her capability for self-control in any circumstance. In the following vignette, ideodynamics are used to suggest, metaphorically, an internal locus of self-control.

Brooke

Sixteen-year-old Brooke has had two years of daily headaches and weekly incapacitating migraines. She has reluctantly attributed a large number of factors—foods, sunlight, second-hand cigarette smoke, heat, loud music—as triggers for her headaches and has thereby been further disabled by trying to avoid them. "I haven't had chocolate in two years!" she complains. On her Imagery/Discomfort Questionnaire she has written that she enjoys traveling and flying kites at the beach. During the initial conversation, her hands are together in her lap. She places the right hand on the arm of the chair as I ask her how her head feels at this moment. "It's about a 3" [*out of 10*].

LS: And how is that arm and hand feeling? [*referring to the right hand and arm*]

Brooke: It's fine [*she replies, curious.*]

LS: Would it like to feel better than "fine?"

Brooke: I guess, [*she smiles and rests back in the chair.*]

LS: That's right. A good start, letting yourself relax more just that way. And does it feel even more comfortable with your eyes open or closed? Whichever is right, let them stay that way. [*She closes her eyes slowly and they stay closed with eye movements beneath the lids.*] Wonderful. I wonder what that hand and arm would enjoy doing next. Would they like to be lighter or heavier?

Brooke: Lighter.

LS: So can there be a kite … catching the wind … on the beach … high up … with a string … all the way … down to that hand? [*She nods to this and all the subsequent questions.*] And can you feel it and enjoy feeling it?

Brooke: Yes.

LS: And can you feel the power of the winds aloft as you watch the kite and its colors?

Brooke: Yes.

LS: Can you feel it jerk and sway? What happens when you jerk back? Does the kite go up? Does it loop around? You don't really know each time, do you?

Brooke: Yes.

LS: It is unpredictable. You are playing with powerful forces in the wind and the Earth's rotation. And even though you cannot control those forces, that arm and hand get to enjoy feeling them … and you can feel your own control … and power through them. Is that a wonderful feeling?

Brooke: Yes.

LS: It is so good to know that you can use your experiences and knowledge to change how your body feels. [*During this set of suggestions-as-questions, Brooke's right hand and arm have lifted off the chair and moved subtly in seemingly random directions. This part of the interaction continues for some minutes in silence then closes with the following*]: So, Brooke, as you finish this experience for now, let that arm and hand continue to enjoy what they are learning. Whenever you need to know that you can control and change how your body is feeling, making it more comfortable and powerful, that arm and hand can remember the pull of the kite and remind you. And you know what happens the more you practice … right?

This ideodynamic process becomes the starting point for self-hypnosis and, at subsequent visits, for further exploration of other sources of comfort.

Prescriptive Strategies

There are volumes of metaphors, prescriptive imagery, stories, and other strategies designed to help children, adolescents, and adults with recurrent and chronic pain (Olness & Kohen, 1996; Hammond, 1990; Rossi & Cheek, 1988; Mills & Crowley, 1986; Sugarman, 1996; Thomson, 2005). As a general rule, however, these lists and referenced texts are best considered reports of what is possible for children and useful for us in order to stimulate our own hypnotic potential, but not as recommended strategies to "do to children." As Olness and Kohen (1996) have observed, there is a tendency for hypnotherapists to approach the child in pain "...in a trial-and-error fashion, randomly trying hypnoanalgesic techniques with which they are most familiar with little thought as to why one method might be preferable to another in a particular instance" (p. 191). When I teach hypnosis workshops, invariably participants ask, "What do you do with kids who have" this kind of pain or that kind of pain? This is the wrong question. It is not a matter of what kind of pain the child or adolescent has. It is about what kind of young person has a particular pain. Because the perception and meaning of pain in each youngster is the singular product of his or her past experience and understanding, each hypnotherapeutic approach must be evocative of that person's uniquely applicable resources. Therefore, rather than selecting metaphors or preconceived strategies, I use the general approaches illustrated above as entry points. Then, I follow the patient's lead while building rapport that lends them the courage to change.

Caveats

A number of caveats have already been addressed in this chapter but bear repeating in summary.

1. *The importance of a thorough evaluation of organic, psychosocial, and lifestyle contributors to recurrent pain syndromes in young people cannot be underestimated.* Not only is the regular review of these factors necessary in order to consider other avenues of

treatment, but the process of such a review reassures the child and family of the care and thoroughness of the clinician.

2. *Avoid direct suggestions for symptom removal.* It is tempting to believe that the hypnotic relationship is powerful enough to support such commands, and, at times they may actually be effective. Certainly the lay belief that the all-powerful hypnotist can take away pain derives in part from a cultural wish that someone else can fix our problems. But in truth, the only person who can do that is the one who "owns the trance" (Olness, 2006). Telling the patient that "The pain will be gone" or "You will feel no pain" is risky. First, it is unlikely to work or work for long. Second, when it is ineffective it undermines the therapeutic relationship: either the therapist or, worse, the patient is inadequate. It also creates a strong "demand characteristic" for the child or adolescent in that he or she risks disappointing the therapist if he or she does not report less pain. Most importantly, while ordering a patient not to have pain may (arguably) be hypnosis, it is not hypnotherapy. Hypnotherapy, especially with young people, is primarily about investing in their own capacities.

3. *Do not "cast spells."* Clinicians tend to have favorite metaphors, stories, and hypnotic techniques, and risk believing that those favorites are the best fit for a given problem, ignoring the unique characteristics, and resources of a particular boy or girl. The most effective are those evoked in each individual child. Hypnosis for recurrent pain is not about the pain but the child who learns to dissociate from it.

4. *When the child or adolescent does not respond well or consistently with increasing comfort, return to establishing rapport.* Something is being left out. Sometimes, despite our best intentions and skills, we are not the right therapist for that young person. As one mother explained to me when her daughter would not return for a third appointment, "Everything you taught my daughter about her headaches made sense and she knows she could do it (benefit from hypnosis) but she is just not ready to get well yet."

Conclusion

Despite the ongoing revolution in addressing pain in children and adolescents in medical settings that began in the 1970s, there is still a primary reliance on medication for the control of recurrent pain rather than a more balanced approach that combines allopathic treatments with inner resources. Certainly there are cost-savings to be realized by investing in young people's abilities to help themselves with less medication, especially when treating recurrent pain. Increased utilization of hypnotherapy ought to decrease medication-induced problems and our expensive cultural bias towards pills over skills. More importantly, the evidence indicates that the most effective way to reduce the development of recurrent pain is to provide effective support of pain relief for acute pain. In order to promote the use of hypnosis in pediatric clinical settings, we need more prospective, controlled trials of hypnosis in the mainstream professional literature demonstrating efficacy and cost-effectiveness. This is the proof that third-party payers require in order to support this work.

The therapist who helps young people with recurrent pain learns a lot in the process. He or she must honestly question his or her own beliefs about the patients, their pain, and their motivation. For those of us trained originally within a model of Cartesian duality (separating mind from body, and body from mind), these young people who possess the courage to change their complex recurrent pain need us to support their ability to do so. If we do not believe that their pain is real, they do not heal. There is no greater reward in hypnotherapy than when a young person frees himself or herself from the tyranny of recurrent pain. Perhaps this is because we know that each young person we see will inevitably encounter more pain, both physical and emotional, in his or her life. We also know that, as a result of this achievement in self-regulation, they will suffer less.

References

Abu-Arafeh, I., & Russell, G. (1994). Prevalence of headache and migraine in school children. *British Medical Journal*, 309, 795–769.

Appel, P. R., & Bleiberg, J. (2006) Pain reduction is related to hypnotizability but not to relaxation or to reduction in suffering: a preliminary investigation. *American Journal of Clinical Hypnosis*, 48(2–3), 153–162.

Bauer, A. M. (1993). Lizards. In Harold G. Cogger, Joseph Forshaw, Edwin Gould, George McKay, consultant editors, *Encyclopedia of animals*. Sydney, Australia: Weldon Owen Pty Limited.

Bennett-Branson, S. M, & Craig, K. D. (1993). Post-operative pain in children: Developmental and family influences on spontaneous coping strategies. *Canadian Journal of Behavioral Science*, 25, 355–383.

Boyce, W. T. (1992). The vulnerable child: New evidence, new approaches. *Advances in Pediatrics*, 39, 1–33.

Brown, D. P., & Fromm, E. (1987). *Hypnosis and behavioral medicine*. New Jersey: Lawrence Erlbaum.

Dubner, R., & Ren, K. (1999). Endogenous mechanisms of sensory modulation. *Pain*, 6 [supplemental] S45–S54.

Fitzgerald, M. (1991). The development of descending brainstem control of its final cord sensory processing. In M. A. Hanson (Ed.), *The fetal and neonatal brainstem* (pp. 127–136). Cambridge: Cambridge University Press.

Fitzgerald, M. (1994). Neurobiology of fetal and neonatal pain. In P. D. Wall & R. Melzack (Eds.), *Textbook of Pain* (pp. 153–164). Edinburgh: Churchill-Livingstone.

Fitzgerald, M., & Howard R. (2003). The neurobiologic basis of pediatric pain. In *Pain in infants, children, and adolescents* (2nd ed., pp. 26–37). Philadelphia: Lippincott, Williams, and Wilkins.

Fordyce, W. E. (2001). Learned pain: Pain as behavior. In J. D. Loeser, S. H. Butler, C. Capman, et al. *Bonica's management of pain* (3rd ed.). Philadelphia: Lippincott Williams and Wilkins.

International Association for the Study of Pain, Subcommittee on Taxonomy. (1979). *Pain*. Seattle: IASP Press.

Gidron, Y., McGrath, P. J., & Goodday, R. (1995). The physical and psychosocial predictors of adolescents' recovery from oral surgery. *Journal of Behavioral Medicine*, 18, 385–399.

Goldstein, A., & Hilgard, E. R. (1975) Lack of influence of the morphine antagonist naloxone on hypnotic analgesia. *Proceedings of the National Academy of Sciences*, 72, 2041–2043.

Hammond, C. D. (Ed.). (1990). Handbook of hypnotic suggestions and metaphors. New York: W.W. Norton.

Hilgard, E. (1974). Toward a neo-dissociation theory: Multiple cognitive controls in human functioning. *Perspectives in Biology and Medicine*, 17, 301–316.

Hilgard, E. R., & Hilgard, J. R. (1994). *Hypnosis in the relief of pain*. New York: Brunner/Mazel, Inc.

Hilgard, J. R., & LeBaron S. (1984). *Hypnotherapy of pain in children with cancer*. Los Altos: William Kaufman.

Holden, E. W., Deichmann, M. M., & Levy, J. D. (1999). Empirically supported treatments in pediatric psychology: Recurrent pediatric headache. *Journal of Pediatric Psychology*, 24(2), 91–109.

Janet, P. (1925). *Psychological healing: A historical and clinical study.* English translation (Eden Paul & Cedar Paul, trans.), New York: Macmillan (French original) (Vols. 1–2).

Kane, S., & Olness, K. (Eds.). (2004). *The art of therapeutic communication: The collected works of Kay F. Thompson*. Carmarthen, Wales, U.K.: Crown House

Katz, E. R., Sharp, B., Kellerman, J., Marston, A. R., Hershman, J. M., & Siegel, S. E. (1982) Beta-endorphin immunoreactivity and acute behavioral distress in children with leukemia *Journal of Nervous and Mental Disease*, 170, 72–77.

Keller, H. (1903). *Optimism, an essay by Helen Keller*. New York: T.Y. Cowell.

Kohen, D. P., & Zajac, R. (in press). Self-hypnosis for headaches: Experience with 178 consecutive children and adolescents: I: Clinical outcomes. *Journal of Pediatrics.*

Kuttner, L. (1996). *A child in pain: How to help, what to do.* Vancouver: Hartley and Marks.

Mather, L., & Mackie, J. (1983). The incidence of postoperative pain in children. *Pain*, 15, 271–282.

McGrath, P. A., & Hillier L. M. (2003). Modifying psychological factors that intensify children's pain and prolong disability. In *Pain in infants, children, and adolescents* (2nd ed.), pp. 85–104. Philadelphia: Lippincott, Williams and Wilkins.

McGrath, P. J. (1999). Commentary: Recurrent headaches: Making what works available to those who need it. *Journal of Pediatric Psychology*, 24(2), 111–112.

Miller, M., Barabasz, A., & Barabasz, M. (1991). Effects of active alert and relaxation hypnotic inductions on cold pressor pain. *Journal of Abnormal Psychology*, 100(2), 223–226.

Mills, J. C., & Crowley, R. J. (1986). *Therapeutic metaphors for children and the child within.* New York: Brunner/Mazel.

Olness, K. (2006). *Hypnosis in pediatric practice: Imaginative medicine in action* [DVD]. Carmarthen, Wales, U.K.: Crown House.

Olness, K., & Kohen, D. P. (1996). Hypnosis and hypnotherapy with children (3rd ed., pp. 197–198). New York: Guilford Press.

Olness, K. N., & Kohen, D. P. (1996). Pain Control. In *Hypnosis and hypnotherapy with children* (pp. 192–193). New York: Guilford Press.

Olness, K., & Libbey, P. (1987). Unrecognized biologic bases of behavioral symptoms in patients and referred for hypnotherapy. *American Journal of Clinical Hypnosis*, 30, 1–8.

Olness, K., McDonald, J. T., & Uden, D. L. (1987). Comparison of self-hypnosis and propranolol in the treatment of juvenile classic migraine. *Pediatrics*, 79(4), 593–597.

Palermo, T. M., & Drotar, D. (1996). Prediction of children's postoperative pain: the role of presurgical expectations and anticipatory emotions. *Journal of Pediatric Psychology*, 21, 683–698.

Poole, S. R., Schmitt, B. D., & Mauro, R. D. (1995). Recurrent pain syndromes: A streamlined approach. *Contemporary Pediatrics*, 12(1), 47–77.

Porter, F. L., German, R. E., & Anand, K. J. (1999). Long-term effects of pain in infants. *Journal of Developmental and Behavioral Pediatrics*, 20, 253–261.

Rainville, P., Carrier, B., Hofbauer, R. K., Bushnell, M. C., & Duncan, G. H. (1999). Dissociation of sensory and affective dimensions of pain using hypnotic modulation. *Pain*, 82(2), 159–171.

Rainville, P., Duncan, G. H., Price, D. D., Carrier, B., & Bushnell, M. C. (1997). Pain affect encoded in human anterior cingulated but not somatosensory cortex. *Science*, 277, 968–971.

Raz, A., Fan J., & Posner, M. I. (2005). Hypnotic suggestion reduces conflict in the human brain. *PNAS*: 10.1073/pnas.0503064102.

Rossi, E. L. (2002). The psychobiology of gene expression: Neuroscience and neurogenesis in hypnosis and the healing arts. New York: W.W. Norton.

Rossi, E. L., & Cheek, D. B. (1988). *Mind-body therapy: Methods of ideodynamic healing in hypnosis*. New York: W.W. Norton.

Schechter, N.L., Berde, C.B., & Yaster M. (2003). *Pain in infants children and adolescents*, 2nd ed., (pp 26–27). Philadelphia: Lippincott, Williams and Wilkins.

Stafstrom, C. E., Goldenholz, S. R., & Dulli, D. A. (2005). Serial headache drawings by children with migraine: Correlation with clinical headache status. *Journal of Child Neurology*, 20(10), 809–813.

Sugarman, L. I. (1996). Hypnosis: teaching children self-regulation. *Pediatrics in Review*, 17(1), 5–11.

Swafford, L., & Allen, D. (1968). Relief in pediatric patients. *Medical Clinics in North America*, 52, 131–136.

Taddio, A., Katz, J., Ilersich, A. L., et al. (1997). Effect of neonatal circumcision on pain response during subsequent routine vaccination. *Lancet*, 349, 599–603.

Thomson, L. (2005). *Harry the hypno-potamus: Metaphorical tales for the treatment of children*. Carmarthen, Wales, U.K.: Crown House

Woolf, C. J., & Costigan, M. (1999). Transcriptional and post-translation will plasticity and the generation of inflammatory pain. *Proceedings of the National Academy of Sciences, USA*, 96, 7723–7730.

Woolf, C. J., & Manion, R. J. (1999). Neuropathic pain: Aetiology, symptoms, mechanisms, and management. *Lancet*, 353, 1959–1964.

Chapter Nineteen

Hypnosis and Palliative Care

Leora Kuttner, PhD (RegPsyc)

I feel I'm stuck in the middle of a doughnut.
> 10-year old child relapsed with a brain tumor
> and struggling with the dilemma
> of whether or not to take chemotherapy

My house is a haunted house. Everyone who goes in dies.
All the daddy's in my family die.
> 7-year-old child whose father
> was dying at home

My Grandad came to visit. He was standing at the door waiting for me.
He told me that he'll look after me.
> 4-year-old child dying of neuroblastoma

Hypnosis is a natural fit for seriously ill children in palliative care (Gardener, 1976; Kuttner & Stutzer, 1995; Kuttner, 2006; Sourkes, 2006). As a therapeutic technique it is gentle, non-intrusive, and child-centered. It can tolerate and work with mystery, paradox, and uncertainty. If incorporated early in treatment it becomes part of the therapeutic scaffold that the seriously ill child relies on to deal with life and death concerns (Gardener, 1976; Kuttner & Stutzer 1995; Kuttner, 2006). As a therapy, hypnosis and self-hypnosis have the capability to sustain the child's inner strength, or to conserve energy as the child's life force diminishes. As an imaginative process, it provides a child with the experience of loved activities that can no longer be accessed. By engaging the child's imagination, hypnosis can be used to imbue meaning, sustain hope, ease despair, lessen pain, and help transport the child to places and experiences that diminish the threat of death, and add clarity to his or her present experience. It is also an adjunctive method that combines well with pharmacological options to address distressing end of life symptom, such as nausea, discomfort, anxiety, pain, and existential distress (Kuttner & Stutzer, 1995; Kuttner, 2006).

This chapter will cover the current and evolving philosophy and practice of pediatric palliative care (PPC). We'll explore how this emerging field of pediatric palliative care and hypnosis are a good fit, and how to use hypnosis to:

- Help children deal with loss and anticipatory loss
- Enliven the role of hope
- Help a child live fully, making every moment count, until they die

A Classic Example of Hypnosis at End of Life

David

In the first published article using hypnosis with a child approaching death, "Hypnotherapy for David," Dr. Gail Gardner (1976) reported initially using hypnosis to control David's nausea and vomiting. When the family learned that hypnosis can be used to enhance positive experiences such as safety and joy, Dr. Gardner suggested that David have a pleasant hypnotic dream that he could repeat as often as he liked:

> He dreamed he was an eagle who enjoyed flying from one safe and peaceful place to another; whenever anything disturbed him, he'd simply fly off to another, even safer and happier place. (p. 130)

He learned to use this at home and following his mother's suggestion: "David, just find your peaceful place," he was able to quickly move from negative to more positive states.

Later, Dr. Gardner used reverse hand-levitation in which she began by lifting the child's hand so that it was suspended in the air, and then gave hypnotic suggestions for the hand to lower to the bed, and for David to go into a peaceful focused state. With this as the

---

induction, she then invited David to engage with his familiar eagle dream so that he could achieve quietness and calm enjoyment. In considering their therapeutic goal she wrote:

> For David and his family it became more possible to tolerate gradual physical deterioration and to avert the threat of psychological deterioration by learning to achieve a feeling of emotional ease and dignity. The sense of threat gradually gave way to a sense of challenge...enhancing his growing trust in himself [*so that he could turn*] his attention to solving problems rather than enduring them. (p. 130)

Most children who are living with a terminal or life-limiting condition will benefit from an ongoing therapeutic relationship in which an experienced clinician engages with the threat of the illness and death with the child, and accompanies the child along the journey towards ultimate separation (Sourkes, 2006; Carter & Levetown, 2004; Field & Behrman, 2001). This is delicate and difficult work requiring training in palliative care issues, and experience in psychotherapy with seriously ill children. Central to this process is knowing how to create contained safety for the child; knowing how to listen, ask, and answer questions in an age-appropriate fashion; and knowing how to use creative play and art activities to promote self-expression. It is key in this work not to take the lead but to bear witness to this exceptional experience. In so doing, a clinician's role is: to accompany the child, to help clarify the medical and psychological processes, to sustain hope, and to provide opportunities for the child to complete the aspects of living that he or she desires.

Definition of Pediatric Palliative Care

Pediatric palliative care is both a philosophy of care and an organised program for delivering care to children with life-threatening and life-limiting conditions (Carter & Levetown, 2004).

The World Health Organization (WHO) Definition

Palliative care for children is the active total care of the child's body, mind and spirit and also involves giving support to the family. It begins when illness is diagnosed, and continues regardless of whether or not a child receives treatment directed at the disease. Health providers must evaluate and alleviate a child's physical, psychological, and social distress. Effective palliative care requires a broad multidisciplinary approach that includes the family and makes use of available community resources, and can be successfully implemented even if resources are limited. It can be provided in hospitals, in community health centres and even in children's homes. (1998)

The pioneering Children's' International Project on Palliative and Hospice Services (ChIPPS) statement adds further therapeutic breadth (2000):

Each child living with a life-threatening condition and his or her family deserve to have their pain and suffering ameliorated to the extent possible by the application of child and family-centered palliative care…The application of the principles of palliative care is a right. Palliative care is about living as well as possible despite the presence of a life-threatening condition. It is about bolstering families' strengths and capacity to cope, and maximizing the quality of their time together. Dying happens on the last day. (ChIPPPS, 2000, section 1, p. 1)

There is a consensus that PPC is an active, total, holistic approach that affirms life by supporting the child's and family's goals for the future and hopes for either cure or life prolongation. To do so, PPC provides:

- Physical and practical support,
- Emotional and bereavement support,
- Spiritual care,
- Social support, and
- Complex symptom management.

Hypnosis is naturalistic, flexible and creative. It can be interwoven in all those aspects of treatment: physical (such as suggestions for pain relief and added ease (Gardner, 1976; Kuttner & Stutzer, 1995; Kuttner, 2006), emotional (creating meaning, connection, feeding hope and providing experiences of joy (Gardner, 1976; Kuttner & Stutzer, 1995; Kuttner, 2006; Sourkes, 2006) and spiritual (promoting prayer and peaceful connections with God in whatever forms the child is comfortable (Kuttner & Stutzer 1995; Carter & Levetown, 2004; Field & Behrman, 2001).

There is further agreement that PPC involves the whole family, including siblings of the affected child, and that care focuses on enhancing quality of life for the child and family.

At best PPC begins at diagnosis and continues throughout the entire course of the child's life and beyond. *There is an attempt to avoid the dichotomy of cure versus treatment* [Italics added] (Carter & Levetown, 2004; Field & Behrman, 2001).

Palliative care for children differs in a number of respects from adult palliative care:

- First and foremost, as a society we are not prepared for children's death; it is contrary to our perceived order of things. Unlike the greater acceptance that, with age, adults die, learning that a child has a terminal condition is a nightmare come true for parents. Moreover, children's diseases are rarer and thus may have a less certain course.
- Physiologically, children's bodies are often more resilient, and they often live longer than do adults with the same condition (Carter & Levetown, 2004).
- The entire family is affected by the child's illness, treatments, hospitalizations, and separation of family members—all of whom are affected by the roller-coaster treatment process (Walsh & McGoldrick, 2004; Sourkes, 1987; Contro, Larson, Scofield, Sourkes, & Cohen, 2002.; Contro, Larson, Scofied, Sourkes, & Cohen, 2004).) Siblings in particular grieve in anticipation and often feel helpless, isolated, and sometimes neglected. While not specifically addressed in this chapter, it's important to underscore that psychological interventions,

such as hypnosis, could be of significant benefit to parents and siblings (Sourkes, 1987).

The Statistics—Incidence

Statistics from the USA indicate a steady decline in childhood death: 85,135 in 1980; 69,429 in 1990; and 53,728 in 2000. The majority of these deaths (52%) occur in infancy, and over half of these (26.6%) occur within the first week, mostly within the first 24 hours of life. The remaining (23.6%) occur within the first year of life (Carter & Levetown, 2004, p. 8). Despite the reduced incidence of childhood death, the impact of one child in palliative care is wide. It has been estimated that for one child who dies, there are at least 300 people affected. The grief and bereavement issues for family, friends, school, and community are significant and are being recognized as part of comprehensive pediatric palliative care (Carter & Levetown, 2004).

Tremendous strides have been made in the management and treatment of life threatening and life limiting pediatric illnesses and disorders, such as cystic fibrosis, the leukemias and lymphomas, and neuromuscular degenerative conditions (Field & Behrman, 2001). Many children and teens thus live through years of intensive and demanding medical treatments, which are both physically and emotionally draining. Living while knowing you're dying, or are at risk to die, is an extremely heavy burden on a child or teen. "These children live with many levels of awareness, and their pain and suffering both physical and psychic, can be great." (Sourkes, 2006, p. 96). Hypnosis has a unique role to play in the therapies for these children to help navigate the downturns, such as a relapse, and to provide comfort, solace, and peace at the end of life.

Despite this, psychological treatment is not universally necessary when a child who is facing death already has comprehensive emotional support from many different sources. Nonetheless, the ability to identify "high-risk" children and intervene in a timely fashion is often missed (Sourkes, 2006). The child's expressed need for support beyond the family, or the quality of relationship with the PPC team, provide some indications that intervention may be appropriate. Furthermore, not all children can or want to talk as they approach the end of their lives. Some may be fatigued, withdrawn, or irritable. Those days and weeks as death approaches and the child's energy diminishes *may* be a poor time to introduce hypnosis to a seriously ill child. The guiding principle is that *when a child is diagnosed with a life-threatening condition,* a comprehensive assessment of the child's and family's needs should direct all appropriate referrals, including psychotherapy and hypnosis.

When first approaching a seriously ill child, a lot depends on the relationship, skill, judgment, and attunement of the clinician. Little is demanded of the child when a naturalistic approach is adopted in response to some indication of interest. An initial trance can lay the groundwork for subsequent and more receptive hypnotic experiences. Initially a primary goal is to derive comfort and safety in present time, thereby investing in the familiar, predictable, ongoing experience of hypnosis for the next time.

Billy

This naturalistic, responsive approach is exemplified in how I first approached 9-year-old Billy, who had severe neurological complications following a leukemia relapse. He was now no longer able to walk. The oncology staff asked me to help as he had become withdrawn and his Mom was in despair. Mom was sitting at the foot of his bed, rubbing his legs. Billy's eyes were closed and the sheets pulled up tightly underneath his chin.

> I began talking quietly to him, inviting him to notice as his eyes were already closed so that he could see inside so clearly, how interesting it would be for him to experience a surprise, a wonderful surprise. "Imagine right now Billy, that you're at a party with friends, family and here in front you've been given a present. [*Pause.*] See it? [*Billy nods imperceptibly.*] Would you like to open it up? It's something you want right now. I wonder what it could be." Billy remained still and then softly said his first words, "It's a teddy bear." "Good! That's exactly what you need for right now. Hold your teddy bear and feel how good

459

that feels, your prize surprise and… I wouldn't be surprised that now as you hold your teddy and cuddle with it, how much stronger it begins to make you feel…..so much a surprise that you may even want to walk around the party and not be bothered by any of the bothers and worries that have been bothering you. Would you like to do that in your imagination so that it makes everything easier? [*Billy's nod was definite*].

Ducky

Children have an awareness of impending death—even the very young child. Dr. Barbara Sourkes (2006) gives a simple and dramatic example of this:

A 3-year-old boy played the same game with a stuffed duck and ambulance each time he came to hospital. At what turned out to be his terminal admission, she reported that this occurred:

Psychologist: How is the duck?

Child: Sick.

Psychologist: Is he going to get better?

Child: [*shook head slowly*] Ducky not get better. Ducky die. (p. 157)

During the terminal phase of life, the child's metaphors can become more symbolic, with archetypal images (e.g., heavenly gates) or catastrophic with their stories and language carrying a sense of impending disaster, or of increased fear. At these times many children and adolescents have become highly attuned to their bodies and more sensitive to physiological changes within it.

Judy

Judy, diagnosed with Ewing's Sarcoma, had undergone bone marrow transplantation. Prior to that she had learned to use sensory-based imagery in her trance to ease her pain and discomfort. She would use her breath to travel inwards and track her breath as it moved around her body. Over the years this evolved into her "scanner" in which she would systemically go through her body, inwardly scanning, easing, and releasing. One of the benefits of this self-regulatory technique was that Judy became highly attuned to her typical body sensations. This gave her an authority and confidence. One day she announced that she had felt this kind of pain before but not in this part of her body. She said, "It's…scary…because it feels different." We were very concerned. She went into trance and described it "...as sort of dense…I don't know…hotter and swollen. I don't like it." Nor did we! To the dismay of the team, the bone scan showed metastases to her lumbar spine. Judy had a certain calm—after all she had discovered it. With her hypnotic techniques fully integrated in her coping, she continued to use them through her remaining 18 months of life, enabling her to maintain self-control and dignity.

Clinical Hypnosis with Children Living While Knowing They Are Dying

Children near the end of life can have spontaneous visions that can provide direction for the entire palliative care team.

Brett

The neuroblastoma in 4-year-old Brett's belly had grown bigger. Staff and parents recognized that his disease had reached a stage at which treatment was no longer helpful. To relieve pain and discomfort intravenous opioid was put in place around the clock. He spent much time "spaced-out" and looking at cartoons on TV. But one day when I came for a session he told me that he had a "good dream. My Grandpa came to visit. He stood at the doorway and told me that he'll look after me." This provided an opportunity for us to discuss his death in the context of the vision he had shared, and, in turn, granted significant comfort to him, his parents, and his Grandma, who had lost her husband three years previously.

Hypnosis with seriously ill children evolves with increasing contact. It's often focused, seemingly simple, and it is central to the process that the child or teen takes the lead in developing personally relevant metaphors so that healing can occur.

Isabel

In the last months of her life, Isabel, a 15-year-old with osteogenic sarcoma, longed to ride a horse bare-back through sea-waves along the beach. While undergoing treatment she recurrently chose this as her favorite place and activity. She entered the trance easily and would feel the freshness of the salt breeze on her face, experience the exhilaration of the power of the horse beneath her carrying her along the open beach and soft sand, and feel at peace with herself and the world. This experience grew so strong that when she was offered through the Make-A-Wish Foundation (a charitable organization that arranges and funds wished-for trips and activities for seriously ill children and adolescents) to have a wish come true, she chose to go to Mexico where she could experience this before she died. She reported how people stared at her thin body and commented on her surgical scars, but she had the holiday of her life and returned more at peace than she had ever been.

Hypnotic imagery has a power and gentleness consistent with the psyche's best ability to heal itself. It is an aspect of the self that is generated by the adolescent. Over time it gains a power that empowers the young person to take creative delight in using it for whatever he or she needs to heal, and to deal with whatever lies ahead.

Caveats

Start early—Don't leave it for later. If the child or teen has not experienced hypnosis before, it is often more difficult to introduce, interest, and engage a child in the terminal stages of life. The child's energy is at a minimum, often the child is naturally withdrawing, and the capacity or desire to learn new material or processes is reduced.

Teach parents or other close family members. Many children and teens prefer to be at home rather than the hospital in their last months of life. As a result, parents and others become the main caregivers (Contro, Larson, Scofield, Sourkes, & Cohen, 2002; Contro, Larson, Scofied, Sourkes, & Cohen, 2004). Even if home visits are a regular part of the PPC program, it empowers those at home to know that they can help their child through a difficult time by going away to a peaceful or favorite place with hypnosis. It gives added support to the child to know that mom and dad also know how to take him or her there.

Inductions using breathing or large ideomotor responses become limited. With physiological deterioration, it may no longer be easy for the child or teen to go into trance using abdominal breathing or techniques such as coin dropping, an enacted balloon and sand-pail, or extended arms coming together. Sometimes the simplest induction, such as staring at a point ahead, or closing eyes and moving inwards, is all the focus and intensification required to induce trance.

Lastly, a general caveat: Know that many children who know they are dying are surprisingly calm. Their primary concern is often for the suffering and anguish of their parents. They will go to extraordinary length to minimize their parents' and siblings' distress, including withholding information and questions. Hypnosis can be a means to begin to open some of these doors.

Conclusion

Hypnosis is a good fit and a clinically sensitive technique for children facing life-threatening or life-limiting illness when it is used by pediatric professionals trained in palliative care issues. Specifically, hypnosis helps develop personal metaphors that can (1) transform anxiety, pain, uncertainty, and despair; (2) work with the paradox of living fully until one dies; (3) sustain hope; and, (4) maximize the opportunities and possibilities. For young people who are capable, hypnosis even helps them to envision an optimal death and memorial service. When introduced early, at diagnosis or the commencement of treatment, the hypnotic experience can play a significant role in the development of coping skills, to help navigate the course of treatment downturns, providing comfort, solace, and peace at the end of life.

> *My motto in life is to live and love it up. You live as long as you can*
> *and all you have left is to love it up, 'cause love never ends.*
> *You can love forever and ever....*
>
> 10-year-old Mikaela
> living with a terminal brain tumor

Resources

Videotapes

- *Making Every Moment Count* (2003)—Documentary (38 minutes) on pediatric palliative care that examines the experiences of five children (birth–19 yrs) who are facing death. Available through National Film of Canada (www.nfb.ca) or 1-800-267-7710, or Fanlight Productions, Boston MA, 1-800-937-4113.

- The Initiative for Pediatric Palliative Care (IPPC) has a comprehensive set of interdisciplinary and interactive educational resources. Available at: www.ippcweb.org

---

* From the documentary on Pediatric Palliative Care, *Making Every Moment Count* (2003).

Books and Materials

- ChIPPS (2000)—Children's International Project on Palliative/ Hospice Services: Compendium of Pediatric Palliative Care. Alexandria, VA: National Hospice and Palliative Care Organization.

- Goldman, A., Hain R., & Liben, S. (2006). *Oxford Textbook of Palliative Care for Children.* Oxford. UK: Oxford University Press.

- Hilden, J., Tobin, D., Lindsay, K. (2003). *Shelter from the Storm.* Cambridge, MA: Perseus. A helpful book for parents.

- Kübler-Ross, E. (1983). *On Children and Death.* New York: Macmillan.

- Sourkes, B. M. (1995). *Armfuls of Time. The Psychological Experience of the Child with a Life-Threatening Illness.* Pittsburgh, PA: University of Pittsburgh Press.

- The National Hospice and Palliative Care Organization: NCHPO Available at: www.nhpco.org

References

Carter, B.S., & Levetown, M. (2004). *Palliative care for infants, children and adolescents: A practical handbook.* Baltimore and London: The Johns Hopkins University Press.

Children's International Project on Palliative/Hospice Services (ChIPPS). (2000). Compendium of Pediatric Palliative Care. Alexandria, VA: National Hospice and Palliative Care Organization.

Contro, N., Larson, J., Scofield, S., Sourkes, B., & Cohen, H. (2002). Family perspectives on the quality of pediatric palliative care. *Archives of Pediatric & Adolescent Medicine,* 156:12–19.

Contro, N., Larson, J., Scofied, S., Sourkes, B., & Cohen, H.J. (2004). Hospital staff and family perspectives regarding quality of pediatric palliative care. *Pediatrics,* 114:1248–1252.

Field, M.J., Behrman, R.E. (Eds.) (2001). *When children die: Improving palliative and end-of-life care for children and their families*. Washington, D.C.: The National Academies Press.

Gardner, G.G. (1976). Childhood, death and human dignity: Hypnotherapy for David. *International Journal of Clinical and Experimental Hypnosis*, Vol. XX1V, 2, 122–139.

Kuttner, L. & Stutzer, C. (1995). Imagery for children in pain, experiencing threat to life and the approach of death. In D. W. Adams & E. J. Deveau (Eds.) *Beyond the Innocence of Childhood* Vol. 2. New York: Baywood.

Kuttner, L. (2006). Pain—An integrative approach. In Goldman, A., Hains, R., & Liben, S. (Eds.) *Oxford textbook of palliative care for children*. Oxford UK: Oxford University Press.

Sourkes, B. (1987). Siblings of the child with a life-threatening illness. *Children in Contemporary Society*, 19:158–184.

Sourkes, B. (2006). Psychological impact of life-limiting conditions on the child. In Goldman, A., Hains, R., & Liben, S. (Eds.) *Oxford textbook of palliative care for children*. Oxford UK: Oxford University Press.

Walsh, F., & McGoldrick, M. (2004). *Living beyond loss: Death in the family*, 2nd ed. New York and London: W.W. Norton.

World Health Organization (WHO). (1998). WHO Definition of Palliative Care. Available at: http://www/who/int/cancer/palliative/definition/en/

Author Index

Subject Index

Abdominal pain, 9, 184, 219, 227, 228, 232, 236, 237, 239, 304, 314, 323, 324, 347, 359, 360, 361, 362, 382, 399, 419, 430
Abreaction, 11, 146, 151, 159
Absorption, 5, 26, 146
Abused children (*see* Child Abuse)
Achenbach Child Behavioral Checklist, 185, 195
"Acting out" behavior, 260
Acute care settings, 301–330, 418
Acute pain, 23, 42, 369, 418, 422, 467
Acute stress disorder (ASD), 140
Adult attitudes, 423
Affect bridge, 151, 159
Age regression, 19, 57, 82, 106, 258
Agoraphobia, 202, 205
Allergies, 18, 233, 415
Altered states of consciousness, 143
Alternative cognitive controls, 428
American Academy of Child and Adolescent Psychiatry, 182, 195
American Psychiatric Association, 154, 176, 202, 208, 209, 210, 212, 214, 218, 237, 246, 263
American Psychological Association, 4, 60, 61, 109, 110, 129, 130, 131, 251, 278, 296, 297, 298
American Society of Clinical Hypnosis (ASCH), iv, v, vii, xii, 108, 115, 131, 157, 176, 234
Amnesia, 67, 68, 69, 106, 143, 212, 340
Analgesia (*see* Hypnoanalgesia)
Anchoring signal/technique/gesture, 375, 442
Anesthesia, 67, 68, 106, 107, 204, 333, 334, 342, 346, 347, 352, 353, 354, 355, 366, 367, 422, 428
Animal magnetism, xiii
Animal phobia, 206

Anorexia nervosa (*see also* Eating disorders), 172
Anterior cingulate cortex, 220, 421, 429, 451
Antisocial behavior, 390
Anxiety, 7, 10, 18, 20, 27, 34, 35, 36, 42, 43, 44, 45, 46, 52, 55, 56, 93, 95, 123, 126, 128, 136, 140, 144, 145, 146, 147, 165, 170, 171, 179, 181, 182, 186, 188, 191, 199–215, 221, 227, 249, 257, 286, 303, 304, 306–310, 314, 316, 319, 324, 327, 334, 338, 340, 352, 355, 357, 359, 363, 364, 365, 367, 369, 376, 377, 382, 384, 385, 387, 400, 403, 405, 454, 464
Anxiety control, 207, 210, 211, 365
Anxiety disorders, 93, 199, 214
Arm techniques, 8, 66, 67–69, 80, 94, 97, 102–104, 349
  catalepsy, 97, 349
  levitation, 8, 66, 67, 68, 69, 80, 97, 103–104
  lowering, 94, 104
  rigidity, 94, 102
Arousal, 127, 140, 142, 143, 151, 212, 274, 307, 320
Assessing hypnotic responsiveness, 85, 110, 127, 232
Asthma, 17, 18, 22, 42, 75, 88, 105, 318, 319, 321, 330, 357, 358, 359, 364, 366, 376, 382, 383, 384, 385
Attention-deficit/hyperactivity disorder (ADHD), 46, 191–193, 241, 243, 246–248, 263, 266, 269, 415
Attitudes about pain, 424–425
Attitudes towards hypnosis, 230
Auditory imagery, 93, 126
Autism, 180

Subject Index

Hypnotherapy (*see also* Hypnosis, Imagery techniques, Self-hypnosis), xiii, 6, 12, 14, 16, 17, 20, 21, 22, 23, 24, 41, 43, 59, 60, 61, 63, 67, 80, 83, 85, 108, 109, 110, 112, 124, 129, 131, 151, 155, 156, 157, 158, 176, 177, 196, 206, 214, 217, 219, 221, 222, 223, 225, 226, 227, 229, 231, 232, 233, 234, 235, 237, 238, 239, 245, 246, 249, 250, 252, 253, 254, 257, 260, 262, 264, 265, 269, 273, 282, 283, 296, 303, 329, 331, 354, 355, 369, 383, 384, 385, 387, 392, 395, 399, 403, 405, 410, 412, 417, 418, 425, 430, 431, 432, 440, 446, 447, 449, 450, 454, 466

authoritarian versus permissive approach, 11, 12, 13, 16, 87, 94, 96, 98, 212, 213, 232, 346

boundaries of, 112, 403

contraindications, 16, 17

and coping skills, 12,

general principles, 112

goals, 80, 254, 369, 387, 405,

guidelines, 112, 131, 239, 303, 430

habit disorders, 176, 177

pain control, 21, 67, 80, 176, 214, 369, 384, 447, 450

psychological disorders, 231

research, 12, 109, 131, 222, 262, 418, 425,

results of, 226, 399,

role of child, 454

Hypnotic abilities, 53, 63–89

Hypnotic conversation, 24, 86, 273–298

Hypnotic induction, 7, 8, 66, 91–108, 110, 126, 172, 175, 191, 202, 220, 226, 230, 232, 234, 304, 314, 318, 355, 406

arm catalepsy, 97, 349

arm levitation technique, 8, 66, 67, 68, 69, 80, 97, 103–104

arm lowering, 94, 104

arm rigidity, 94, 102

auditory imagery techniques, 93, 126

autistic children, 180

biofeedback, 21, 189, 248, 249, 264, 269, 270, 331, 403, 410, 412

breathing, 4, 10, 38, 56, 99, 105, 107, 150, 166, 193, 207, 234, 235, 274, 301, 304, 306, 311, 314, 317, 318, 319, 320, 321, 325, 345, 349, 358, 364, 376, 377, 433, 463

choice of technique, 55

cloud gazing, 38, 94

coin, 39, 94, 102, 103, 254, 463

counting, 100, 106, 107, 169, 205, 209

distraction, 93, 104–106, 249, 274, 369

eye fixation, 39, 93, 102

favorite activity, 462

favorite place, 38, 39, 94, 100, 105, 126, 170, 173, 211, 213, 349, 350, 351, 352, 462, 463

favorite song, 370

floppy Raggedy Ann/Andy, 36, 102, 148

hand levitation, 68, 102

ideomotor techniques, 102

mighty oak tree, 102

movement imagery techniques, 100

permissive methods, 94

progressive relaxation in, 98, 377

questionnaire for, 196, 414, 437, 438, 443

and self-hypnosis (*see* Self-Hypnosis)

sports activity (*see also* Sports Imagery/Metaphors), 100

storytelling technique, 93, 146, 150, 151

teddy bear, 66, 99, 102, 459

483

Self-hypnosis (*see also* Hypnosis; Hypnotherapy; Imagery techniques), 14, 15, 38, 39, 91, 95, 163, 175, 193, 201–203, 210, 228, 232, 319, 327–328, 344, 347, 348, 351, 370, 382, 392, 395–396, 403, 405, 412, 432, 450
  anxiety, 202–203
  asthma, 319
  encopresis, 403, 405
  enuresis, 392
  for the care-giver, 327–328
  parental roles, 14, 370
  recordings for, 15, 39, 163
  self-talk, 210
Self-monitoring, 70, 395, 402, 432–436
Self-stimulatory behaviors, 163, 172–173
Separation anxiety, 207, 208
Severely disturbed, 59
Sexual abuse (*see also* Child abuse), 130, 258
Siblings, 230, 379, 457–458, 463, 466
Sick role, 219
Simple phobia, 206, 209
Sleep disorders (*see also* Night Terrors and Nightmares), 126, 140, 142, 188, 191, 389
Sleepwalking, 143
Sneezing, 221, 231, 237
Social phobia, 207
Society for Clinical and Experimental Hypnosis (SCEH), xii, 412
Society for Developmental and Behavioral Pediatrics (SDBP), xii, 31, 44
Soiling, fecal (*see also* Encopresis), 397–407, 412
Somatoform disorders, 217–239, 383
Specific phobia (*see also* Simple phobia), 206, 209
Speech problems (*see also* Stammering and stuttering), 163, 173–174

Spontaneous hypnosis, 21, 146, 187, 192
Sports imagery/metaphors, 75, 94–95, 100, 153, 208, 348, 394, 404
Stammering and stuttering (*see also* Speech problems), 163, 173–174
Stop sign strategies, 191–193
Stories and storytelling, 11–12, 23, 33–34, 41–42, 69, 93, 94, 146, 150, 151, 153, 157, 341, 343, 346, 445–446, 460
  induction, 93, 94
  palliative care, 445–446, 460
  trauma, 151, 153, 157
Stress (*see also* Posttraumatic stress disorder (PTSD), vii, 18, 24, 54, 55, 140, 141, 154–159, 209, 211, 212, 217, 219, 221, 229, 233, 237, 238, 250, 270, 327–328, 340, 368–370, 374, 389, 398, 409, 422,
  acute stress disorder, 140, 141, 154–159
  anxiety, 209, 211, 212
  care-givers, 327–328
  chronic disease, 368–370, 374
  enuresis, 389, 398, 404
  hypothalamic-pituitary-adrenal (HPA) axis, 18, 24, 422
  somatoform disorders, 217, 219, 221
  trauma, 135, 140
Stress-coping model, 219
Stuttering (*see also* Speech problems, Stammmering and stuttering), 163, 173–174
Subconscious abilities, 64–69, 71, 77, 80, 83
Substance abuse, 142, 182, 253, 367
Suggestibility, 82, 340
Suggestion, 22, 29, 32–33, 34, 51, 78, 96, 106–107, 152–153, 170, 175, 313 334, 342, 345–347, 350, 351, 354, 364, 374–375, 434, 444, 446
  anchoring, 375